Dedication

This book is dedicated to my beloved family for all their love and support as well as their understanding during my endless hours of working on this edition:

To my husband Dan, who is my rock and my constant support whom I could not live without;

To my three wonderful children: Patrick, Jamie, and Christi who give me moral support, make me laugh, and who constantly try to keep me up to date on all the modern technologies that have helped me communicate with them, communicate with my colleagues, and write this book. They keep me young with their ideas and assistance; they constantly have a "joie de vivre";

To my two dogs: Sparky and Bear who kept my feet warm while I sat for hours at the computer working on this edition but demanded daily play, and provided a wonderful mental break from writing;

To my brother-in-law George, who was an inspiration to everyone he knew and met with his positive attitude and fighting spirit that he had up until the day he died from pancreatic cancer.

And,

In loving memory of my parents, John and Norma, who kept me busy as their daughter and caregiver while they were alive, and were always proud of everything I did.

In addition, I dedicate this edition:

To my colleagues who keep me informed, give me moral and intellectual support, and who keep me inspired to maintain my passion for the field of cardiovascular and pulmonary physical therapy. I have enjoyed being a mentor to many rising cardiopulmonary specialists as well as all my students, and have especially enjoyed being a resident mentor to my first resident, Erica Colclough, and my current residents Tiffany Haney and Stephen Ramsey. I also especially rely on the support and inspiration of some very dear friends/colleagues including Dianne Jewell, Andrew Ries, Claire Rice, and Joanne Watchie.

And finally, I can never forget my very special friends/mentors to whom I am forever grateful and whose memories and teachings are with me always: Michael Pollock (1937–1998), Linda Crane (1951–1999), and Gary Dudley (1952–2006).

Contributors

Erinn Barker, DPT
Cardiovascular and Pulmonary Physical Therapist Resident
Department of Physical Therapy
Duke University Hospital
Durham, North Carolina

Pamela Bartlo, PT, DPT, CCS
Clinical Associate Professor
Physical Therapy
D'Youville College
Buffalo, New York

Staff PT in Cardiac and Pulmonary Rehabilitation
Rehabilitation Department
Mount St. Mary's Hospital
Lewiston, New York

Traci Tiemann Betts, PT, DPT, CCS
Physical Therapist - Cardiopulmonary Clinical Specialist
Physical Medicine and Rehabilitation
Baylor Institute for Rehabilitation - Baylor University
Medical Center - Baylor Scott & White Healthcare
Dallas, Texas

Tamara L. Burlis, PT, DPT, CCS
Associate Director of Clinical Education, Assistant Professor, Program in
Physical Therapy and Internal Medicine, Washington University,
St. Louis, Missouri

Rohini K. Chandrashekar, PT, MS, CCS
Guest Lecturer, Physical Therapy
Texas Woman's University
Houston, Texas
Physical Therapist, Rehabilitation
Triumph Hospital Clear Lake
Webster, Texas

Meryl Cohen, DPT, MS, CCS
Assistant Professor
Department of Physical Therapy
Miller School of Medicine
University of Miami
Coral Gables, Florida
Adjunct Instructor
Massachusetts General Hospital
Institute of Health Professions
Boston, Massachusetts

Kelley Crawford, DPT
Level III Clinician, Rehabilitation, Medicine
Maine Medical Center
Portland, Maine

Rebecca Crouch, PT, DPT, CCS
Adjunct Faculty
Doctoral Program in Physical Therapy
Duke University
Durham, North Carolina
Coordinator of Pulmonary Rehabilitation,
PT/OT Duke University Medical Center
Durham, North Carolina

Nicole DeLuca, DPT, CCS
Program Coordinator, Cardiopulmonary Rehabilitation
Physical Medicine and Rehabilitation
Miami VA Healthcare System
Miami, Florida

Konrad J. Dias, PT, DPT, CCS
Associate Professor
Physical Therapy Program
Maryville University
St. Louis, Missouri

Christen DiPerna, PT, DPT
Physical Therapist
Indiana University Health Methodist Hospital
Indianapolis, Indiana

Anne Mejia-Downs, PT, CCS
Assistant Professor
Krannert School of Physical Therapy
University of Indianapolis
Indianapolis, Indiana
Physical Therapist
Department of Rehabilitation Services
Clarian Health Partners
Indianapolis, Indiana

Jennifer Edelschick, PT, DPT
Coordinator of Pediatric Acute PT/OT Services
Physical and Occupational Therapy
Duke Medicine
Durham, North Carolina

Tara Marie Dickinson Fahrner, PT, DPT, CCS
Physical Therapist
Physical Medicine
Sacred Heart Hospital
Pensacola, Florida

Ann Winkel Fick, PT, DPT, MS, CCS
Director of Clinical Education Associate Professor
Physical Therapy
Maryville University
St. Louis, Missouri
PRN Physical Therapist
Physical Therapy
Barnes-Jewish Hospital
St. Louis, Missouri

Danielle L. Fioriello, PT, MPT, CCS
Physical Therapist
Cardiac and Pulmonary Rehabilitation
Mount Sinai Beth Israel
New York, New York

Courtney Frankel, PT, MS, CCS
Clinical Research Coordinator II
Department of Medicine
Duke University
Durham, North Carolina

Susan L. Garritan, PT, PhD, CCS
Clinical Assistant Professor
Rehabilitation Medicine, Acute Care Physical Therapy Coordinator
Tisch Hospital
New York University
Langone Medical Center
New York, New York

Natalie M. Goldberg, PT, DPT, CCS
Adjunct Professor
Department of Physical Therapy
University of Hartford
Hartford, Connecticut

Physical Therapist
Department of Rehabilitation
Hartford Hospital
Hartford, Connecticut

Kate Grimes, MS, PT, CCS
Clinical Assistant Professor
Massachusetts General Hospital
Institute of Health Professions
Boston, Massachusetts

Ellen Hillegass, PT, EdD, CCS, FAACVPR, FAPTA
President, Cardiopulmonary Specialists, Inc
A Consulting Corporation,
Partner in PT CARDIOPULMONARY EDUCATORS, LLC
A webinar-based continuing education company
www.ptcardiopulmonaryeducators.com
Adjunct Professor
Department of Physical Therapy
Mercer University
Atlanta, Georgia
And
Adjunct Professor
Department of Physical Therapy
Western Carolina University
Cullowhee, North Carolina

Morgan Johanson, PT, MSPT, CCS
Coordinator of Inpatient and Outpatient
Cardiac and Pulmonary Physical Therapy
Co-Director
Cardiovascular and Pulmonary Physical Therapy Residency Program
Physical Medicine and Rehabilitation
Ann Arbor VA Healthcare System
Ann Arbor, Michigan

Tamara Klintwork-Kirk, PT, CCS
Clinical Services Coordinator
Department of Physical and Occupational Therapy
Duke University Hospital
Durham, North Carolina

Meghan Lahart, PT, DPT, CCS
Physical Therapist II
Rehabilitation Services
Advocate Christ Medical Center
Oak Lawn, Illinois

Kristin M. Lefebvre, PT, PhD, CCS
Assistant Professor
Institute for Physical Therapy Education
Widener University
Chester, Pennsylvania

Ana Lotshaw, PT, PhD, CCS
Rehabilitation Supervisor
Physical Medicine and Rehabilitation
Baylor University Medical Center
Dallas, Texas

Sean T. Lowers, PT, DPT, CCS
Senior Physical Therapist
Department of Physical Therapy and Occupational Therapy
Duke University Health System
Durham, North Carolina

Kate MacPhedran, PT, PhDc, CCS
Instructor
Doctor of Physical Therapy
Gannon University
Erie, Pennsylvania

Frailty Consultant
Consultants in Cardiovascular Diseases, Inc.
Saint Vincent Hospital
Erie, Pennsylvania

Susan Butler McNamara, MMSc, PT, CCS
Team Leader
Division of Rehabilitation Medicine
Maine Medical Center
Portland, Maine

Harold Merriman, PT, PhD, CLT
Associate Professor
Department of Physical Therapy
University of Dayton
Dayton, Ohio

Andrew Mills, PT, DPT
Assistant Professor
School of Physical Therapy
Touro University Nevada
Henderson, Nevada

Amy Pawlik, PT, DPT, CCS
Program Coordinator
Cardiopulmonary Rehabilitation Therapy Services
The University of Chicago Hospitals
Chicago, Illinois

Christiane Perme, PT, CCS
Senior Physical Therapist
Department of Physical Therapy and Occupational Therapy
The Methodist Hospital
Houston, Texas

Karlyn J. Schiltgen, PT, DPT, OCS, CCS
Physical Therapist
Department of Inpatient PT/OT
Duke University Hospital
Durham, North Carolina

Alexandra Sciaky, PT, DPT, MS, CCS
Adjunct Faculty
Department of Physical Therapy
University of Michigan-Flint
Flint, Michigan
Senior Physical Therapist
Coordinator of Clinical Education, Physical Medicine and Rehabilitation
Physical Therapy Section
Veterans Affairs Ann Arbor Healthcare System
Ann Arbor, Michigan

Debra Seal, PT, DPT
Senior Pediatric Physical Therapist
Acute Therapy
Cedars-Sinai Medical Center
Los Angeles, California

Joanne Watchie, MA, PT, CCS
Owner
Joanne's Wellness Ways
Pasadena, California

Preface

Originally this text was developed to meet the needs of the physical therapy community, as cardiopulmonary was identified as one of the four clinical science components in a physical therapy education program as well as in clinical practice. Those aspects of physical therapy commonly referred to as "cardiovascular and pulmonary physical therapy" are recognized as fundamental components of the knowledge base and practice base of all entry-level physical therapists. Therefore this text was developed for entry-level physical therapists, as well as individuals in practice who need more in-depth knowledge of cardiopulmonary content. This text is also utilized by many clinicians studying for advanced practice board certification as well as those involved in residency programs. Although intended primarily for physical therapists, this text has been useful to practitioners in various disciplines who teach students or who work with patients who suffer from primary and secondary cardiopulmonary dysfunction. This fourth edition can also be used by all practitioners who teach entry-level clinicians, work with residents as well as to help in clinical practice of patients with cardiopulmonary dysfunction.

This fourth edition has gone through update and revision from the third edition to make the text more user friendly and provide more interactive learning. The same six sections exist: *Anatomy and Physiology; Pathophysiology; Diagnostic Tests and Procedures; Surgical Interventions, Monitoring and Support; Pharmacology;* and *Cardiopulmonary Assessment and Intervention.* The six sections were kept as they facilitate the progression of understanding of the material in order to be able to perform a thorough assessment and provide an optimal intervention as well as provide measurable outcomes to assess change.

The revisions you should notice include both major and minor changes. All chapters have been revised as well as supplemented with many figures and tables and some videos to help the learner visualize the written information. Additional figures, case studies, and resource material can also be found on the Evolve website that accompanies this text. The number of clinical notes was increased to help clinicians and students understand certain clinical findings and help them relate them to the pathophysiology of cardiovascular and pulmonary disease. All chapters were updated with new information, technology, and research.

Each chapter had specific revisions that should be highlighted. Chapters 1 and 2, which explain anatomy and physiology, increased the number of figures to help the learner relate the pathophysiology to the normal anatomy and physiology. In addition, the developmental and maturational anatomy was moved to the pediatrics chapter (Chapter 20) to help the learner compare the pathophysiology to the normal in this population. Chapter 3, *Ischemic Cardiovascular Conditions and Other Vascular Pathologies,* underwent revision particularly in areas that were lacking such as venous dysfunction including deep vein thrombosis. New material was added, so that you will now find hypertension, peripheral arterial disease, cerebrovascular disease, renal disease, and aortic aneurysm in this chapter, in addition to ischemic disease. Chapter 4, *Cardiac Muscle Dysfunction and Failure,* was restructured and revised to improve the flow and understanding of this important pathologic condition as well as all new figures and tables to help understand heart dysfunction and failure.

Due to the complexities and number of conditions of restrictive lung dysfunction many more tables were created in Chapter 5 to separate the material and assist the learner to identify key information quickly. Chapter 6, *Chronic Obstructive Pulmonary Diseases,* was updated and revised to emphasize the importance of this disease and the fact that COPD is the third leading cause of death. Revisions in Chapter 7, *Cardiopulmonary Implications of Specific Diseases,* emphasize information on obesity, diabetes, and metabolic syndrome, as well as cancer and neuromuscular diseases.

New technologies and advancements in diagnostic tests and surgical procedures were added to Chapters 8, 9, 10, and 11. Chapter 11, *Cardiovascular and Thoracic Interventions* underwent major overhaul with many new figures and text. The advances in transplantation were discussed in Chapter 12 and *Monitoring and Life Support* (Chapter 13) was revised to increase the depth of information on ventilators as well as other monitoring equipment found in intensive care units and used by PTs when mobilizing patients earlier.

As advances in health care and diagnostics occur, so do improvements and changes in medications, so both *Cardiovascular Medications* (Chapter 14) and *Pulmonary Medications* (Chapter 15) required updating. Chapter 16 (*Examination and Assessment Procedures*) was revised with addition of new tables to help organize assessments and improve the understanding of this material. Chapter 17, *Interventions for Acute Cardiopulmonary Conditions* added a greater emphasis on early mobility and Chapter 18, *Interventions and Prevention Measures for Individuals with Cardiovascular Disease, or Risk of Disease* had major updating and revision, new clinical notes and many new figures and tables. Chapter 19, *Pulmonary Rehabilitation* was revised to correspond with changes in the new pulmonary rehabilitation (PR) definition and in the changing practice since Medicare revised payment for PR. Chapter 20, *Pediatric Cardiopulmonary Physical Therapy* and Chapter 21, *The Lymphatic System* were two wonderful additions to the third edition of *Cardiopulmonary Physical Therapy* and were updated with some new figures. And, finally, the text ends with the outcomes chapter which was totally revamped and provides great information for measurement of improvement in the cardiopulmonary patient population.

Whenever possible, case studies are provided to exemplify the material being presented. Additional case studies are found on Evolve.

No matter how well you understand the material in this book, it will not make you a master clinician, skilled in the assessment and treatment of cardiovascular and pulmonary disorders. To become even a minimally competent clinician, you will have to practice physical therapy under the tutelage of an experienced clinician. *Essentials of Cardiopulmonary Physical Therapy* cannot provide you with everything there is to know about the assessment and treatment of cardiovascular and pulmonary disorders. It will provide the essentials as the title indicates. Learning is a continuous process, and technology and treatment are forever improving; therefore this text provides clinicians as well as educators with the most current information at the time of publication.

It is my true hope that you appreciate this edition and are able to learn from all the wealth of information provided by such wonderful contributors. Without heart and breath there is no therapy!

Acknowledgments

"Change is good and change equals opportunity!" This statement explains how I have approached each edition, but most especially this edition! Hopefully you will gain knowledge and insight from all the changes as there are many excellent contributions from my colleagues, who are THE experts in cardiovascular and pulmonary physical therapy and who poured their passion into their chapters. This edition is what I consider the "Mentoring" edition….many of the co-authors in the chapters are newly recognized cardiopulmonary specialists and past Residents of Cardiopulmonary Residency programs and new to writing. They were mentored along the way, and what they provided to this edition was amazing content, figures, videos, and updated material that makes this text stand out. We can all learn from these experts and you will as you dig into the material in the following pages.

Learning does not stop with this text. Continuing education is a vital component of lifelong learning so I would also encourage all of my readers to continue their lifelong learning in cardiopulmonary physical therapy by utilizing always updated webinars from www.ptcardiopulmonaryeducators.com.

During the publication phase of the first edition of the *Essentials of Cardiopulmonary Physical Therapy*, I was always worried about new developments in the field of Cardiovascular and Pulmonary diagnosis and treatment that were not going to be covered in the book. My very first editor, Margaret Biblis, kept saying "that's what the next edition is for" and that is how I approached the second edition and again the third and fourth edition. I have saved comments and suggestions along the way as well as attended conferences regularly to stay current with new developments in the field. And, with the age of the internet, you have access to the new Evolve site that accompanies this text. Instructional material including PowerPoint presentations and a test bank are available to instructors in the course, as well as updated information.

So, I would like to thank all the amazing experts who have helped with this fourth edition, including each of the wonderful contributors as well as all those clinicians, students, and faculty members who provided feedback on previous editions and who continue to use this book in their courses and their every day practice. I would like to especially thank the contributors for their ability to work under my constant nagging to achieve their deadlines and for providing great material including figures, tables, and clinical notes. I would also like to acknowledge and thank Angela Campbell and Meryl Cohen, who kept pressing me to get this edition going and make it interactive, as it was their comments that pushed me to finally initiate the fourth edition.

Of course my family and my dogs need to be acknowledged for all the time I spent at the computer working on this edition instead of spending time with them.

Lastly, this edition truly would not be published were it not for my wonderful editor, Brian Loehr, who called me weekly, joked with me about content and figures, and learned a lot of cardiopulmonary along the way while pushing this edition to a timely completion. He has become a friend and the best editor ever! Thanks, Brian!

Contents

1

Anatomy of the cardiovascular and pulmonary systems

Konrad J. Dias

This chapter describes the anatomy of the cardiovascular and pulmonary systems as it is relevant to the physical therapist. Knowledge of the anatomy of these systems provides clinicians with the foundation to perform the appropriate examination and provide optimal treatment interventions for individuals with cardiopulmonary dysfunction. An effective understanding of cardiovascular and pulmonary anatomy allows for comprehension of function and an appreciation of the central components of oxygen and nutrient transport to peripheral tissue. A fundamental assumption is made; namely, that the reader already possesses some knowledge of anatomic terms and cardiopulmonary anatomy.

Thorax

The bony thorax covers and protects the major organs of the cardiopulmonary system. Within the thoracic cavity exist the heart, housed within the mediastinum centrally, and laterally are two lungs. The bony thorax provides a skeletal framework for the attachment of the muscles of ventilation.

The thoracic cage (Fig. 1-1) is conical at both its superior and inferior aspects and somewhat kidney shaped in its transverse aspect. The skeletal boundaries of the thorax are the 12 thoracic vertebrae dorsally, the ribs laterally, and the sternum ventrally.

Sternum

The sternum, or breastbone, is a flat bone with three major parts: *manubrium, body,* and *xiphoid process* (see Fig. 1-1). Superiorly located within the sternum, the manubrium is the thickest component articulating with the clavicles and first and second ribs. A palpable jugular notch or suprasternal notch is found at the superior border of the manubrium of the sternum. Inferior to the manubrium lies the body of the sternum, articulating laterally with ribs three to seven. The sternal angle, or "angle of Louis," is the anterior angle formed by the junction of the manubrium and the body of the sternum. This easily palpated structure is in level with the second costal cartilage anteriorly and thoracic vertebrae T4 and T5 posteriorly. The most caudal aspect of the sternum is the xiphoid process, a plate of hyaline cartilage that ossifies later in life.

The sternal angle marks the level of bifurcation of the trachea into the right and left main stem bronchi and provides for the pump-handle action of the sternal body during inspiration.[1]

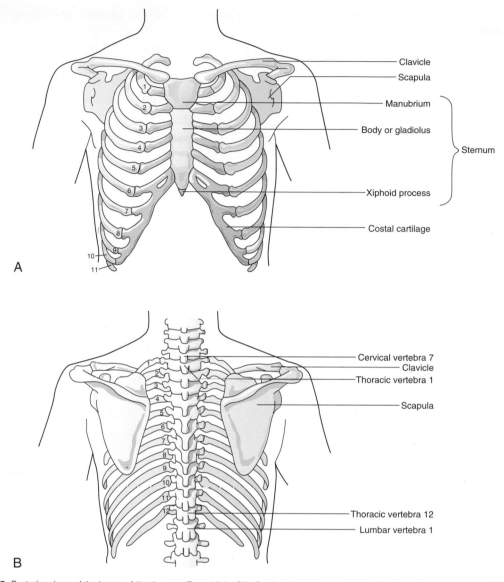

Figure 1-1 A, Anterior. **B,** Posterior views of the bones of the thorax. (From Hicks GH: *Cardiopulmonary Anatomy and Physiology,* Philadelphia, 2000, Saunders.)

Pectus excavatum is a common congenital deformity of the anterior wall of the chest in which several ribs and the sternum grow abnormally (see Fig. 5-25). This produces a caved-in or sunken appearance of the chest. It is present at birth, but rapidly progresses during the years of bone growth in the early teenage years. These patients have several pulmonary complications, including shortness of breath caused by altered mechanics of the inspiratory muscles on the caved-in sternum and ribs, and often have cardiac complications caused by the restriction (compression) of the heart.[2]

To gain access to the thoracic cavity for surgery, including coronary artery bypass grafting, the sternum is split in the median plane and retracted. This procedure is known as a *median sternotomy.* Flexibility of the ribs and cartilage allows for separation of the two ends of the sternum to expose the thoracic cavity.[3]

Ribs

The ribs, although considered "flat" bones, curve forward and downward from their posterior vertebral attachments toward their costal cartilages. The first seven ribs attach via

their costal cartilages to the sternum and are called the *true ribs* (also known as the *vertebrosternal ribs*); the lower five ribs are termed the *false ribs*—the eighth, ninth, and tenth ribs attach to the rib above by their costal cartilages (the vertebrochondral ribs), and the eleventh and twelfth ribs end freely (the vertebral ribs; see Fig. 1-1). The true ribs increase in length from above downward, and the false ribs decrease in length from above downward.

Each rib typically has a vertebral end separated from a sternal end by the body or shaft of the rib. The head of the rib (at its vertebral end) is distinguished by a twin-faceted surface for articulation with the facets on the bodies of two adjacent thoracic vertebrae. The cranial facet is smaller than the caudal, and a crest between these permits attachment of the interarticular ligament.

Fig. 1-2 displays the components of typical ribs three to nine, each with common characteristics, including a head, neck, tubercle, and body. The neck is the 1-inch long portion of the rib extending laterally from the head; it provides attachment for the anterior costotransverse ligament along its cranial border. The tubercle at the junction of the neck and the

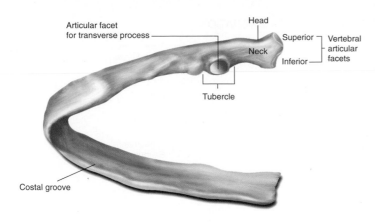

Articular facet
for transverse process

Head

Superior ⌐ Vertebral
Neck   │ articular
Inferior ⌐   └ facets

Tubercle

Costal groove

Figure 1-2 Typical middle rib as viewed from the posterior. The head end articulates with the vertebral bones, and the distal end is attached to the costal cartilage of the sternum. (From Wilkins RL: *Egan's Fundamentals of Respiratory Care*, ed 9, St. Louis, 2009, Mosby.)

body of the rib consists of an articular and a nonarticular portion. The articular part of the tubercle (the more medial and inferior of the two) has a facet for articulation with the transverse process of the inferior-most vertebra to which the head is connected. The nonarticular part of the tubercle provides attachment for the ligament of the tubercle.

The shaft, or body, of the rib is simultaneously bent in two directions and twisted about its long axis, presenting two surfaces (internal and external) and two borders (superior and inferior). A costal groove for the intercostal vessels and nerve extends along the inferior border dorsally but changes to the internal surface at the angle of the rib. The sternal end of the rib terminates in an oval depression into which the costal cartilage makes its attachment.

Although rib fractures may occur in various locations, they are more common in the weakest area where the shaft of the ribs bend—the area just anterior to its angle. The first rib does not usually fracture, as it is protected posteroinferiorly by the clavicle. When it is injured, the brachial plexus of nerves and subclavian vessel injury may occur.[4] Lower rib fractures may cause trauma to the diaphragm resulting in a diaphragmatic hernia. Rib fractures are extremely painful because of their profound nerve supply. It is important for all therapists to recommend breathing, splinting, and coughing strategies for patients with rib fractures. Paradoxical breathing patterns and a flail chest may also need to be evaluated in light of multiple rib fractures in adjacent ribs.[3]

Chest tubes are inserted above the ribs to avoid trauma to vessels and nerves found within the costal grove. A chest tube insertion involves the surgical placement of a hollow, flexible drainage tube into the chest. This tube is used to drain blood, air, or fluid around the lungs and effectively allow the lung to expand. The tube is placed between the ribs and into the space between the inner lining and the outer lining of the lung (pleural space).

The first, second, tenth, eleventh, and twelfth ribs are unlike the other, more typical ribs. The first rib is the shortest and most curved of all the ribs. Its head is small and rounded and has only one facet for articulation with the body of the first thoracic vertebra. The sternal end of the first rib is larger and thicker than it is in any of the other ribs. The second rib, although longer than the first, is similarly curved. The body is

not twisted. There is a short costal groove on its internal surface posteriorly. The tenth through twelfth ribs each have only one articular facet on their heads. The eleventh and twelfth ribs (floating ribs) have no necks or tubercles and are narrowed at their free anterior ends. The twelfth rib sometimes is shorter than the first rib.

The Respiratory System

The respiratory system includes the bony thorax, the muscles of ventilation, the upper and the lower airways, and the pulmonary circulation. The many functions of the respiratory system include gas exchange, fluid exchange, maintenance of a relatively low-volume blood reservoir, filtration, and metabolism, and they necessitate an intimate and exquisite interaction of these various components. Because the thorax has already been discussed, this section deals with the muscles of ventilation, the upper and lower airways, and the pulmonary circulation.

Muscles of Ventilation

Ventilation, or breathing, involves the processes of inspiration and expiration. For air to enter the lungs during inspiration, muscles of the thoracic cage and abdomen must move the bony thorax to create changes in volume within the thorax and cause a concomitant reduction in the intrathoracic pressure. Inspiratory muscles increase the volume of the thoracic cavity by producing bucket-handle and pump-handle movements of the ribs and sternum, as depicted in Fig. 1-3. The resultant reduced intrathoracic pressure generated is below atmospheric pressure, forcing air into the lungs to help normalize pressure differences. The essential muscles to achieve the active process of inspiration at rest are the diaphragm and internal intercostals. To create a more forceful inspiration during exercise or cardiopulmonary distress, accessory muscles assist with the inspiration. The accessory muscles include the sternocleidomastoid, scalenes, serratus anterior, pectoralis major and minor, trapezius, and erector spinae muscles.

Diaphragm

The diaphragm is the major muscle of inspiration. It is a musculotendinous dome that forms the floor of the thorax and separates the thoracic and abdominal cavities (Fig. 1-4). The diaphragm is divided into right and left hemidiaphragms. Both hemidiaphragms are visible on radiographic studies from the front or back. The right hemidiaphragm is protected by the liver and is stronger than the left. The left hemidiaphragm is more often subject to rupture and hernia, usually because of weaknesses at the points of embryologic fusion. Each hemidiaphragm is composed of three musculoskeletal components, including the sternal, costal, and lumbar portions that converge into the central tendon. The central tendon of the diaphragm is a thin but strong layer of tendons (aponeurosis) situated anteriorly and immediately below the pericardium. There are three major openings to enable various vessels to traverse the diaphragm. These include the vena caval opening for the inferior vena cava; the esophageal opening for the esophagus and gastric vessels; and the aortic opening containing the aorta, thoracic duct, and azygos veins. The phrenic nerve arises from the third, fourth, and fifth cervical spinal nerves (C3 to C5) and is involved in contraction of the diaphragm.

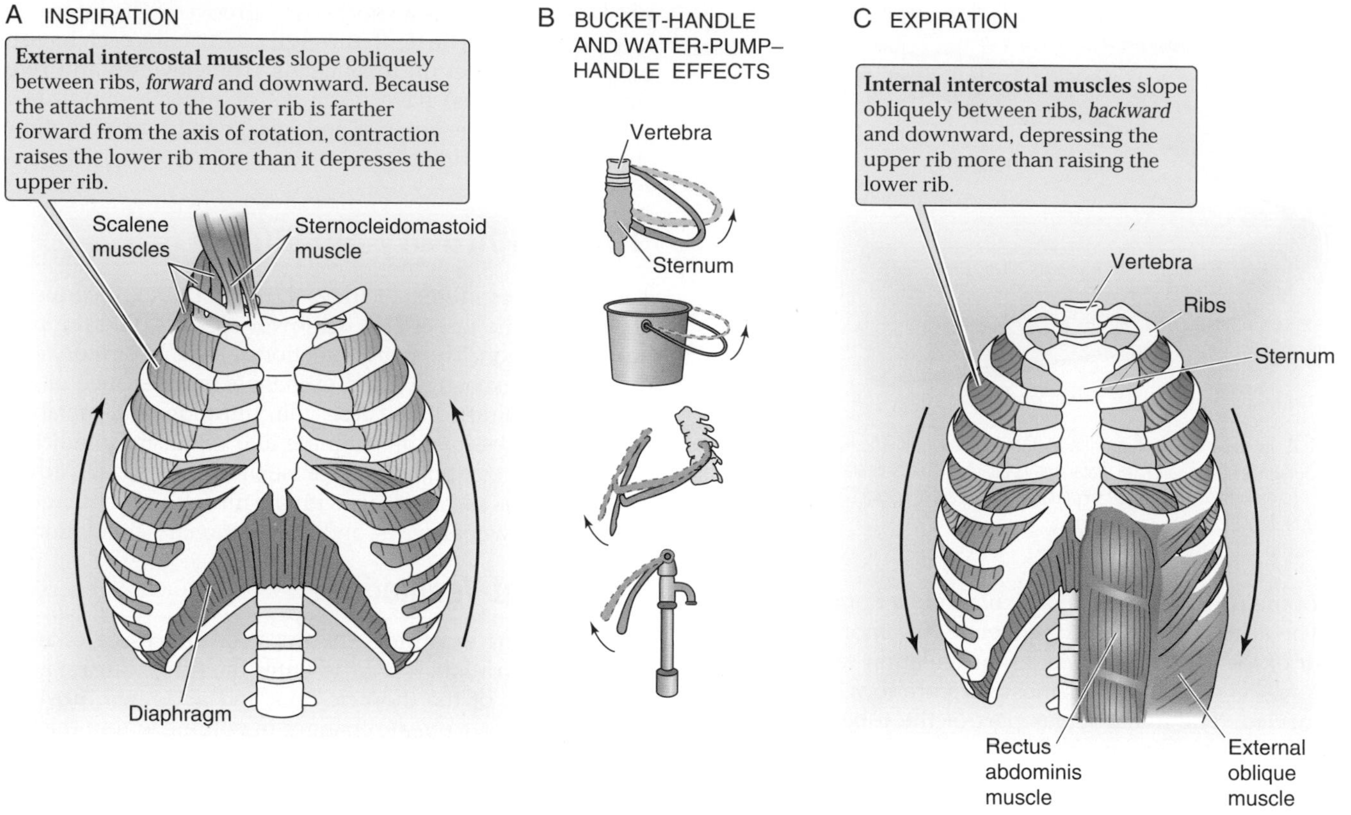

A INSPIRATION

External intercostal muscles slope obliquely between ribs, *forward* and downward. Because the attachment to the lower rib is farther forward from the axis of rotation, contraction raises the lower rib more than it depresses the upper rib.

Scalene muscles

Sternocleidomastoid muscle

Diaphragm

B BUCKET-HANDLE AND WATER-PUMP–HANDLE EFFECTS

Vertebra

Sternum

C EXPIRATION

Internal intercostal muscles slope obliquely between ribs, *backward* and downward, depressing the upper rib more than raising the lower rib.

Vertebra

Ribs

Sternum

Rectus abdominis muscle

External oblique muscle

Figure 1-3 A-C, Actions of major respiratory muscles. (From Boron WF: *Medical Physiology*, updated ed, St. Louis, 2005, Saunders.)

The resting position of the diaphragm is an arched position high in the thorax. The level of the diaphragm and the amount of movement during inspiration vary as a result of factors such as body position, obesity, and size of various gastrointestinal organs present below the diaphragm. During normal ventilation or breathing, the diaphragm contracts to pull the central tendon down and forward. In doing so, the resting dome shape of the diaphragm is reversed to a flattening of the diaphragm. Contraction of this muscle increases the dimensions of the thorax in a cephalocaudal, anterior posterior, and lateral direction.[1] The increase in volume decreases pressure in the thoracic cavity and simultaneously causes a decrease in volume and an increase in pressure within the abdominal cavity. The domed shape of the diaphragm is largely maintained until the abdominal muscles end their extensibility, halting the downward displacement of the abdominal viscera, essentially forming a fixed platform beneath the central tendon. The central tendon then becomes a fixed point against which the muscular fibers of the diaphragm contract to elevate the lower ribs and thereby push the sternum and upper ribs forward. The right hemidiaphragm meets more resistance than the left during its descent, because the liver underlies the right hemidiaphragm and the stomach underlies the left; it is therefore more substantial than the left.

In patients with chronic obstructive pulmonary disease (COPD), there is compromised ability to expire. This results in a flattening of the diaphragm as a result of the presence of hyperinflated lungs.[1,5] It is essential for therapists to reverse hyperinflation and restore the normal resting arched position of the diaphragm using any exercise aimed at strengthening the diaphragm muscle. A flat and rigid diaphragm cannot be strengthened and will cause an automatic firing of the accessory muscles to trigger inspiration.

Body position in supine, upright, or side lying alters the resting position of the diaphragm, resulting in concomitant changes in lung volumes.[6] In the supine position, without the effects of gravity, the level of the diaphragm in the thoracic cavity rises. This allows for a relatively greater excursion of the diaphragm. Despite a greater range of movement of the diaphragm, lung volumes are low as a consequence of the elevated position of the abdominal organs within the thoracic cavity. In an upright position, the dome of the diaphragm is pulled down because of the effects of gravity. The respiratory excursion is less in this position; however, the lung volumes are larger. In the side-lying position, the hemidiaphragms are unequal in their positions: the uppermost side drops to a lower level and has less excursion than that in the sitting position; the lowermost side rises higher in the thorax and has a greater excursion than in the sitting position. In quiet breathing, the diaphragm normally moves about two-thirds of an inch; with maximal ventilatory effort, the diaphragm may move from 2.5 to 4 inches.[5]

Clinical tip

Stomach fullness, obesity with presence of a large pannus, ascites with increased fluid in the peritoneal space from liver disease, and pregnancy are additional factors affecting the normal excursion of the diaphragm during inspiration.

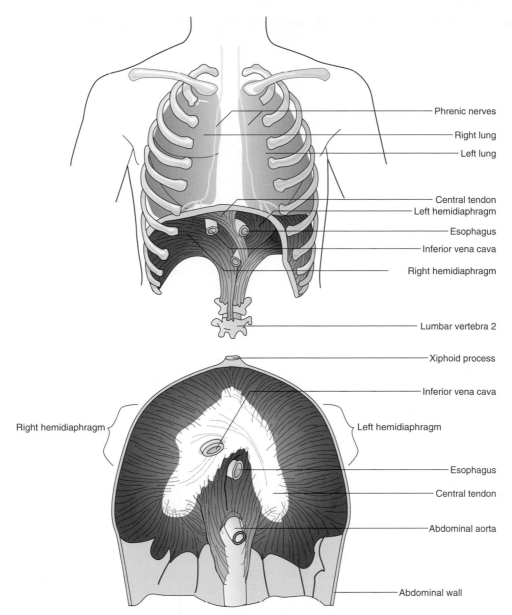

Figure 1-4 The diaphragm originates from the lumbar vertebra, lower ribs, xiphoid process, and abdominal wall and converges in a central tendon. Note the locations of the phrenic nerves and openings for the inferior vena cava, esophagus, and abdominal aorta. (From Hicks GH: *Cardiopulmonary Anatomy and Physiology,* Philadelphia, 2000, Saunders.)

External Intercostal Muscles

The external intercostal muscles originate from the lower borders of the ribs and attach to the upper border of the ribs below (Fig. 1-5). There are 11 external intercostal muscles on each side of the sternum. Contraction of these muscles pull the lower rib up and out toward the upper rib, thereby elevating the ribs and expanding the chest.

Accessory Muscles

Fig. 1-6 explains the anatomy of the accessory muscles.

Sternocleidomastoid Muscle

The sternocleidomastoid arises by two heads (sternal and clavicular from the medial part of the clavicle), which unite to extend obliquely upward and laterally across the neck to the mastoid process. For this muscle to facilitate inspiration, the head and neck must be held stable by the neck flexors and extensors. This muscle is a primary accessory muscle and elevates the sternum, increasing the anteroposterior diameter of the chest.

Scalene Muscle

The scalene muscles lie deep to the sternocleidomastoid, but may be palpated in the posterior triangle of the neck. These muscles function as a unit to elevate and fix the first and second ribs:

- The *anterior* scalene muscle passes from the anterior tubercles of the transverse processes of the third or fourth to the sixth cervical vertebrae, attaching by tendinous insertion into the first rib.
- The *middle* scalene muscle arises from the transverse processes of all the cervical vertebrae to insert onto the first rib (posteromedially to the anterior scalene, the brachial plexus and subclavian artery pass between the anterior scalene and middle scalene).
- The *posterior* scalene muscle arises from the posterior tubercles of the transverse processes of the fifth and sixth

cervical vertebrae, passing between the middle scalene and levator scapulae, to attach onto the second or third rib.

Upper Trapezius

The trapezius (upper fibers) muscle arises from the medial part of the superior nuchal line on the occiput and the ligamentum nuchae (from the vertebral spinous processes between the skull

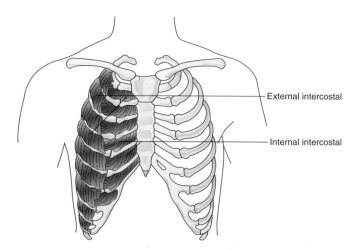

Figure 1-5 The external intercostal muscles lift the inferior ribs and enlarge the thoracic cavity. The internal intercostal muscles compress the thoracic cavity by pulling together the ribs. (From Hicks GH: *Cardiopulmonary Anatomy and Physiology*, Philadelphia, 2000, Saunders.)

and the seventh cervical vertebra) to insert onto the distal third of the clavicle. This muscle assists with ventilation by helping to elevate the thoracic cage.

Pectoralis Major and Minor

The pectoralis major arises from the medial third of the clavicle, from the lateral part of the anterior surface of the manubrium and body of the sternum, and from the costal cartilages of the first six ribs to insert upon the lateral lip of the crest of the greater tubercle of the humerus. When the arms and shoulders are fixed, by leaning on the elbows or grasping onto a table, the pectoralis major can use its insertion as its origin and pull on the anterior chest wall, lifting the ribs and sternum, and facilitate an increase in the anteroposterior diameter of the thorax.

The pectoralis minor arises from the second to fifth or the third to sixth ribs upward to insert into the medial side of the coracoid process close to the tip. This muscle assists in forced inspiration by raising the ribs and increasing intrathoracic volume.

Serratus Anterior and Rhomboids

The serratus anterior arises from the outer surfaces of the upper eight or nine ribs to attach along the costal aspect of the medial border of the scapula. The primary action of the serratus is to abduct, rotate the scapula, and hold the medial border firmly over the rib cage. The serratus can only be utilized as an accessory muscle in ventilation, when the rhomboids stabilize

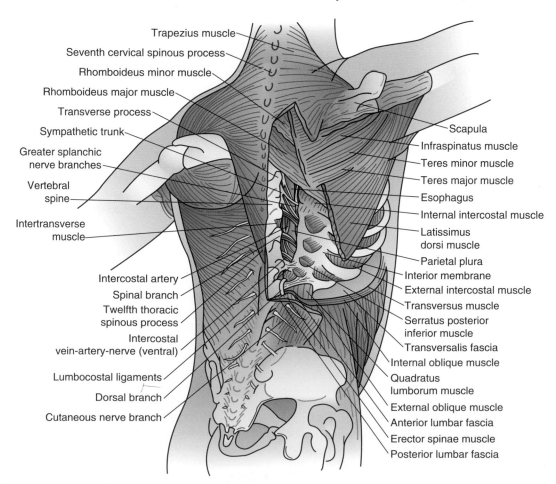

Figure 1-6 Musculature of the chest wall. (From Ravitch MM, Steichen FM: *Atlas of General Thoracic Surgery*, Philadelphia, 1988, Saunders.)

the scapula in adduction.[7] The action of the rhomboids fixes the insertion, allowing the serratus to expand the rib cage by pulling the origin toward the insertion.

Latissimus Dorsi

The latissimus dorsi arises from the spinous processes of the lower six thoracic, the lumbar, and the upper sacral vertebrae, from the posterior aspect of the iliac crest, and slips from the lower three or four ribs to attach to the intertubercular groove of the humerus.[7] The posterior fibers of this muscle assist in inspiration as they pull the trunk into extension.

Serratus Posterior Superior

The serratus posterior superior passes from the lower part of the ligamentum nuchae and the spinous processes of the seventh cervical and first two or three thoracic vertebrae downward into the upper borders of the second to fourth or fifth ribs. This muscle assists in inspiration by raising the ribs to which it is attached and expanding the chest.

Thoracic Erector Spinae Muscles

The erector spinae is a large muscle group extending from the sacrum to the skull. The thoracic erector spinae muscles extend the thoracic spine and raise the rib cage to allow greater expansion of the thorax.

Muscles of Expiration

Abdominal Muscles

The abdominal muscles include the rectus abdominis, transversus abdominis, and internal and external obliques. These muscles work to raise intraabdominal pressure when a sudden expulsion of air is required in maneuvers such as huffing and coughing. Pressure generated within the abdominal cavity is transmitted to the thoracic cage to assist in emptying the lungs.

Internal Intercostal Muscles

Eleven internal intercostal muscles exist on each side of the sternum. These muscles arise on the inner surfaces of the ribs and costal cartilages and insert on the upper borders of the adjacent ribs below (see Fig. 1-5). The posterior aspect on the internal intercostal muscles is termed the *interosseus portion* and depresses the ribs to aid in a forceful expiration. The intercartilaginous portion of the internal intercostals elevates the ribs and assists in inspiration.

Pulmonary Ventilation

Pulmonary ventilation, commonly referred to as *breathing*, is the process in which air is moved in and out of the lungs. Inspiration, an active process at rest and during exercise, involves contraction of the diaphragm and external intercostal muscles. The muscle that contracts first is the diaphragm, with a caudal movement and resultant increase within the volume of the thoracic cavity. The diaphragm eventually meets resistance against the abdominal viscera, causing the costal fibers of the diaphragm to contract and pull the lower ribs up and out—*the bucket-handle movement.* The outward movement is also facilitated by the external intercostal muscles. In addition, a pump-handle movement of the upper ribs

is achieved through contraction of the external intercostals and the intercartilaginous portion of the internal intercostal muscles. The actions of the inspiratory muscles expand the dimensions of the thoracic cavity and concomitantly reduce the pressure in the lungs (intrathoracic pressure) below the air pressure outside the body. With the respiratory tract being open to the atmosphere, air rushes into the lungs to normalize the pressure difference, allowing inspiration to occur and the lungs to fill with air.

During forced or labored breathing, additional accessory muscles need to be used to increase the inspiratory maneuver. The accessory muscles raise the ribs to a greater extent and promote extension of the thoracic spine. These changes facilitate a further increase in the volume within the thoracic cavity and a subsequent drop in the intrathoracic pressure beyond that caused by the contraction of the diaphragm and external intercostals. This relatively lower intrathoracic pressure will promote a larger volume of air entering the lung.

At rest, expiration is a passive process and achieved through the elastic recoil of the lung and relaxation of the external intercostal and diaphragm muscle. As the external intercostals relax, the rib drops to its preinspiratory position and the diaphragm returns to its elevated dome position high in the thorax. To achieve a forceful expiration, additional muscles can be used, including the abdominals and internal intercostal muscles. The internal intercostals actively pull the ribs down to help expel air out of the lungs. The abdominals contract to force the viscera upward against the diaphragm, accelerating its return to the dome position.

Clinical tip

The changes in intraabdominal and intrathoracic pressure that occur with forced breathing assist with venous return of blood back to the heart. The drop in pressure allows for a filling of the veins, and the changing pressure within the abdomen and thorax cause a milking effect to help return blood back to the heart.

Pleurae

Two serous membranes, or pleurae, exist that cover each lung (Fig. 1-7). The pleura covering the outer surface of each lung is the visceral pleura and is inseparable from the tissue of the lung. The pleura covering the inner surface of the chest wall, diaphragm, and mediastinum is called the *parietal pleura*. The parietal pleura is frequently described with reference to the anatomic surfaces it covers: the portion lining the ribs and vertebrae is named the *costovertebral pleura*; the portion over the diaphragm is the *diaphragmatic pleura*; the portion covering the uppermost aspect of the lung in the neck is the *cervical pleura*; and that overlying the mediastinum is called the *mediastinal pleura.*[8] Parietal and visceral pleurae blend with one another where they come together to enclose the root of the lung. Normally, the pleurae are in intimate contact during all phases of the ventilatory cycle, being separated only by a thin serous film. There exists a potential space between the pleurae called the *pleural space* or *pleural cavity.* A constant negative pressure within this space maintains lung inflation.

Surface anatomy of pleurae and lungs

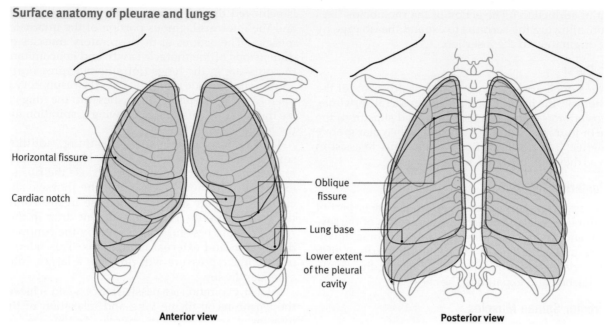

Figure 1-7 Pleurae of the lungs. (From Craven J: The lungs and their relations. *Anaesth Intensive Care Med*, 9(11):459-512, 2008.)

The serous fluid within the pleural space serves to hold the pleural layers together during ventilation and reduce friction between the lungs and the thoracic wall.[6,8]

The parietal pleura receives its vascular supply from the intercostal, internal thoracic, and musculophrenic arteries. Venous drainage is accomplished by way of the systemic veins in the adjacent parts of the chest wall. The bronchial vessels supply the visceral pleura. There exists no innervation to the visceral pleura and therefore no sensation.[5] The phrenic nerve innervates the parietal pleura of the mediastinum and central diaphragm, whereas the intercostal nerves innervate the parietal pleura of the costal region and peripheral diaphragm.

Irritation of the intercostally innervated pleura may result in the referral of pain to the thoracic or abdominal walls, and irritation of the phrenic-supplied pleura can result in referred pain in the lower neck and shoulder.[9]

Several complications can affect pleural integrity. Infection with resultant inflammatory response within the pleura is termed *pleuritis* or *pleurisy* and is best appreciated through the presence of pleural chest pain and an abnormal pleural friction rub on auscultation.[9] A pleural effusion refers to a buildup of fluid in the pleural space commonly seen after cardiothoracic surgery or with cancer. This is evidenced by diminished or absent breath sounds in the area of the effusion, is more likely to be in gravity-dependent areas, and is accompanied by reduced lung volumes. Blood in the pleural space is termed a *hemothorax*, whereas air in the pleural space from a collapsed lung is termed a *pneumothorax*. Finally, a bacterial infection with resultant pus in the pleural space is referred to as *empyema*.

Management for several of these complications of the pleural space is achieved through insertion of a chest tube into the pleural space to drain pleural secretions or to restore a negative pressure within the space and allow for lung inflation. A needle aspiration of fluid from the space, a thoracocentesis, may be performed for patients with large pleural effusions.

Lungs

The lungs are located on either side of the thoracic cavity, separated by the mediastinum. Each lung lies freely within its corresponding pleural cavity, except where it is attached to the heart and trachea by the root and pulmonary ligament. The substance of the lung—the parenchyma—is normally porous and spongy in nature. The surfaces of the lungs are marked by numerous intersecting lines that indicate the polyhedral (secondary) lobules of the lung. The lungs are basically cone shaped and are described as having an apex, a base, three borders (anterior, inferior, and posterior), and three surfaces (costal, medial, and diaphragmatic).

The apex of each lung is situated in the root of the neck, its highest point being approximately 1 inch above the middle third of each clavicle. The base of each lung is concave, resting on the convex surface of the diaphragm. The inferior border of the lung separates the base of the lung from its costal surface; the posterior border separates the costal surface from the vertebral aspect of the mediastinal surface; the anterior border of each lung is thin and overlaps the front of the pericardium. Additionally, the anterior border of the left lung presents a cardiac notch. The costal surface of each lung conforms to the shape of the overlying chest wall. The medial surface of each lung may be divided into vertebral and mediastinal aspects. The vertebral aspect contacts the respective sides of the thoracic vertebrae and their intervertebral disks, the posterior intercostal vessels, and nerves. The mediastinal aspect is notable for the cardiac impression; this concavity is larger on the left than on the right lung to accommodate the projection of the apex of the heart toward the left. Just posterior to the cardiac impression is the hilus, where the structures forming the root of the lung enter and exit the parenchyma. The extension of the pleural covering below and behind the hilus from the root of the lung forms the pulmonary ligament.

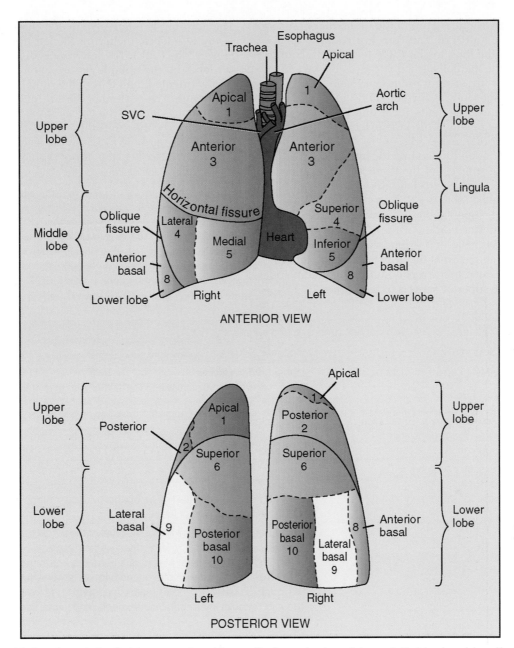

Figure 1-8 Topography of the lung demonstrating the lobes, segments, and fissures. The fissures (or chasms) demarcate the lobes in each lung. Numbers refer to specific bronchopulmonary segments. *SVC*, Superior vena cava. (From Koeppen B, Stanton B: *Berne and Levy Physiology*, ed 6, Philadelphia, 2010, Mosby.)

Hila and Roots

The point at which the nerves, vessels, and primary bronchi penetrate the parenchyma of each lung is called the *hilus*. The structures entering the hila of the lungs and forming the roots of each of the lungs are the principal bronchus, the pulmonary artery, the pulmonary veins, the bronchial arteries and veins, the pulmonary nerve plexus, and the lymph vessels. They lie next to the vertebral bodies of the fifth, sixth, and seventh thoracic vertebrae. The right root lies behind the superior vena cava and a portion of the right atrium, below the end of the azygos vein; the left root lies below the arch of the aorta and in front of the descending thoracic aorta. The pulmonary ligament lies below the root; the phrenic nerve and the anterior pulmonary plexus lie in front of the root; the vagus nerve and posterior pulmonary plexus lie behind the root.

Lobes, Fissures, and Segments

The right lung consists of three lobes, including the right upper lobe (RUL), right middle lobe (RML), and right lower lobe (RLL). Two fissures separate these three lobes from one another. The upper and middle lobes of the right lung are separated from the lower lobe by the oblique (major) fissure (Fig. 1-8). Starting on the medial surface of the right lung at the upper posterior aspect of the hilus, the oblique fissure runs upward and backward to the posterior border at about the level of the fourth thoracic vertebra; it then descends anteroinferiorly across the anterior costal surface to intersect the lower border of the lung approximately 5 inches from the median plane and then passes posterosuperiorly to rejoin the hilus just behind and beneath the upper pulmonary vein. The RML is separated from the RUL by the horizontal (minor) fissure that joins the oblique fissure at the midaxillary line at about the level of the fourth rib and runs horizontally across the costal surface of the lung to about the level of the fourth costal cartilage; on the medial surface, it passes backward to join the hilus near the upper-right pulmonary vein.

Each lobe of the right lung is further subdivided into segments. The RUL has three segments, including the apical, posterior, and anterior segments. This lobe extends to the level of the fourth rib anteriorly and is adjacent to ribs three to five posteriorly. The RML is subdivided into the lateral and medial lobes. This lobe is the smallest of the three lobes. Its inferior border is adjacent to the fifth rib laterally and the sixth rib medially. The lowermost lobe, the RLL, consists of four segments (anterior basal, superior basal, lateral basal, and posterior basal). The superior border of the RLL is at the level of the sixth thoracic vertebra and extends inferiorly down to the diaphragm. During maximal inspiration, the inferior border of the RLL may extend to the second lumbar vertebra and superimpose over the superior aspects of the kidney.

The left lung is relatively smaller than the right lung and has only two lobes, including the left upper lobe (LUL) and left lower lobe (LLL). The left lung is divided into upper and lower lobes by the oblique fissure, which is somewhat more vertically oriented than that of the right lung; there is no horizontal fissure. The portion of the left lung that corresponds to the right lung is termed the *lingular segment* and is a part of the LUL. Posteriorly, the inferior border of the LUL is at the level of the sixth rib, and the LLL is at the level of the eleventh rib.

Table 1-1 describes the topographic boundaries for the bronchopulmonary segments of each lung.

> ### Clinical tip
>
> An understanding of the various lobes and segments and their anatomic orientation is essential for appropriate positioning and removal of secretions from various aspects of the lung during bronchopulmonary hygiene procedures.

Table 1-1 Topographic boundaries for the bronchopulmonary lung segments

Lobe	Segment	Borders
Upper Lobe	Anterior segment (right or left)	Upper border: clavicle Lower border: a horizontal line at the level of the third intercostal space (ICS), or fourth rib, anteriorly
	Apical segment (R) or apical aspect, apicoposterior segment (L)	Anteroinferior border: clavicle Posteroinferior border: a horizontal line at the level of the upper lateral border of the spine of the scapula
	Posterior segment (R) or posterior aspect, apicoposterior segment (L)	Upper border: a horizontal line at the level of the upper lateral border of the spine of the scapula Lower border: a horizontal line at, or approximately 1 inch below, the inferomedial aspect of the spine of the scapula
Middle Lobe (R) or Lingula (L)		Upper border: a horizontal line at the level of the third ICS, or fourth rib, anteriorly Lower and lateral borders: the oblique fissure (a horizontal line at the level of the sixth rib anteriorly) extending to the anterior axillary line; from the anterior axillary line, angling upward to approximately the fourth rib at the posterior axillary line The midclavicular line separates the medial and lateral segments of the right middle lobe A horizontal line at the level of the fifth rib, anteriorly, separates the superior and inferior lingular segments
Lower Lobe	Superior (basal) segment (right or left)	Upper border: a horizontal line at, or approximately 1 inch below, the inferomedial aspect of the spine of the scapula Lower border: a horizontal line at, or approximately 1 inch above, the inferior angle of the scapula
	Posterior (basal) segment (right or left)	Upper border: a horizontal line at, or approximately 1 inch above, the inferior angle of the scapula Lateral border: a "plumb line" bisecting the inferior angle of the scapula Lower border: a horizontal line at the level of the tenth ICS, posteriorly
	Lateral (basal) segment (right or left)	Upper border: a horizontal line at, or approximately 1 inch above, the inferior angle of the scapula Medial border: a "plumb line" bisecting the inferior angle of the scapula Lateral border: the midaxillary line Lower border: a horizontal line at the level of the tenth ICS, posteriorly
	Anterior (basal) segment (R) or anterior aspect, anteromedial (basal) segment (L)	Upper border: the oblique fissure (a horizontal line at the level of the sixth rib anteriorly, extending to the anterior axillary line; from the anterior axillary line, angling upward to approximately the fifth rib at the midaxillary line Lateral border: the midaxillary line

Upper Respiratory Tract

Nose.

The nose is a conglomerate of bone and hyaline cartilage. The nasal bones (right and left), the frontal processes of the maxillae, and the nasal part of the frontal bone combine to form the bony framework of the nose. The septal, lateral, and major and minor alar cartilages combine to form the cartilaginous framework of the nose. The periosteal and perichondral membranes blend to connect the bones and cartilages to one another.

Three major muscles assist with movement of the bony framework of the nose. The procerus muscle wrinkles the skin of the nose. The nasalis muscle has two parts, including the transverse and alar portions, and assists in flaring the anterior nasal aperture.[8] Finally, the depressor septi muscle works with the nasalis muscle to flare the nostrils.[8] Skin covers the external nose.

The nasal cavity is a wedge-shaped passageway divided vertically into right and left halves by the nasal septum and compartmentalized by the paranasal sinuses (Fig. 1-9). Opening anteriorly via the nares (nostrils) to the external environment, the nasal cavity blends posteriorly with the nasopharynx. The two halves are essentially identical, having a floor, medial and lateral walls, and a roof divided into three regions: the vestibule, the olfactory region, and the respiratory region.

The primary respiratory functions of the nasal cavity include air conduction, filtration, humidification, and temperature control; it also plays a role in the olfactory process.

Three nasal conchae project into the nasal cavity from the lateral wall toward the medial wall; they are named the *superior, middle,* and *inferior conchae.* The conchae serve to increase the respiratory surface area of the nasal mucous membrane for greater contact with inspired air. The vestibule of the nasal cavity is lined with skin containing many coarse hairs and sebaceous and sweat glands. Mucous membrane lines the remainder of the nasal cavity. Fig. 1-10 depicts examples of some selected types of mucosal coverings in the upper and lower respiratory tracts.

The olfactory region of the nasal cavity is distinguished by specialized mucosa. This pseudostratified olfactory epithelium is composed of ciliated receptor cells, nonciliated sustentacular cells, and basal cells that help to provide a sense of smell.[8] Sniffing increases the volume of inspired air entering the olfactory region, allowing the individual to smell something specific.[4]

The respiratory region is lined with a mixture of columnar or pseudostratified ciliated epithelial cells, goblet cells, nonciliated columnar cells with microvilli, and basal cells. Serous and mucous glands, which open to the surface via branched ducts, underlie the basal lamina of the respiratory epithelium.[10] The submucosal glands and goblet cells secrete an abundant quantity of mucus over the mucosa of the nasal cavity, making it moist and sticky. Turbulent airflow, created by the conchae, causes inhaled dust and other particulate matter larger than approximately 10 μm to "rain out" onto this sticky layer, which is then moved by ciliary action backward and downward out of the nasal cavity into the nasopharynx at an average rate of about 6 mm per minute.[11,12]

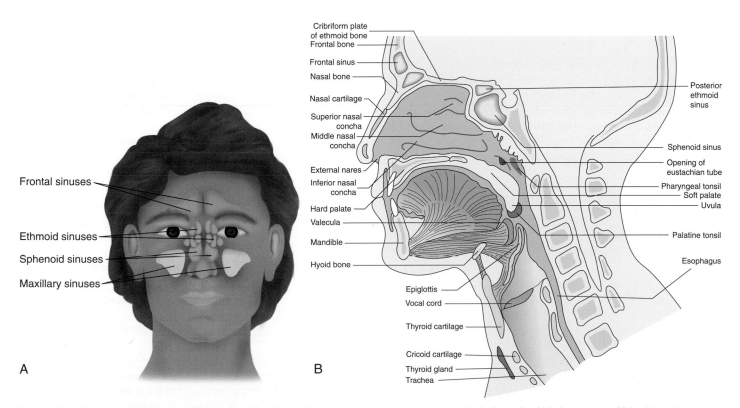

Figure 1-9 A, Positions of the frontal, maxillary, sphenoid, and ethmoid sinuses; the nasal sinuses are named for the bones in which they occur. **B,** Midsagittal section through the upper airway. (From Wilkins RE: *Fundamentals of Respiratory Care,* ed 9, St. Louis, 2009, Mosby.)

SQUAMOUS

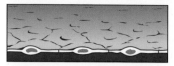

including mesothelium–lining coelomic surfaces; endothelium–lining vascular channels. Structural variants include continuous, discontinuous, and fenestrated endothelia.

CUBOIDAL

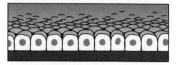

COLUMNAR

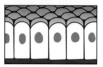
Without surface specialization

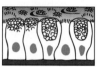
Glandular

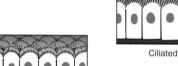
With microvilli (brush/striated border)

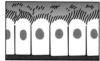
Ciliated

Pseudostratified (distorted columnar)

STRATIFIED CUBOIDAL/COLUMNAR

TRANSITIONAL

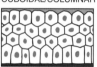
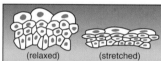
(relaxed)　　(stretched)

Figure 1-10 Types of cells composing the mucosal lining of the upper and lower respiratory tracts. (Modified from Williams PI, Warwick R, Dyson M, et al, editors: *Gray's Anatomy*, ed 37, New York, 1989, Churchill Livingstone.)

Clinical tip

Nasotracheal suctioning must be performed with caution in individuals with low platelet counts because of the likelihood of trauma and bleeding to superficial nasal conchae and cells within the nasal cavity. The placement of a nasopharyngeal airway or nasal trumpet may reduce trauma with recurrent blind suctioning procedures in these patients.

Individuals with seasonal allergies who are prone to developing sinus infections are also prone to developing bronchitis if the infection leaves the sinus cavities and drops down the throat to the bronchioles.

Pharynx.

The pharynx is a musculomembranous tube approximately 5 to 6 inches long and located posterior to the nasal cavity. It extends from the base of the skull to the esophagus that corresponds with a line extending from the sixth cervical vertebra to the lower border of the cricoid cartilage. The pharynx consists of three parts: the nasopharynx, the oropharynx, and the laryngopharynx.

Nasopharynx.

The nasopharynx is a continuation of the nasal cavity, beginning at the posterior nasal apertures and continuing backward and downward. Its roof and posterior wall are continuous; its lateral walls are formed by the openings of the eustachian tubes; and its floor is formed by the soft palate anteriorly and the pharyngeal isthmus (the space between the free edge of the soft palate and the posterior wall of the pharynx), which marks the transition to the oropharynx. The epithelium of the nasopharynx is composed of ciliated columnar cells.

Oropharynx.

The oropharynx extends from the soft palate and pharyngeal isthmus superiorly to the upper border of the epiglottis inferiorly. Anteriorly, it is bounded by the oropharyngeal isthmus (which opens into the mouth) and the pharyngeal part of the tongue. The posterior aspect of the oropharynx is at the level of the body of the second cervical vertebra and upper portion of the body of the third cervical vertebra. The epithelium in the oropharynx is composed of stratified squamous cells.

Laryngopharynx.

The laryngopharynx extends from the upper border of the epiglottis to the inferior border of the cricoid cartilage and the esophagus. The laryngeal orifice and the posterior surfaces of the arytenoid and cricoid cartilages form the anterior aspect of the laryngopharynx. The posterior aspect is at the level of the lower portion of the third cervical vertebra, the bodies of the fourth and fifth cervical vertebrae, and the upper portion of the body of the sixth cervical vertebra. The epithelium in the laryngopharynx is composed of stratified squamous cells.

Larynx.

The larynx, or voice box, is a complex structure made up of several cartilages and forms a connection between the pharynx and the trachea. The position of the larynx depends on the age and sex of the individual, being opposite the third to sixth cervical vertebrae in the adult male and somewhat higher in adult females and children.

The larynx consists of the endolarynx and its surrounding cartilaginous structures. The endolarynx is made of two sets of folds, including the false vocal cords (supraglottis) and true vocal cords.[8] Between the true cords are slit-shaped spaces that form the glottis. A space exists above the false vocal cords and is termed the *vestibule*. Six supporting cartilages, including three large (epiglottis, thyroid, cricoid) and three smaller (arytenoid, corniculate, cuneiform), prevent food, liquids, and foreign objects from entering the airway. Two sets of laryngeal muscles (internal and external) play important roles in swallowing, ventilation, and vocalization. The larynx controls airflow and closes to increase intrathoracic pressure to generate an effective cough. Sounds with speech are created as expired air vibrates over the contracting vocal cords.

Clinical tip

Endotracheal intubation may cause damage to structures within the larynx, producing an inflammatory response—laryngitis—where patients present with hoarseness and pain during speech.

Lower Respiratory Tract

The lower respiratory tract extends from the level of the true vocal cords in the larynx to the alveoli within the lungs. Generally, the lower respiratory tract may be divided into two

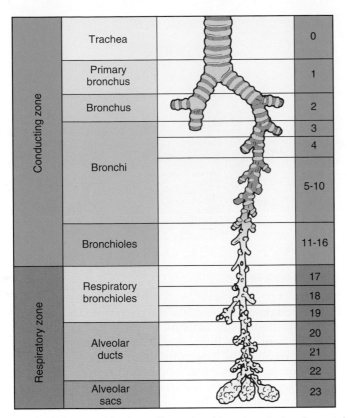

Conducting zone	Trachea		0
	Primary bronchus		1
	Bronchus		2
	Bronchi		3
			4
			5-10
	Bronchioles		11-16
Respiratory zone	Respiratory bronchioles		17
			18
			19
	Alveolar ducts		20
			21
			22
	Alveolar sacs		23

Figure 1-11 Structure of the airways. The number of the various structures is reported for two lungs. (From Costanzo LS: *Physiology*, ed 3, St. Louis, 2007, Saunders.)

parts: the tracheobronchial tree, or conducting airways, and the acinar or terminal respiratory units.

Tracheobronchial tree or conducting airways.

The conducting airways are not directly involved in the exchange of gases in the lungs. They simply conduct air to and from the respiratory units. Airway diameter progressively decreases with each succeeding generation of branching, starting at approximately 1 inch in diameter at the trachea and reaching 1 mm or less at the terminal bronchioles. The cartilaginous rings of the larger airways give way to irregular cartilaginous plates, which become smaller and more widely spaced with each generation of branching, until they disappear at the bronchiolar level.[13] There may be as many as 16 generations of branching in the conducting airways from the mainstem bronchi to the terminal bronchioles (Fig. 1-11).[14]

Trachea.

The trachea is a tube approximately 4 to 4.5 inches long and approximately 1 inch in diameter, extending downward along the midline of the neck, ventral to the esophagus. As it enters the thorax, it passes behind the left brachiocephalic vein and artery and the arch of the aorta. At its distal end, the trachea deviates slightly to the right of midline before bifurcating into right and left mainstem bronchi. Between 16 and 20 incomplete rings of two or more hyaline cartilages are often joined together along the anterior two-thirds of the tracheal circumference, forming a framework for the trachea. Fibrous and elastic tissues and smooth muscle fibers complete the ring posteriorly. The first and last tracheal cartilages differ somewhat from the others: the first is broader and is attached by the cricotracheal

ligament to the lower border of the cricoid cartilage of the larynx. The last is thicker and broader at its middle, where it projects a hook-shaped process downward and backward from its lower border—the carina—between the two mainstem bronchi. The carina is located at the fifth thoracic vertebra or sternal notch and represents the cartilaginous wedge at the bifurcation of the trachea into the right and left mainstem bronchi.

Mainstem and lobar bronchi.

The right mainstem bronchus is wider and shorter than its left counterpart, and it diverges at approximately a 25-degree angle from the trachea. It passes laterally downward behind the superior vena cava for approximately 1 inch before giving off its first branch—the upper lobe bronchus—and entering the root of the right lung. Approximately 1 inch farther, it gives off its second branch—the middle lobe bronchus—from within the oblique fissure. Thereafter, the remnant of the mainstem bronchus continues as the lower lobe bronchus.

The left mainstem bronchus leaves the trachea at an angle of approximately 40 to 60 degrees and passes below the arch of the aorta and behind the left pulmonary artery, proceeding for a little more than 2 inches before it enters the root of the left lung, giving off the upper lobe bronchus and continuing on as the lower lobe bronchus. The left lung has no middle lobe, which is a major distinguishing feature in the general architecture of the lungs.

Segmental and subsegmental bronchi.

Each of the lobar bronchi gives off two or more segmental bronchi; an understanding of their anatomy is essential to the appropriate assessment and treatment of pulmonary disorders (Fig. 1-12). The RUL bronchus divides into three segmental bronchi about a half inch from its own origin: the first—the apical segmental bronchus—passes superolaterally toward its distribution in the apex of the lung; the second—the posterior segmental bronchus—proceeds slightly upward and posterolaterally to its distribution in the posteroinferior aspect of the upper lobe; the third—the anterior segmental bronchus—runs anteroinferiorly to its distribution in the remainder of the upper lobe. The RML bronchus divides into a lateral segmental bronchus, which is distributed to the lateral aspect of the middle lobe, and a medial segmental bronchus to the medial aspect. The RLL bronchus first gives off a branch from its

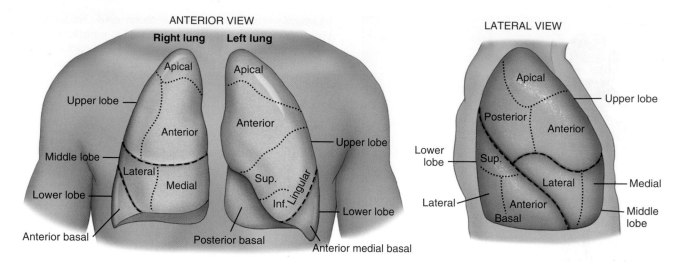

Figure 1-12 Anterior and lateral views of the bronchopulmonary segments as seen projected to the surface of the lungs.

posterior surface—the superior segmental bronchus—which passes posterosuperiorly to its distribution in the upper portion of the lower lobe. Then, after continuing to descend posterolaterally, the lower lobe bronchus yields the medial basal segmental bronchus (distributed to a small area below the hilus) from its anteromedial surface. The next offshoots from the lower lobe bronchus are the anterior basal segmental bronchus, which continues its descent anteriorly, and a very small trunk that almost immediately splits into the lateral basal segmental bronchus (distributed to the lower lateral area of the lower lobe) and the posterior basal segmental bronchus (distributed to the lower posterior area of the lower lobe).

The LUL bronchus extends laterally from the anterolateral aspect of the left mainstem bronchus before dividing into correlates of the right upper and middle lobar bronchi. However, these two branches remain within the LUL because there is no left middle lobe. The uppermost branch ascends for approximately one-third of an inch before yielding the anterior segmental bronchus, and then continues its upward path as the apicoposterior segmental bronchus before subdividing further into its subsegmental distribution. The caudal branch descends anterolaterally to its distribution in the anteroinferior area of the LUL, a region called the *lingula*. This lingular bronchus divides into the superior lingular and inferior lingular segmental bronchi.

The LLL bronchus descends posterolaterally for approximately one-third of an inch before giving off the superior segmental bronchus from its posterior surface (its distribution is similar to that of the RLL superior segmental bronchus). After another one-half to two-thirds of an inch, the lower lobe bronchus splits in two: the anteromedial division is called the *anteromedial basal segmental bronchus*, and the posterolateral division immediately branches into the lateral basal and posterior basal segmental bronchi. The distributions of these segmental bronchi are similar to those of their right-lung counterparts.

The epithelium of the upper regions of the conducting airways is pseudostratified and, for the most part, ciliated. The epithelium of the terminal and respiratory bronchioles is single layered and more cuboidal in shape, and many of the cells are nonciliated. The lamina propria, to which the epithelial basal lamina is attached, contains longitudinal bands of elastin throughout the length of the tracheobronchial tree that spread into the elastin network of the terminal respiratory units. The framework thus created is responsible for much of the elastic recoil of the lungs during expiration.

The most abundant types of cells in the bronchial epithelium are the ciliated cells. Ciliated cells are found in all levels of the tracheobronchial tree down to the level of the respiratory bronchioles. The cilia projecting from their luminal surfaces are intimately involved in the removal of inhaled particulate matter from the airways via the "mucociliary escalator" mechanism.

Two of the bronchial epithelial cells are mucus secreting: the mucous cells and serous cells.[15] Mucous cells, formerly called *goblet cells*, are normally more numerous in the trachea and large airways, becoming less numerous with distal progression, until they are infrequently found in the bronchioles. Serous cells are much less numerous than mucous cells and are confined predominantly to the extrapulmonary bronchi. Both types of cells are nonciliated, although both exhibit filamentous surface projections.

Clinical tip

Smoking paralyzes ciliated epithelial cells. These cilia will be paralyzed for 1 to 3 hours after smoking a cigarette, or will be permanently paralyzed in chronic smokers.[16] The inability of the mucociliary escalator to work increases the individual's risk for developing respiratory infections.

Terminal respiratory (acinar) units.

The conducting airways terminate in gas-exchange airways made up of respiratory bronchioles, alveolar ducts, and alveoli (Fig. 1-13). These structures together are termed the *acinus* and participate in gas exchange. The functional unit of the lung is the alveoli, where gas exchange occurs. The acinus is connected to the interstitium through a dense network of fibers. Two major types of epithelial cells exist along the alveolar wall. Squamous pneumocytes (type I) cells are flat and thin and cover approximately 93% of the alveolar surface.

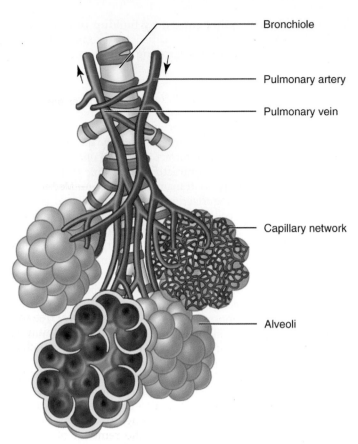

Bronchiole

Pulmonary artery

Pulmonary vein

Capillary network

Alveoli

Figure 1-13 A view of the terminal respiratory unit showing the alveolar sac and blood supply surrounding. (From Malamed SF: *Sedation*, ed 4, Mosby, St. Louis, 2010.)

Granular pneumocytes (type II) cells are thick, are cuboidal shaped, cover 7% of the alveolar wall, and are involved in the production of surfactant.[13] Surfactant is a lipoprotein that lowers alveolar surface tension at end expiration and thereby prevents the lung from collapsing. The alveoli, like the bronchi, contain cellular components of inflammation and immunity. The alveolar macrophage engulfs and ingests foreign material in the alveoli and provides a protective function against disease.

Capillaries composed of a single layer of endothelial cells deliver blood in close proximity to the alveoli. Capillaries can distend and accommodate to the volume of blood being delivered to the lung. The alveolar capillary interface is where exchange of gases occurs. The thickness of the alveolar capillary membrane is between 0.5 and 1.0 μm.

Innervation of the Lungs

The lungs are invested with a rich supply of afferent and efferent nerve fibers and specialized receptors. Parasympathetic fibers are supplied by preganglionic fibers from the vagal nuclei via the vagus nerves to ganglia around the bronchi and blood vessels. Postganglionic fibers innervate the bronchial and vascular smooth muscle, as well as the mucous cells and submucosal bronchial glands. The parasympathetic postganglionic fibers from thoracic sympathetic ganglia innervate essentially the same structures. Posterior and anterior pulmonary plexuses are formed by contributions from the postganglionic sympathetic and

parasympathetic fibers at the roots of the lungs. Generally, stimulation of the vagus nerve results in bronchial constriction, dilation of pulmonary arterial smooth muscle, and increased glandular secretion.[17] Stimulation of the sympathetic nerves causes bronchial relaxation, constriction of pulmonary arterial smooth muscle, and decreased glandular secretion.[17]

Bronchodilators enhance sympathetic stimulation to the lungs to cause relaxation of bronchial smooth muscle cells and reduce secretions.

The Cardiovascular System

Mediastinum

The mediastinum lies between the right and left pleura of the lungs and near the median sagittal plane of the chest. From an anteroposterior perspective, it extends from the sternum in front to the vertebral column behind and contains all the thoracic viscera except the lungs.[8] It is surrounded by the chest wall anteriorly, the lungs laterally, and the spine posteriorly. It is continuous with the loose connective tissue of the neck and extends inferiorly onto the diaphragm. It is the central compartment of the thoracic cavity and contains the heart, the great vessels of the heart, esophagus, trachea, phrenic nerve, cardiac nerve, thoracic duct, thymus, and lymph nodes of the central chest.[8,13]

A shifting of the structures within the mediastinum (mediastinal shift) is appropriate to consider and examine on the chest radiograph in patients who have air trapped in the pleural space (pneumothorax) or after removal of a lung (pneumonectomy).[3] In a tension pneumothorax or pneumonectomy, the mediastinum shift away from the affected or operated side.

Heart

The heart is the primary pump that circulates blood through the entire vascular system. It is closely related to the size of the body and is roughly the size of the individual's closed fist. It lies obliquely (diagonally) in the mediastinum, with two-thirds lying left of the midsagittal plane. The superior portion of the heart formed by the two atria is termed the *base* of the heart. It is broad and exists at the level of the second intercostal space in adults. The apex of the heart, defined by the tip of the left ventricle, projects into the fifth intercostal space at the midclavicular line.

The heart moves freely and changes its position during its contraction and relaxation phase, as well as during breathing. As the heart contracts, it moves anteriorly and collides with the chest wall. The portion of the heart that strikes the chest wall is the apex of the heart and is termed the *point of maximum impulse*.[1] Normally, this point is evidenced at the anatomic landmark of the apex, which is the fifth intercostal space at the midclavicular line. In terms of ventilation, quiet resting breathing does not alter the point of maximum impulse because of minimal excursion of the diaphragm. However, with deep inspiration, there is more significant inferior depression of the diaphragm, causing the heart to descend and rotate to the right, displacing the point of maximum impulse away from the normal palpable position.[1]

The point of maximum impulse is relatively more lateral in patients with left ventricular hypertrophy caused by an increase in left ventricular mass. Also, patients with a pneumothorax and resultant mediastinal shift will demonstrate an altered point of maximum impulse away from the normal anatomic position of the apex of the heart.

Tissue Layers

Pericardium

The heart wall is made up of three tissue layers (Fig. 1-14). The outermost layer of the heart is a double-walled sac termed the *pericardium*, anchored to the diaphragm inferiorly and the connective tissue of the great vessels superiorly. The two layers of the pericardium include an outer parietal pericardium and an inner visceral pericardium, also referred to as the *epicardium*.[8] The parietal pericardium is a tough, fibrous layer of dense, irregular connective tissue, whereas the visceral pericardium is a thin, smooth, and moist serous layer. Between the two layers of the pericardium is a closed space termed the *pericardial space* or *pericardial cavity* filled with approximately 10 to 20 mL of clear pericardial fluid.[18] This fluid separates the two layers and minimizes friction during cardiac contraction.

In patients with inflammation of the pericardium, fluid may accumulate in the closed pericardial space, producing cardiac tamponade, evidenced as compromised cardiac function and contractility caused by buildup of fluid in the pericardial space. Finally, pericarditis is also commonly noted after a coronary artery bypass grafting procedure.

Myocardium

The middle layer of the heart is termed the *myocardium*. It is the layer of the heart that facilitates the pumping action of the heart as a result of the presence of contractile elements. Myocardial cells are unique, as they demonstrate three important traits: automaticity (the ability to contract in the absence of stimuli); rhythmicity (the ability to contract in a rhythmic manner); and conductivity (the ability to transmit nerve impulses).[17] Myocardial cells may be categorized into two groups based on their function: mechanical cells contributing to mechanical contraction and conductive cells contributing to electrical conduction.[1,17] Mechanical cells, also termed *myocytes*, are large cells containing a larger number of actin and myosin myofilaments, enabling a greater capacity for mechanical shortening needed for pump action. In addition, these cells have a large number of mitochondria (25% of cellular volume) to provide sufficient energy in the form of adenosine triphosphate (ATP) to the heart, an organ that can never rest.[5,17] The conducting myocardial cells are joined by intercalated disks forming a structure known as a *syncytium*. A syncytium characterizes a group of cells in which the protoplasm of one cell is continuous with that of adjacent cells.[8] Intercalated disks contain two junctions: desmosomes attaching one cell to another and connexins that allow the electrical flow to spread from one cell to another. These two junctions work together to move the impulse through a low-resistance pathway.

Injured myocardial cells cannot be replaced, as the myocardium is unable to undergo mitotic activity. Thus death of cells from an infarction or a cardiomyopathy may result in a significant reduction in contractile function.

Endocardium

The innermost layer of the heart is termed the *endocardium*. This layer consists of simple squamous endothelium overlying a thin areolar tissue layer.[18] The tissue of the endocardium forms the inner lining of the chambers of the heart and is continuous with the tissue of the valves and the endothelium of the blood vessel.

Because the endocardium and valves share similar tissue, patients with endocarditis must be ruled out for valvular dysfunction. Endocardial infections can spread into valvular tissue, developing vegetations on the valve.[19] Bronchopulmonary hygiene procedures, including percussions and vibrations, are contraindicated for patients with unstable vegetations, as they may dislodge, move as emboli, and cause an embolic stroke.

Chambers of the Heart

The heart is divided into right and left halves by a longitudinal septum (Fig. 1-15). The right side of the heart receives deoxygenated venous blood (returning from the body), and the left side of the heart receives oxygenated blood (returning from the lungs). Each half of the heart is made up of two chambers: superiorly the atria and inferiorly the ventricles. Thus the four chambers of the heart include the right atrium (Fig. 1-16, *A*), right ventricle

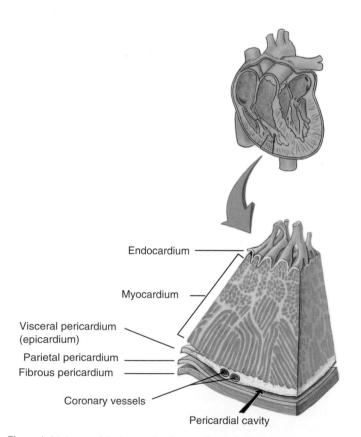

Endocardium

Myocardium

Visceral pericardium (epicardium)

Parietal pericardium

Fibrous pericardium

Coronary vessels

Pericardial cavity

Figure 1-14 Layers of the heart wall. (From Applegate E: *The Anatomy and Physiology Learning System*, ed 3, St. Louis, 2007, Saunders.)

(see Fig. 1-16, *A*), left atrium (see Fig. 1-16, *B*), and left ventricle (see Fig. 1-16, *B*). The atria receive blood from the systemic and pulmonary veins and eject blood into the ventricles. The ventricles eject blood that is received from the atria into arteries that deliver blood to the lungs and the systemic circulation.

Right Atrium

The chamber of the right atrium (see Fig. 1-16, *A*) consists of a smooth posterior and medial inner wall. Parallel muscle bundles known as *pectinate muscles* exist anteriorly and laterally. Both right and left atria have small earlike extensions called *auricles* that help to increase volume within the chambers. The right atrium receives deoxygenated blood from three major vessels. The superior vena cava collects venous blood from the head and upper extremities; the inferior vena cava collects blood from the trunk and lower extremities; and the coronary sinus collects venous blood specifically from the heart. The coronary sinus empties into the right atrium above the tricuspid valve. Normal

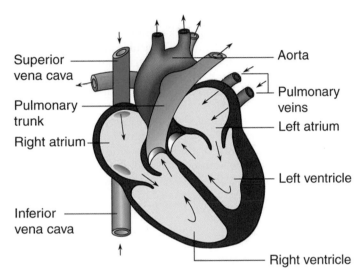

Figure 1-15 View of heart showing all four chambers and forward blood flow through right and left sides. (From Khanna N: *Illustrated Synopsis of Dermatology and Sexually Transmitted Diseases*, New Delhi, 2005, Peepee Publishers and Distributors.)

diastolic pressure to enable filling ranges from 0 to 8 mm Hg and is clinically referred to as the *central venous pressure*.

The effective contraction of the pectinate muscles of the atria accounts for approximately 15% to 20% of cardiac output—the atrial kick.[19] In patients with abnormal electrical conduction causing a quivering of the atria (atrial fibrillation), the mechanical contractile ability of the pectinate muscles is reduced, resulting in a low atrial kick and compromised cardiac output.[1,5]

Right Ventricle

The right ventricle is shaped like a crescent or triangle, enabling it to eject large volumes of blood through a small valve into a low-pressure pulmonary system. Blood within the right ventricle is received from the right atrium through a one-way valve present between the atrium and ventricle termed the *tricuspid atrioventricular valve*. It ejects blood to the lungs via the pulmonic semilunar valve into the pulmonary artery. The right ventricle (see Fig. 1-16, *A*), like the right atrium, may be considered in two parts: (1) a posteroinferior inflow tract, termed the *body*, which contains the tricuspid valve, chordae tendineae, papillary muscles, and trabeculated myocardium; and (2) an anterosuperior outflow tract, called the *infundibulum*, from which the pulmonary trunk arises.[8] Four muscular bands separate the inflow and outflow portions of the right ventricle, including the infundibular septum, the parietal band, the septal band, and the moderator band. Pressures within the right ventricle are relatively lower compared with the left ventricle, with diastolic pressures ranging from 0 to 8 mm Hg and systolic pressures ranging from 15 to 30 mm Hg.[17]

During periods of exacerbation, patients with chronic lung pathologies, including COPD and pulmonary fibrosis, often present with hypoxemia and increased pressure within the pulmonary vasculature, termed *pulmonary artery hypertension*, caused by compromised perfusion capacity to the lung.[19,20] The increased pressure within the pulmonary artery increases the workload on the right ventricle, causing cor pulmonale, or right ventricular hypertrophy, and resultant right ventricular failure.

Left Atrium

The left atrium is divided from the right atrium by an interatrial septum. It has a relatively thicker wall compared with

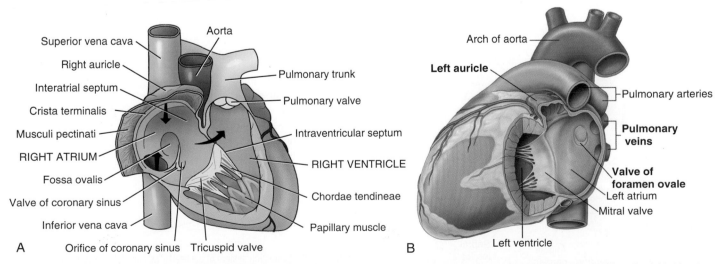

Figure 1-16 Schematic of the heart. **A,** Right atrium and ventricle. The arrows indicate the flow of blood from the venae cavae to the right atrium and from the right atrium to the right ventricle. **B,** Left atrium and ventricle. The blood flows from the pulmonary veins to the left atrium, through the mitral valve into the left ventricle, and from there into the systemic circulation. (From Snopek AM: *Fundamentals of Special Radiographic Procedures*, ed 5, St. Louis, 2007, Saunders.)

the right atrium to adapt to higher pressures of blood entering the chamber from the lung. Oxygenated blood from the lungs enters the left atrium posteriorly via the pulmonary veins. These vessels have no valves; instead, pectinate muscles extend from the atria into the pulmonary veins and exert a sphincterlike action to prevent backflow of blood during contraction of the atria. The normal filling pressure of the left ventricle is between 4 and 12 mm Hg. Oxygenated blood is ejected out of the left atrium through the mitral atrioventricular (bicuspid) valve to enter the left ventricle.

Regurgitation, or insufficiency of the mitral valve, causes blood to accumulate in the left atrium and elevate left atrial pressures. These chronically elevated pressures alter the integrity of the atrial wall and predispose the individual to developing a quivering of the atria wall (atrial fibrillation) and potential blood clots within the left atrium.

Left Ventricle

The almost conical left ventricle (see Fig. 1-16, *B*) is longer and narrower than the right ventricle. The walls of the left ventricle are approximately three times thicker than those of the right, and the transverse aspect of the cavity is almost circular. In contrast to the inflow and outflow orifices of the right ventricle, those of the left are located adjacent to one another, being separated only by the anterior leaflet of the mitral valve and the common fibrous ridge to which it and the left and posterior cusps of the aortic valve are attached. The interventricular septum forms the medial wall of the left ventricle and creates a separation between the left and right ventricle.

This chamber receives oxygenated blood from the left atrium via the mitral valve and ejects blood through the aortic valve and into the aorta to the peripheral systemic vasculature. Normal systolic pressures within the left ventricle are 80 to 120 mm Hg, and diastolic pressures are 4 to 12 mm Hg. Because of the elevated pressures within this chamber, the wall thickness of the left ventricle is the greatest compared with the three other chambers of the heart.

Pathologic thickening of the left ventricular wall is evidenced in patients with various cardiovascular complications, including but not limited to, hypertension, aortic stenosis, and heart failure, as a consequence of an increase in the afterload. This pathologic thickening alters the contractile ability of the ventricle and reduces its filling capacity, causing a reduction in cardiac output.

Heart Valves

Four heart valves (Fig. 1-17) ensure one-way blood flow through the heart. Two atrioventricular valves exist between the atria and the ventricle, including the tricuspid valve on the right and the mitral or bicuspid valve on the left between the left atrium and ventricle. The semilunar valves lie between the ventricles and arteries and are named based on their corresponding vessels: pulmonic valve on the right in association with the pulmonary artery, and aortic valve on the left relating to the aorta.

Flaps of tissue called *leaflets* or *cusps* guard the heart valve openings. The right atrioventricular valve has three cusps and therefore is termed *tricuspid*, whereas the left atrioventricular valve has only two cusps and hence is termed *bicuspid*. These leaflets are attached to the papillary muscles of the myocardium by chordae tendineae. The primary function of the atrioventricular valves is to prevent backflow of blood into the atria during ventricular contraction or systole, and the semilunar valves prevent backflow of blood from the aorta and pulmonary artery into the ventricles during diastole. Opening and closing of each valve depends on pressure gradient changes within the heart created during each cardiac cycle.

An initial disturbance of valvular function may be picked up through auscultation of the heart sounds and evidenced by variety of murmurs. It must be noted that the identification of a murmur would warrant the need for additional testing, including echocardiography, to accurately diagnose pathology within a particular valve.

Conduction System

In a normal conduction system (Fig. 1-18), electrical impulses arise in the sinoatrial (SA), or sinus, node. The SA node is

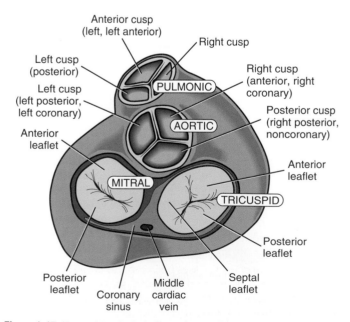

Figure 1-17 Nomenclature for the leaflets and cusps of the principal valves of the heart.

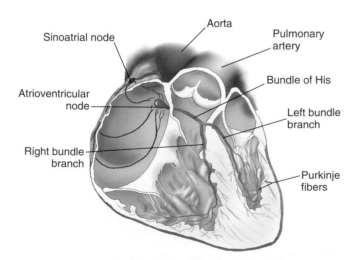

Figure 1-18 Conduction system of the heart. The electrical impulse originates in the heart, and contraction of the heart's chambers is coordinated by specialized heart tissues. (From Leonard PC: *Building a Medical Vocabulary: With Spanish Translations*, ed 7, St. Louis, 2009, Saunders.)

located at the junction of the right atrium and superior vena cava. The P cells of the SA node are the sites for impulse generation; consequently, the SA node is termed the *pacemaker* of the heart, as it makes or creates the impulses that pace the heart.[8] The normal pacing ability of the SA node is between 60 and 100 beats per minute (bpm) at rest. The impulse generated at the SA node travels down one of three internodal tracts to the atrioventricular (AV) node. The three conduction pathways that exist between the SA and AV node include an anterior tract of Bachman, a middle tract of Wenckebach, and a posterior tract of Thorel.[8]

The AV node is located at the inferior aspect of the right atrium, near the opening of the coronary sinus and above the tricuspid valve. Posterior to the AV node are several parasympathetic autonomic ganglia that serve as receptors for the vagus nerve and cause slowing of the cardiac cycle. The major function of the AV node during each cardiac cycle is to slow down the cardiac impulse to mechanically allow time for the ventricles to fill.

Conducting fibers from the AV node converge to form the bundle of His to carry the impulse into the ventricles. The bundle of His appears as a triangle of nerve fibers within the posterior border of the interventricular septum. The bundle bifurcates to give rise to the right and left bundle branches carrying the impulse to the right and left ventricles, respectively. The right bundle branch (RBB) is thin, with relatively fewer branches proceeding inferiorly to the apex of the right ventricle. The left bundle branch (LBB) arises perpendicularly and divides into two branches or fascicles.[8] The left anterior bundle branch crosses the left anterior papillary muscle and proceeds along the base of the left ventricle toward the aortic valve. The left posterior bundle branch advances posteriorly through the posterior papillary muscle toward the posterior inferior left ventricular wall.

Both bundles terminate into a network of nerve fibers called the *Purkinje fibers*. These fibers extend from the apex of each ventricle and penetrate the heart wall to the outer myocardium. Electrical stimulation of the Purkinje fibers causes mechanical contraction of the ventricles. It may be important to appreciate that normal electrical conduction through the heart allows for appropriate mechanical activity and maintenance of cardiac output to sustain activity. An alteration in the conduction pathway subsequently alters the mechanical activity of the heart and reduces cardiac output.

Clinical tip

An evaluation of electrocardiographic (ECG) changes is necessary to help a clinician recognize and differentially diagnose reduced exercise tolerance caused from an electrical disturbance producing mechanical alterations that reduce cardiac output and exercise tolerance and not a true mechanical problem within the heart.

Innervation

Although the SA node and conduction pathway have an intrinsic rate of depolarization causing contraction of the myocardium, the autonomic nervous system influences the rate of impulse generation, contraction, relaxation, and strength of contraction.[6,17] Thus autonomic neural transmission creates changes in the heart rate and contractility to allow adjustments in cardiac output to meet metabolic demands. A cardiac plexus contains both sympathetic and parasympathetic nerve fibers and is located anterior to the tracheal bifurcation.

The cardiac plexus receives its parasympathetic input from the right and left vagus nerves.[17] Subsequently, nerves branch off the plexus, follow the coronary vessels, and innervate the SA node and other components of the conduction system. There is relatively less parasympathetic innervation to the ventricles, resulting in a sympathetic dominance on ventricular function. Vagal stimulation is inhibitory on the cardiovascular system and is evidenced by decreased heart rate and blood pressure.[6] The neurohormone involved with parasympathetic stimulation is acetylcholine.

The sympathetic input to the plexus arises from the sympathetic trunk in the neck. Cardiac nerves from the cervical and upper four to five thoracic ganglia feed into the cardiac plexus.[6,17] Sympathetic stimulation releases catecholamines (epinephrine and norepinephrine) that interact with β-adrenergic receptors on the cardiac cell membrane, causing an excitation of the cardiovascular system. This is evidenced by an increase in heart rate, increased contractility through a greater influx of calcium into myocytes, increased blood pressure, a shortening of the conduction time through the AV node, and an increase in rhythmicity of the AV pacemaker fibers.

Sympathetic nervous system stimulation is cardioexcitatory and increases heart rate and contractility—the fight-or-flight response. Conversely, parasympathetic stimulation is cardioinhibitory and slows down heart rate and contractility.

Cardiac and Pulmonary Vessels

Aorta

The ascending aorta begins at the base of the left ventricle and is approximately 2 inches long. From the lower border of the third costal cartilage at the left of the sternum, it passes upward and forward toward the right as high as the second right costal cartilage. The aorta exhibits three dilations above the attached margins of the cusps of the aortic valve at the root of the aorta—the aortic sinuses (of Valsalva). The coronary arteries (Fig. 1-19) open near these aortic sinuses of Valsalva. Three branches typically arise from the upper aspect of the arch of the aorta: the brachiocephalic trunk (innominate artery), the left common carotid artery, and the left subclavian artery. The openings of the coronary arteries block blood from entering into the arteries when the aortic valve is open (during systole). Therefore the part of the cardiac cycle when the coronary arteries receive their blood is during diastole, when the aortic valves are closed.

Right Coronary Artery

The right coronary artery arises from the right anterolateral surface of the aorta and passes between the auricular appendage of the right atrium and the pulmonary trunk, typically giving off a branch to the sinus node and yielding two or three right anterior ventricular rami as it descends into the coronary sulcus to come around the right (acute) margin of

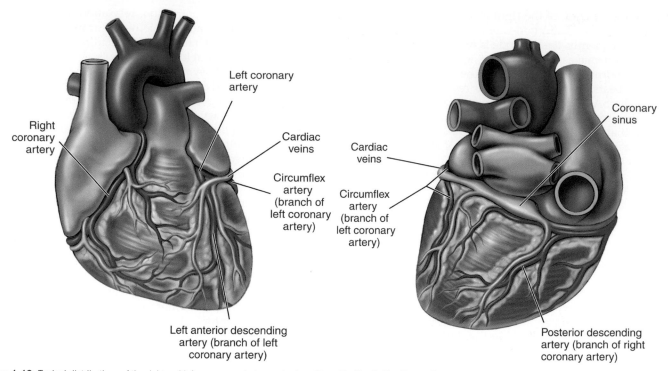

Figure 1-19 Typical distributions of the right and left coronary arteries and veins (From Herlihy B: *The Human Body in Health and Illness*, ed 4, St. Louis, 2011, Saunders.)

the heart into the posterior aspect of the sulcus. As the right coronary artery crosses the right margin of the heart, it gives off the right (acute) marginal artery before continuing as far as the posterior interventricular sulcus, where it usually turns to supply the diaphragmatic surfaces of the ventricles as the posterior interventricular (posterior descending) artery. In approximately 70% of hearts, an atrioventricular nodal artery is given off just before the posterior interventricular artery.[21]

Left Coronary Artery

The left coronary artery originates from the left anterolateral aspect of the aorta and splits into two major branches: the anterior interventricular and circumflex arteries. The anterior interventricular, or left anterior descending artery (LAD), traverses the anterior interventricular groove to supply sternocostal aspects of both ventricles. In its course, the anterior interventricular artery gives off right and left anterior ventricular and anterior septal branches. The larger left anterior ventricular branches vary in number from two to nine, with the first being designated the *diagonal artery*. Approximately 70% of the left ventricle is fed by the LAD artery. The circumflex artery runs in the coronary sulcus between the left atrium and ventricle, crosses the left margin of the heart, and usually continues to its termination, just short of the junction of the right coronary and the posterior interventricular arteries. In many instances, as the circumflex artery crosses the left margin of the heart, it gives off a large branch that supplies this area—the left marginal (obtuse) artery.

The right coronary artery is the primary supply route for blood to the majority of the right ventricle and the inferior and posterior portions of the left ventricle. In addition, specialized conduction tissue within the right atrium, including the SA node and AV node, are nourished by the right coronary artery. The LAD supplies blood to the anterior and septal aspects of the left ventricle, and the circumflex artery supplies blood to the lateral aspect of the left ventricle.

Occlusion of a coronary artery produces an infarction in a defined region within the heart. Right coronary artery occlusions cause inferior or posterior infarctions and affect the functioning of the SA node in the right atrium. Left anterior descending artery occlusions produce anterior septal infarctions, also termed the *widow maker*, whereas circumflex occlusions are responsible for generating lateral infarctions.

Distribution of blood supply within the heart is variable from one individual to another because of the presence of collateral circulation involving the formation of new blood vessels (angiogenesis) in areas of the heart that are partially occluded.

Pulmonary Artery

The pulmonary trunk runs upward and backward (first in front of and then to the left of the ascending aorta) from the base of the right ventricle; it is approximately 2 inches in length. At the level of the fifth thoracic vertebra, it splits into right and left pulmonary arteries. The right pulmonary artery runs behind the ascending aorta, superior vena cava, and upper pulmonary vein, but in front of the esophagus and right primary bronchus to the root of the lung. The left pulmonary artery runs in front of the descending aorta and the left primary bronchus to the root of the left lung. It is attached to the arch of the aorta by the ligamentum arteriosum.

Clinical tip

A saddle embolus is life threatening and involves an embolus dislodged at the bifurcation of the right and left pulmonary arteries.

Pulmonary Veins

The pulmonary veins, unlike the systemic veins, have no valves. They originate in the capillary networks and join together to ultimately form two veins—a superior and an inferior pulmonary vein—from each lung, which open separately into the left atrium (see Fig. 1-19).

Vena Cava and Cardiac Veins

The superior vena cava is approximately 3 inches long from its termination in the upper part of the right atrium opposite the third right costal cartilage to the junction of the two brachiocephalic veins. The inferior vena cava extends from the junction of the two common iliac veins, in front of the fifth lumbar vertebra, passing through the diaphragm to open into the lower portion of the right atrium. The vena cavae have no valves.

The cardiac veins can be categorized into three groups: the coronary sinus and its supplying veins, the anterior cardiac veins, and the thebesian veins. Most of the veins of the heart drain into the coronary sinus, which runs into the posterior aspect of the coronary sulcus and empties through the valve of the coronary sinus, a semilunar flap, into the right atrium between the opening of the inferior vena cava and the tricuspid valve. As Fig. 1-19 shows, the small and middle cardiac veins, the posterior vein of the left ventricle, the left marginal vein, and the great cardiac vein feed the coronary sinus.

The anterior cardiac veins are fed from the anterior part of the right ventricle. They originate in the subepicardial tissue, crossing the coronary sulcus as they terminate directly into the right atrium. The right marginal vein runs along the right border of the heart and usually opens directly into the right atrium. Occasionally, it may join the small cardiac vein.

The thebesian veins (venae cordis minimae) vary greatly in their number and size. These tiny veins open into all the cavities of the heart, but are most numerous in the right atrium and ventricle, are found occasionally in the left atrium, and are rare in the left ventricle.

Systemic Circulation

Oxygenated blood ejected out of the heart flows through the aorta into systemic arteries. These arteries branch into smaller vessels called *arterioles*, which further branch into the smallest vessels, the capillaries primarily involved in the exchange of nutrients and gases. Deoxygenated blood from the capillaries enters venules that join together to form larger veins that return blood back to the right heart and lungs. Blood vessels have three layers: the innermost tunica intima, middle tunica media, and outermost tunica adventitia.

Arteries

The wall of the artery is composed of elastic and fibrous connective tissue and smooth muscle. Anatomically, arteries can be categorized into two types depending on the structural components along their wall. Elastic arteries, including the aorta and pulmonary trunk, have a thick tunica media with more elastic fibers than smooth muscle cells, allowing for a greater stretch as blood is ejected out

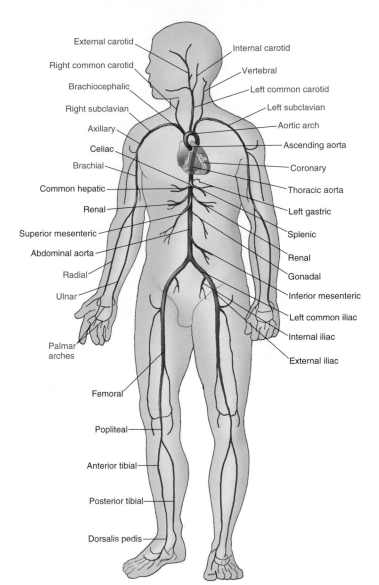

Figure 1-20 Anterior view of the aorta and its principal arterial branches. Labels for the ascending, arch, thoracic, and abdominal aorta and their corresponding arteries are shown. (From Leonard PC: *Building a Medical Vocabulary: With Spanish Translations*, ed 7, St. Louis, 2009, Saunders.)

of the heart. During diastole, the elasticity of the vessel promotes recoil of the artery and maintains blood pressure within the vessel. Muscular arteries are present in medium and small arteries and contain more smooth muscle cells within the middle tunica media layer. These arteries have the ability of vasoconstriction and vasodilation as a result of the presence of smooth muscles cells to control the amount of blood flow to the periphery.[6] These smooth muscle cells are under autonomic nervous system influence through the presence of α-receptors. As the artery becomes more distal, a greater amount of smooth muscle is evidenced. Arterioles have primarily smooth muscle along their walls, enabling their diameter to alter significantly as needed. Arterioles empty into capillary beds. The density of capillaries within a capillary bed is greater in active tissue, including the muscle. Exchange of nutrients and gases occur within the capillary bed. Fig. 1-20 depicts the major arterial tree within the human body.

Endothelium

Endothelial cells form the endothelium, or endothelial lining, of the blood vessel. These cells have the ability to adjust their number and arrangement to accommodate local requirements. Endothelial cells serve several important functions, including filtration and permeability, vasomotion, clotting, and inflammation.[19] Atherosclerosis is initiated through endothelial dysfunction, evidenced by endothelial cells that are extensively permeable to fat cells and white blood cells.

Veins

Compared with arteries, veins have thinner walls and a larger diameter. Veins also have less elastic tissue and hence are not as distensible. In the lower extremity, veins have valves to assist with unidirectional flow of blood back to the heart. Blood is transferred back to the heart through muscle pump activity, which causes a milking effect on the veins.

Patients with incompetent valves in their veins develop varicosities in their lower extremities. Also, patients on prolonged bed rest are likely to develop deep vein thrombosis from a lack of muscle activity, resulting in a pooling of blood and clot formation within the venous vasculature.

Summary

This chapter provides the reader with an understanding of the anatomy of the cardiovascular and pulmonary systems and its relevance for the therapist. This content provides the basis for an understanding of the pathophysiology of these systems and lays a foundation for the development of relevant examination and treatment strategies to use when managing patients with cardiopulmonary dysfunction. A comprehensive understanding of anatomy is fundamental to the knowledge base of the therapist in understanding the central components involved in the delivery of oxygen and nutrients to peripheral tissue.

References

1. DeTurk W, Cahalin L: *Cardiovascular and Pulmonary Physical Therapy: An Evidenced-Based Approach*, New York, 2004, McGraw-Hill.
2. Townsend CM, Beauchamp RD, Evers BM, et al.: *Sabiston Textbook of Surgery*, ed 18, Philadelphia, 2008, Saunders.
3. Paz J, West M: *Acute Care Handbook for Physical Therapists*, ed 3, Philadelphia, 2009, Saunders.
4. Ganong WF: *Review of Medical Physiology*, ed 21, New York, 2003, McGraw-Hill.
5. Frownfelter D, Dean E: *Cardiovascular and Pulmonary Physical Therapy: Evidence and Practice*, ed 4, St. Louis, 2006, Mosby.
6. Fox S: *Human Physiology*, ed 11, Boston, 2009, McGraw-Hill.
7. Kendall FP, McCreary EP, Provance PG, et al.: *Muscles: Testing and Function*, ed 5, Baltimore, 2005, Lippincott Williams and Wilkins.
8. Gray H, Bannister LH, Berry MM, et al.: *Gray's Anatomy: The Anatomical Basis of Medicine and Surgery*, ed 38, New York, 1996, Churchill Livingstone.
9. Goodman C, Fuller K: *Pathology: Implications for the Physical Therapist*, ed 3, St. Louis, 2009, Saunders.
10. Lund VJ: Nasal physiology: Neurochemical receptors, nasal cycle and ciliary action, *Allergy Asthma Proc* 17(4):179–184, 1996.
11. Richerson HB: Lung defense mechanisms, *Allergy Proc* 11(2):59–60, 1990.
12. Janson-Bjerklie S: Defense mechanisms: Protecting the healthy lung, *Heart Lung* 12(6):643–649, 1983.
13. Moore K, Dalley A: *Clinically Oriented Anatomy*, ed 5, Baltimore, 2006, Lippincott, Williams and Wilkins.
14. Berend N, Woolcock AJ, Marlin GE: Relationship between bronchial and arterial diameters in normal human lungs, *Thorax* 34(3):354–358, 1979.
15. Mason RJ, Broaddus VC, Murray JF, et al.: *Textbook of Respiratory Medicine*, ed 4, Philadelphia, 2006, Saunders.
16. Heuther SE, McCance KL: *Understanding Pathophysiology*, ed 3, St. Louis, 2004, Mosby.
17. Guyton AC, Hall JE: *Textbook of Medical Physiology*, ed 11, Philadelphia, 2006, Saunders.
18. Moore K, Dalley A: *Clinically Oriented Anatomy*, ed 5, Baltimore, 2006, Lippincott Williams and Wilkins.
19. Cheitlin MD: *Clinical Cardiology*, ed 7, Stamford, CT, 2004, Appleton & Lange.
20. Berne RM, Levy MN: *Cardiovascular Physiology*, ed 8, Philadelphia, 2002, Mosby.
21. Abuin G, Nieponice A: New findings on the origin of the blood supply to the atrioventricular node. Clinical and surgical significance, *Tex Heart Inst J* 25(2):113–117, 1998.

2

Physiology of the cardiovascular and pulmonary systems

Konrad J. Dias

This chapter reviews concepts relating to the physiology of the cardiovascular and pulmonary systems and its relevance in physical therapy practice. The cardiopulmonary systems not only share a close spatial relationship in the thoracic cavity, but also have a close functional relationship to maintain homeostasis. Physiologically, these systems must work collaboratively to provide oxygen required for energy production and assist in removing carbon dioxide manufactured as a waste product. A disorder affecting the lungs has a direct effect on the heart and vice versa. An understanding of normal physiology helps the reader better appreciate pathophysiologic changes associated with diseases and dysfunction of these systems that will be discussed in subsequent chapters.

The Pulmonary System

The pulmonary system has several important functions. The most important function of the pulmonary system is to exchange oxygen and carbon dioxide between the environment, blood, and tissue. Oxygen is necessary for the production of energy. If a cell has oxygen, a single molecule of glucose can undergo aerobic metabolism and produce 36 adenosines triphosphate (ATP). However, if a cell is devoid of oxygen, each molecule of glucose undergoes anaerobic metabolism, yielding only 2 ATP. Thus pathology of the pulmonary system

will result in reduced energy production because of decreased oxygen within the tissue and a concomitant reduction in the exercise tolerance of the individual. Carbon dioxide is another gas that must be effectively exchanged at the level of the lung. Through the release of carbon dioxide from the body, the pulmonary system plays an important role in regulating the acid–base balance and maintaining normal blood pH. The second function of the pulmonary system is temperature homeostasis, which is achieved through evaporative heat loss from the lungs. Finally, the pulmonary system helps to filter and metabolize toxic substances, as it is the only organ that receives all blood coming from the heart.

To facilitate comprehension of the physiology of the pulmonary system, three major physiologic components are discussed in this chapter, including (1) the process of ventilation or breathing; (2) the process of gas exchange or respiration; and (3) the transport of gases to peripheral tissue.

Ventilation

Ventilation, or breathing, often misnamed respiration, involves the mechanical movement of gases into and out of the lungs.[1] At rest, an adult breathes at a rate of 10 to 15 breaths/minute, termed the *ventilatory rate* or *respiratory rate*. Approximately 350 to 500 mL of air is inhaled or exhaled at rest with each breath and is termed the *tidal volume* (TV or VT). The amount of effective ventilation, termed the *minute ventilation,* expressed in liters per minute, is calculated by multiplying the ventilatory rate and tidal volume. The minute ventilation represents the total volume of air that is inhaled or exhaled in 1 minute. At rest, the minute ventilation is approximately 5 L/min, whereas at maximum exercise, it increases to a level between 70 and 125 L/min.[2]

Additional Lung Volumes

Before considering the mechanical properties of the lungs during ventilation or breathing, it is helpful to consider the static volumes of the lungs measured via spirometry studies (Fig. 2-1).[2–4] As mentioned earlier, the volume of air normally inhaled and exhaled with each breath during quiet breathing is called the *tidal volume* (TV or VT). The additional volume of air that can be taken into the lungs beyond the normal tidal inhalation is called the *inspiratory reserve volume* (IRV). The additional volume of air that can be let out beyond the normal tidal exhalation is called the *expiratory reserve volume* (ERV). The volume of air that remains in the lungs after a forceful expiratory effort is called the *residual volume* (RV). The inspiratory capacity (IC) is the sum of the tidal and inspiratory reserve volumes; it is the maximum amount of air that can be inhaled after a normal tidal exhalation. The functional residual capacity (FRC) is the sum of the expiratory reserve and RV; it is the amount of air remaining in the lungs at the end of a normal tidal exhalation. The importance of FRC cannot be overstated; it represents the point at which the forces tending to collapse the lungs are balanced against the forces tending to expand the chest wall. The vital capacity (VC) is the sum of the inspiratory reserve, tidal, and expiratory reserve volumes; it is the maximum amount of air that can be exhaled following a maximum inhalation. The total lung capacity (TLC) is the maximum volume to which the lungs can be expanded; it is the sum of all the pulmonary volumes.

Control of Ventilation

Breathing requires repetitive stimulation from the brain, as skeletal muscles required for ventilation are unable to contract without nervous stimulation.[5] Although breathing usually occurs automatically and involuntarily, there are circumstances when individuals hold their breath, take deep breaths, or change ventilation, such as when singing or laughing. In light of this, it is important to review the mechanisms involved in helping to control breathing.

This section describes the neural mechanisms that regulate ventilation. Neurons in parts of the brainstem, including the medulla oblongata and pons, provide control for automatic breathing and adjust ventilatory rate and tidal volume for normal gas exchange (Fig. 2-2).[5] The medulla oblongata contains inspiratory neurons that produce inspiration and expiratory neurons that are triggered with forced expiration. Inspiratory neurons are located in the inspiratory center, or dorsal respiratory group, of the medulla. An enhanced frequency of firing of these neurons increases the motor units recruited and results in a deeper breath.[6] An elongation in the time of firing prolongs each breath and results in a slower respiratory rate.[6] A cessation of neural stimulation of these neurons causes elastic recoil of the lungs and passive expiration.

The expiratory center, or ventral respiratory group, in the medulla contains inspiratory neurons in the midregion and expiratory neurons in the anterior and posterior zones. Neural stimulation of the expiratory neurons causes inhibition of the inspiratory center when a deeper expiration is warranted.

The pons has two major centers that assist with ventilation, including the pneumotaxic center in the upper pons and the apneustic center in the lower pons.[5] The pneumotaxic center maintains the rhythm of ventilation, balancing the time periods of inspiration and expiration by inhibiting the apneustic center or the inspiratory center of the medulla. The apneustic center facilitates apneustic or prolonged breathing patterns when it is uninhibited from the pneumotaxic center.

Breathing concerning a conscious change in pattern involves control from the motor cortex of the frontal lobe of the cerebrum.[6] Here impulses are sent directly down to the corticospinal tracts to the respiratory neurons in the spinal cord, bypassing the respiratory centers in the brainstem to trigger changes in ventilation.

Afferent Connections to the Brainstem

The respiratory centers of the brainstem receive afferent input from various locations, including the limbic system, hypothalamus, chemoreceptors, and lungs.[5]

Hypothalamic and Limbic Influence

Sensations of pain and alterations in emotion alter ventilation through input coming to the brainstem from the limbic system and hypothalamus.[7] For example, anxiety triggers hyperventilation and a concomitant reduction in carbon dioxide levels in blood, as the rate of carbon dioxide elimination out of the lungs exceeds the rate of carbon dioxide production in the body.

> **Clinical tip**
>
> Patients with injuries within the central nervous system from an acute brain injury or stroke demonstrate altered ventilatory patterns following neurologic insult. These patients lose the normal response to breathing, resulting in altered ventilatory rates and volumes.

Chemoreceptors

Chemoreceptors are located in the brainstem and peripheral arteries. These receptors are responsible for sensing alterations in blood pH, carbon dioxide, and oxygen levels.[7] There primarily exist two types of chemoreceptors, including

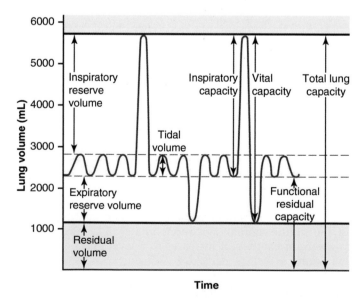

Figure 2-1 Lung volumes and capacities as displayed by a time-versus-volume spirogram. Values are approximate. The tidal volume is measured under resting conditions. (From Seeley RR, Stephens TD, Tate P: *Anatomy & Physiology*, ed 3, New York, 1995, McGraw-Hill.)

central and peripheral chemoreceptors. The receptors found along the anterior lateral surfaces of the upper medulla of the brainstem are called *central chemoreceptors.* These receptors are stimulated when carbon dioxide concentrations rise in the cerebrospinal fluid. Central chemoreceptors facilitate an increased depth and rate of ventilation so as to restore normal carbon dioxide levels and pH in the body.[5,7] Peripheral chemoreceptors are found within the carotid artery and aortic arch. These receptors help to increase ventilation in response to increasing levels of carbon dioxide in blood (hypercapnia), as well as low oxygen levels in blood (hypoxia).[5,7]

In a small percentage of patients with chronically high carbon dioxide levels in blood, such as in patients with severe chronic obstructive pulmonary disease (COPD), the body begins to rely more on oxygen receptors and less on carbon dioxide receptors to regulate breathing. This is termed the *hypoxic drive to breathe* and is a form of respiratory drive in which the body uses oxygen receptors instead of carbon dioxide receptors to regulate the respiratory cycle.[8] Normal ventilation is driven mostly by the levels of carbon dioxide in the arteries, which are detected by peripheral chemoreceptors, and very little by oxygen levels. An increase in carbon dioxide triggers the chemoreceptors and causes a resultant increase in ventilatory rate. In these few patients with COPD who demonstrate the hypoxic drive, oxygen receptors serve as the primary means of regulating breathing rate. For these patients, oxygen supplementation must be prudently administered, as an increase in oxygen within blood (hyperoxemia) suppresses the hypoxic drive and results in a reduced drive to breathe.[8]

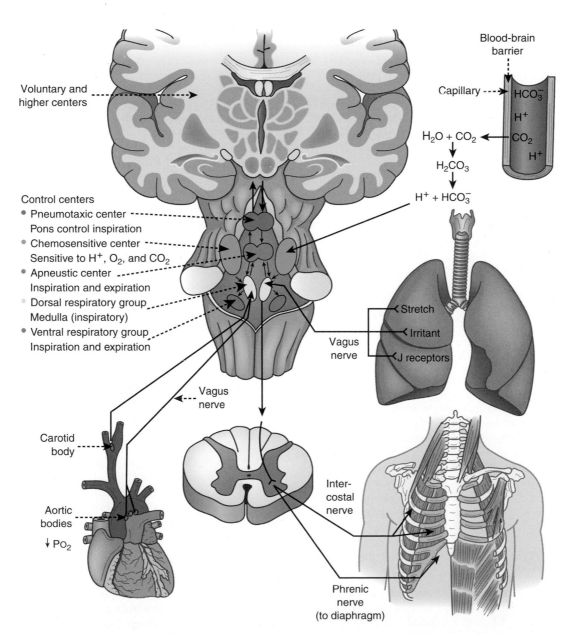

Figure 2-2 Neurochemical respiratory control system. (From McCance KL, Huether SE, Brashers VL, et al, editors: *Pathophysiology: The Biologic Basis for Disease in Adults and Children,* ed 6, St. Louis, 2010, Mosby.)

Lung Receptors

There exist three types of receptors on the lung that send signals to the respiratory centers within the brainstem:

1. *Irritant receptors:* These receptors are found within the epithelial layer of the conducting airways and respond to various noxious gases, particulate matter, and irritants, causing them to initiate a cough reflex. When stimulated, these receptors also cause bronchial constriction and increase ventilatory rate.[5]

2. *Stretch receptors:* These receptors are located along the smooth muscles lining the airways and are sensitive to increasing size and volume within the lung.[6] Hering and Breuer discovered that ventilatory rate and volume was reduced following distention of anesthetized animal lungs. This stimulation of the ventilatory changes in response to increased volume and size is termed the *Hering–Breuer reflex* and is more active in newborns. In adults, this reflex is only active with large increases in the tidal volume, which is especially seen during exercise, and protects the lung from excessive inflation.[6]

3. *J receptor:* The juxtapulmonary receptors (J receptors) are located near the pulmonary capillaries and are sensitive to increased pulmonary capillary pressures. On stimulation, these receptors initiate a rapid, shallow breathing pattern.[7] Additionally, the interstitial J receptors produce a cough reflex with fluid accumulation within the lung in patients with pulmonary edema and pleural effusions.

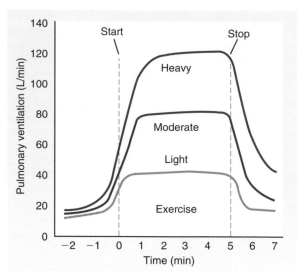

Figure 2-3 Ventilatory response during exercise.

> ### Clinical tip
>
> In patients with acute left-side congestive heart failure and resultant pulmonary edema, the interstitial J receptors within the lung are stimulated. The firing of these receptors causes the patient to breathe in a shallow, tachypneic pattern. This breathing pattern causes a milking of the lymphatic vasculature to facilitate a removal of fluid out of the lungs.[9]

Joint and Muscle Receptors

Receptors within peripheral joints and muscles of the extremities respond to changes in movement and increase ventilation. During exercise, a twofold increase in minute ventilation is noted—an initial abrupt increase in ventilation followed by a secondary gradual increase in ventilation (Fig. 2-3).[10] The initial abrupt increase in ventilation is a result of sensory input conveyed from receptors within peripheral joints and muscles, whereas the secondary gradual increase in ventilation is a result of changes in pH within the blood caused by increased lactic acid production. This is conveyed to the brainstem by the chemoreceptors.

Mechanics of Breathing

Movement of air into and out of the lungs occurs as a result of pressure differences between the two ends of the airway. Airflow through the conducting airway is directly proportional to the pressure difference created between the ends of the airway and inversely proportional to the resistance within the airway. In addition, ventilation is affected by various physical properties of the lungs, including compliance, elasticity, and surface tension. This section focuses on pressure changes that allow breathing to occur and explains how lung compliance, elasticity, and surface tension affect breathing. The physiologic importance for pulmonary surfactant is also discussed.

Intrapulmonary and Atmospheric Pressures

Inspiration is always an active process and involves contraction of the respiratory muscles. When the diaphragm and external intercostals contract they increase the volume of the thoracic cavity and lung. This in turn causes a concomitant reduction in the intrapulmonary pressure, or pressure within the lung (Fig. 2-4).[11] The pressure within the lung is reduced in accordance with Boyle's law, which states that the pressure of a given quantity of gas is inversely proportional to its volume. During inspiration, an increase in lung volume within the thoracic cavity decreases intrapulmonary pressures below atmospheric levels. This is termed a *subatmospheric* or *negative intrapulmonary pressure*. This difference in pressure between the atmosphere and the lungs facilitates the flow of air into the lungs to normalize pressure differences. Conversely, expiration occurs when the intrapulmonary pressure exceeds the atmospheric pressure, allowing the lungs to recoil inward and expel air into the atmosphere.

There exists a primary difference between normal ventilation and mechanical ventilation. In normal ventilation, air is pulled into the lungs because of a negative pressure created through activation of the respiratory muscles. Patients placed on mechanical ventilation lack the ability to generate an effective negative or subatmospheric pressure. In light of this, the mechanical ventilator forces air into the lungs through creation of a positive pressure greater than the atmospheric pressure that exists within the lung.

It is also important to note that patients on mechanical ventilation often demonstrate reduced strength of the inspiratory muscles (including the diaphragm), as the ventilator assists with breathing. These patients may benefit from breathing exercises, positioning, and the use of an inspiratory muscle trainer to improve functioning of the inspiratory muscles.

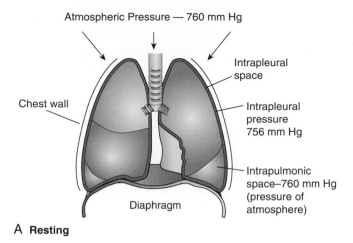

Atmospheric Pressure — 760 mm Hg

Chest wall

Intrapleural space

Intrapleural pressure 756 mm Hg

Intrapulmonic space–760 mm Hg (pressure of atmosphere)

Diaphragm

A Resting

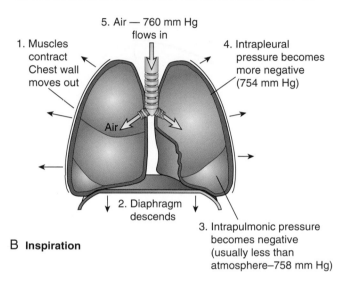

5. Air — 760 mm Hg flows in

1. Muscles contract Chest wall moves out

4. Intrapleural pressure becomes more negative (754 mm Hg)

Air

2. Diaphragm descends

3. Intrapulmonic pressure becomes negative (usually less than atmosphere–758 mm Hg)

B Inspiration

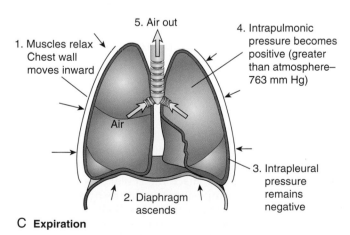

5. Air out

1. Muscles relax Chest wall moves inward

4. Intrapulmonic pressure becomes positive (greater than atmosphere– 763 mm Hg)

Air

3. Intrapleural pressure remains negative

2. Diaphragm ascends

C Expiration

Figure 2-4 A-C, Ventilation: Changes in pressure with inspiration and expiration. (From Gould BE: *Pathophysiology for the Health Professions*, ed 3, St. Louis, 2007, Saunders.)

Intrapleural and Transmural Pressures

Two layers cover each lung, including the outer parietal pleura and inner visceral pleura, separated by an intrapleural space containing a thin layer of viscous fluid. A small amount of viscous fluid within the intrapleural space serves as a lubricant and allows for the lungs to slide relative to the chest during breathing. With ventilation, there exist two opposing forces, including an inward pull from the elastic tension of the lung tissue trying to collapse the lung and an outward pull of the thoracic wall trying to expand the lungs.[1,2,5] These two opposing forces give rise to a subatmospheric (negative) pressure within the intrapleural space, termed the *intrapleural pressure*. This intrapleural pressure is normally lower than the intrapulmonary pressure developed during both inspiration and expiration. In light of these two pressure differences, a transpulmonary or transmural pressure is developed across the wall of the lung.[1,2,5] The transmural pressure considers the difference between the intrapulmonary and intrapleural pressure. The inner intrapulmonary pressure is relatively greater than the outer intrapleural pressure, allowing the difference in pressure (the transmural pressure) to maintain the lung near the chest wall. It is the transmural or transpulmonary pressure that allows changes in lung volume to parallel changes in thoracic excursion during inspiration and expiration.

When changes in lung volume do not parallel the normal outward and inward pull during inspiration and expiration, respectively, and are, in fact, opposite, the breathing pattern is said to be *paradoxical*. This breathing pattern is often seen in patients with multiple rib fractures and a resultant flail chest.

Physical Properties of Lungs

The processes of inspiration and expiration are facilitated by three physical properties of lung tissue. Compliance allows lung tissue to stretch during inspiration; the elastic recoil of the lung allows passive expiration to occur; and surface tension forces with the alveoli allow the lung to get smaller during expiration.

Compliance.

The lung can be compared with a balloon during inspiration, where there exists a tendency to collapse or recoil while inflated. To maintain inflation, the transmural pressure, or pressure difference between the intrapulmonary pressure and intrapleural pressure, must be maintained. A distending force is needed to overcome the inward recoil forces of the lung. This outward force is provided by the elastic properties of the lung and through the action of the inspiratory muscles.

Compliance describes the distensibility of lung tissue. It is defined as the change in lung volume per change in transmural or transpulmonary pressure, expressed symbolically as $\Delta V/\Delta P$ (Fig. 2-5).[12] In other words, a given transpulmonary pressure will cause a greater or lesser degree of lung expansion, depending on the distensibility or compliance of the lung. The compliance of the lung is reduced by factors that produce a resistance to distension. Also, the compliance is reduced as the lung approaches its TLC, where it becomes relatively stiffer and less distensible.

In patients with emphysema, the chronicity of the disease leads to progressive destruction of the elastic recoil, making the compliance high.[13] A reduced inward pull from low recoil allows small changes in transmural pressure to cause large changes in lung volumes and resultant hyperinflation of the lung. The changes seen in individuals with emphysema include a barrel chest and flattened diaphragms. These negative sequelae result in less diaphragm use with breathing, more accessory muscle, and an increase in the work of breathing.

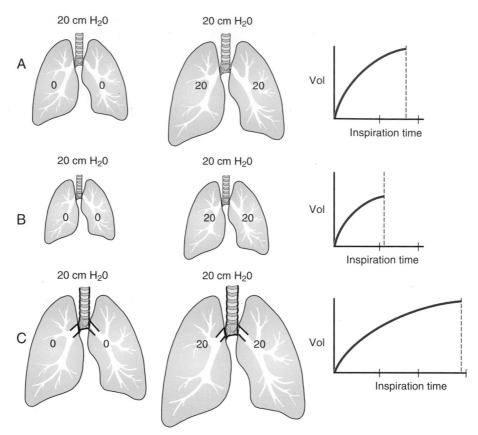

Figure 2-5 A-C, Lung compliance changes associated with disease.

In patients with pulmonary fibrosis, the lung is fibrotic and stiff and thereby has reduced compliance.[13] In these patients, despite large changes in transmural pressure, only small changes in lung volume will occur as a result of the stiffness or lack of distensibility of lung tissue. Consequently, clinically one sees individuals with increased respiratory rates and accessory muscle use because of decreased lung volumes. The work of breathing with activity is greatly increased as a consequence of the inability to increase lung volumes.

Elasticity.

Elasticity refers to the tendency of a structure to return to its initial size after being distended. A network of elastin and collagen fibers within the alveolar wall and surrounding bronchi and pulmonary capillaries provides for the elastic properties of the lung.

Surface tension.

Although the elastic characteristics of the lung tissue itself play a role in resisting lung distension or compliance, the surface tension at the air–liquid interface on the alveolar surface has a greater influence. Anyone who has ever attempted to separate two wet microscope slides by lifting (not sliding) the top slide from the bottom has firsthand experience with the forces of surface tension. In the lung, a thin film of fluid on the alveolus has a surface tension, which is caused by water molecules at the surface being relatively more attracted to other water molecules than to air. This surface tension acts to collapse the alveolus and increase the pressure of air within the alveolus. The law of Laplace states that the pressure created within the

alveolus is directly proportional to the surface tension and inversely proportional to the radius of the alveolus.

For example, consider two alveoli of different sizes, one at either end of a bifurcated respiratory bronchiole (Fig. 2-6); because of the size difference, the smaller alveolus must have a higher pressure than the larger alveolus if the surface tension of each is the same. To keep the air in the smaller alveolus from emptying into the larger, a surface-active agent is needed to decrease the overall surface tension of the alveoli so as to lower wall tension in proportion to the radius of the alveolus (see Fig. 2-6). Moreover, it must do so almost in anticipation of diminishing alveolar size. Only if such a surface-active agent were present could alveoli with different radii coexist in the lungs.

The surface-active agent in the human lung that performs this function is called *surfactant*.[14,15] Pulmonary surfactant is not composed of a single class of molecules, but, rather, is a collection of interrelated macromolecular lipoprotein complexes that differ in composition, structure, and function.[14,15] Nonetheless, the principal active ingredient of surfactant is dipalmitoyl phosphatidylcholine (DPPC). The structure of the surfactant molecule is such that it presents a nonpolar end of fatty acids (two palmitate residues) that is insoluble in water, and a smaller, polar end (a phosphatidylcholine group) that dissolves readily in water. Thus surfactant orients itself perpendicularly to the surface in the alveolar fluid layer, with its nonpolar end projecting toward the lumen. If surfactant were uniformly dispersed throughout the alveoli, its concentration at the air–fluid interface would vary in accordance with the surface area of any individual alveolus. Thus the molecules

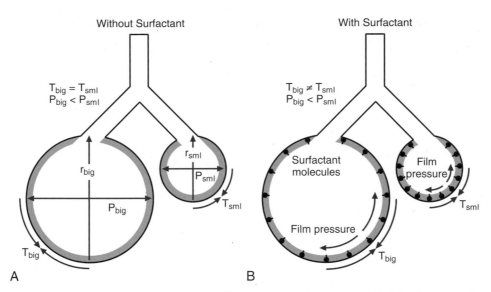

Figure 2-6 Two pairs of unequally filled alveoli arranged in parallel illustrate the effect of a surface-active agent. One pair of alveoli is shown without surfactant **(A)** and the other is shown with surfactant **(B)**. In the alveoli without surfactant, if T_{sml} were the same as T_{big}, P_{sml} would have to be many times greater than P_{big}; otherwise, the smaller alveolus would empty into the larger one. In the alveoli with surfactant, T_{sml} is reduced in proportion to the radius of the alveolus, which permits P_{sml} to equal P_{big}. Thus alveoli of different radii can coexist. Refer to the text for details.

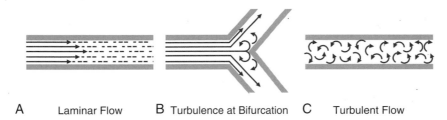

Figure 2-7 Laminar and turbulent airflow in the airways. **A,** At low flow rates, air flows in a laminar pattern, and the resistance to airflow is proportional to the flow rate. **B,** At airway bifurcation, eddy formation creates a transitional flow pattern. **C,** At high flow rates, when a great deal of turbulence is created, the resistance to airflow is proportional to the square of the flow rate. (Redrawn from West JB: *Respiratory Physiology: The Essentials*, ed 9, Baltimore, 2012, Lippincott Williams & Wilkins.)

would be compressed in the smaller alveoli, as depicted in Fig. 2-6. Compressing the surfactant molecules increases their density and builds up a film pressure that counteracts much of the surface tension at the air–fluid interface. The rate of change in the surface tension resulting from compression of the surfactant molecules as the alveolus gets smaller is faster than the rate of change of the decreasing alveolar radius, so that a point is rapidly reached in which the pressure in the small alveolus equals the pressure in the big alveolus.

Surfactant begins to develop in late fetal life. Premature babies may be born with less surfactant, resulting in collapsed alveoli and respiratory distress. In an effort to reduce complications in women likely to go into premature labor (<7 months' gestation), the fetus is injected with amniotic fluid from the placenta of an infant born through cesarean section to mature the fetus's lungs. It is important to note that even under normal circumstances, the first breath of life is more challenging, as the newborn must overcome greater surface tension forces in order to inflate its partially collapsed alveoli.

Resistance to airflow.

The ability to inflate the lungs with air depends on pressure differences and resistance to flow within the airways.[2,5] Poiseuille's law states that flow through a vessel or airway is directly proportional to the pressure difference and radius and inversely proportional to the length of the airway and viscosity of the gas. In addition, it is important to note that the radius is raised to the fourth power, and so small changes in the radius account for large changes in airflow through the airway.[5,7]

The upper airways are responsible for most of the airway resistance. As a result, the lower airways play a much smaller role in influencing airway resistance because of the irregularity of the branching patterns, as well as variations in the diameter of the lumen of the distal airway.[6] In addition, resistance in smaller airways is lower because flow is laminar. This involves only slight resistance between the sides of the airway and resistance caused by collision of air molecules. In the upper airway, airflow is relatively highly turbulent, involving increased resistance as a result of frequent molecular collisions in addition to the resistance along the sides of the tube (Fig. 2-7).

Resistance to airflow is also affected by the diameter of the airway, which is influenced by changes in the transmural pressure within the lung during ventilation. With inspiration, the pressure outside the airway within the lung (transmural pressure) is relatively more negative than the airway pressure, thereby increasing the radius of the airway and reducing resistance to airflow. Conversely, with expiration, the transmural pressure is greater than the airway pressure, reducing the radius and increasing airway resistance.[2]

Finally, resistance to airflow may also be affected by autonomic nervous system control. Increases in parasympathetic nervous system activation cause constriction of the smooth muscle cells of the bronchi and increase airway resistance, whereas sympathetic influence decreases airway resistance. Also, mucus and edema in the airway as a consequence of inflammation increase airway resistance and reduce airflow.[1,2]

Status asthmaticus, an acute asthma attack, is marked by severe airway resistance caused by constriction of bronchial smooth muscle cells and mucus production within the airway (Fig. 2-8). These patients use accessory muscles to increase transmural pressures to increase airway radius. In addition, they benefit from bronchodilators to relieve smooth muscle cell constriction and from steroids to reduce the inflammatory process and mucus production.

Respiration

Respiration refers to the process of gas exchange in the lungs facilitated through the process of simple diffusion. This process serves two major functions, including the replenishment of the blood's oxygen supply used for oxidative energy production and the removal of carbon dioxide returning from venous blood manufactured as a waste product. For diffusion to occur, there are two requirements: air bringing in oxygen to the lungs (alveolar ventilation) and blood to receive the oxygen and give up carbon dioxide (pulmonary perfusion). Air is delivered to the distal alveolus for gas exchange via the process of pulmonary ventilation; blood is brought to the lungs from the right side of the heart through the pulmonary artery and branching pulmonary capillaries. Gas exchange or respiration between the alveoli and pulmonary capillary occurs across the semipermeable alveolar–capillary membrane, also referred to as the *respiratory membrane*.

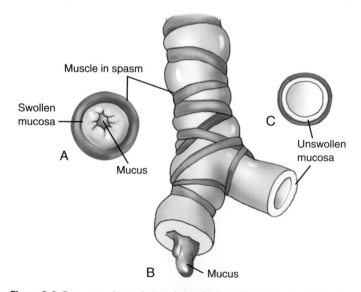

Figure 2-8 Factors causing expiratory obstruction in asthma. **A,** Cross-section of a bronchiole occluded by muscle spasm, swollen mucosa, and mucus. **B,** Longitudinal section of an obstructed bronchiole. **C,** Cross-section of a clear bronchiole. (From Shiland BJ: *Mastering Healthcare Terminology*, ed 3, St. Louis, 2010, Mosby.)

Partial Pressures of Gases

The air delivered to distal alveoli is a mixture of gases. It is important to understand that each gas exerts its own pressure in proportion to its concentration in the gas mixture. The amount of individual pressure exerted by each gas within the mixture is termed the *partial pressure* of that individual gas. According to Dalton's law, the total pressure of a mixture of gases equals the sum of the individual gases within the mixture. Atmospheric air is a mixture of gases containing 79.04% nitrogen, 20.93% oxygen, and 0.03% carbon dioxide.[7] At sea level, the barometric or atmospheric pressure is 760 mm Hg. This is considered the total pressure of the mixture of the three gases present in the atmosphere. Therefore the partial pressure of nitrogen in the atmosphere is 600 mm Hg (79.04% of 760), of oxygen is 159 mm Hg (20.83% of 760), and of carbon dioxide is 0.2 mm Hg (0.03% of 760). Once gases enter the body, Henry's law explains how gases in the body are dissolved in fluids. According to this law, gases dissolve in liquids in proportion to their partial pressure.[16]

Diffusion

To allow for effective gas exchange to occur between the alveoli and pulmonary capillary, different partial pressures of oxygen and carbon dioxide must exist in each of the two areas. The differences in partial pressure of each gas within the alveoli and pulmonary capillary create a pressure gradient across the alveolar capillary interface. This gradient will enable gases to diffuse from areas of high concentration to areas of low concentration across the semipermeable respiratory membrane.

> **Clinical tip**
>
> The diffusing capacity of lung for carbon monoxide (DLCO) is a test of the integrity of the alveolar–capillary surface area for gas transfer.[13] It may be reduced in disorders that damage the alveolar walls (septa), such as emphysema, leading to a loss of effective surface area. The DLCO is also reduced in disorders that thicken or damage the alveolar walls, such as pulmonary fibrosis.

Perfusion

Perfusion refers to blood flow to the lungs available for gas exchange. The driving pressure in the pulmonary circulation is much less than the systemic circulation, yet flow rates in both circulation systems are similar because of reduced vascular resistance within the pulmonary circulation. Thus the pulmonary circulation system is considered a low-resistance, low-pressure pathway. The low pressure allows for relatively lower filtration pressures compared with the systemic vascular system, thereby protecting the lung from pulmonary edema, a dangerous condition where fluid accumulates in the lung, hindering alveolar ventilation and gas exchange.

In addition, perfusion of the lung is affected by alterations in the partial pressures of oxygen within the alveoli.[16] Pulmonary arterioles constrict when partial pressures of oxygen in alveoli are low and dilate when alveolar partial pressures for oxygen increase. These vasomotor changes of the pulmonary and systemic vasculature help to reduce blood flow to areas in the lung that are poorly ventilated and increase blood flow to peripheral tissue that needs more oxygen. The vasoconstriction of the pulmonary vasculature to low oxygen levels is automatic and improves the ability for gas exchange. This phenomenon prevents blood from poorly ventilated alveoli (with low partial pressures of oxygen) from mixing with blood from well-ventilated alveoli (with relatively higher partial pressures of oxygen). If blood did have to mix, then the overall oxygen concentration for blood leaving the lungs and returning to the heart would be lower because of the dilution effect.

Finally, alterations in the pH of blood affect vasomotor tone of the pulmonary vasculature, thereby affecting perfusion required for gas exchange.[6] A low pH, or acidemia, causes pulmonary vasoconstriction. The lung is significantly involved in regulating the acid–base balance in blood. When the pH of blood is reduced as a result of lung pathology, vasoconstriction of the pulmonary vessels is potentiated in response to the altered pH, which, in turn, affects the gas exchange and exacerbates the problem to a higher degree.

Ventilation and Perfusion Matching

For optimal respiration or gas exchange to occur, the distribution of gas (ventilation, abbreviated V) and blood (perfusion, abbreviated Q) at the level of the alveolar capillary interface must be matched. Position plays a vital role in the distribution of ventilation and perfusion to different aspects of the lung. In the upright position, gravity allows for a greater amount of blood flow or perfusion to the base of the lung relative to the apices.[16] In addition, alveoli in the upper portions or apices of the lung have greater RV of gas and are subsequently larger.[16] The larger alveoli have greater surface tension and have relatively more difficulty inflating because of less compliance than the smaller alveoli toward the base of the lung. In light of this, ventilation and perfusion are relatively greater toward the base of the lung, favoring better matching and resultant respiration or gas exchange.[16] A change in the position of the patient changes areas of ventilation and perfusion. Generally, greater ventilation and perfusion occur in gravity-dependent areas, thereby allowing better respiration to occur in the dependent lung when an individual is in the side-lying position (Fig. 2-9).

Often, ventilation and perfusion ratios are not uniform within the lung, which compromises gas exchange. Regions of the lung with relatively greater amounts of perfusion compared with ventilation act as shunts. Conversely, regions of the lung with relatively greater amounts of ventilation compared with perfusion act as dead space. Alterations in the ventilation–perfusion matching lead to hypoxia and reduced oxygen to peripheral tissue.

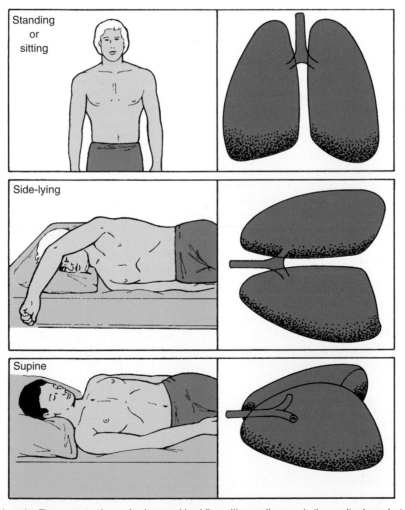

Figure 2-9 Pulmonary blood flow and gravity. The greatest volume of pulmonary blood flow will normally occur in the gravity-dependent areas of the lungs. Body position has a significant effect on the distribution of pulmonary blood flow. (From McCance KL, Huether SE, Brashers VL, et al, editors: *Pathophysiology: The Biologic Basis for Disease in Adults and Children*, ed 6, St. Louis, 2010, Mosby.)

An effective noninvasive tool to measure respiration is the pulse oximeter. It is important for clinicians to monitor pulse oximeter readings and observe for signs of distress when changing patient positions that alter the V/Q matching. Abnormal V/Q ratios cause concomitant reductions in pulse oximetry that are noted in patients with pneumonia, pulmonary embolus, edema, emphysema, bronchitis, and other pulmonary disorders.

Transport of Oxygen and Carbon Dioxide

Following the previous discussions of how air is brought into the lungs through the process of pulmonary ventilation and exchanged within the lungs via respiration, it is important to consider the mechanisms for the delivery of oxygen to peripheral tissue and the removal of carbon dioxide that the tissue produces as a waste product. This section reviews transport of each gas individually.

Transport of Oxygen

A majority of oxygen (98%) is transported to the peripheral tissue bound to hemoglobin within red blood cells of blood. A very small portion of oxygen (<2%) is dissolved in plasma within blood.

Hemoglobin

A hemoglobin molecule consists of four protein chains called *globins* and four iron-containing organic molecules called *hemes*.[2,5] The protein component of the molecule contains two identical α and two identical β protein chains. The α chains contain 141 amino acids, and the β chains contain 146 amino acids.[7] The four-polypeptide chains are connected to each heme molecule. Each heme molecule has a central iron atom that can combine with a single molecule of oxygen. Consequently, as a result of the presence of four heme molecules, one hemoglobin has the ability to carry four oxygen molecules to the peripheral tissue.

Hemoglobin molecules within blood can exist in one of four conditions, depending on the molecule that binds to, unloads from, or is unable to bind to the iron atom within heme. Oxyhemoglobin represents a hemoglobin molecule bound to oxygen, because iron in heme is in its reduced state. Deoxyhemoglobin refers to the oxyhemoglobin molecule that has released its oxygen molecule to peripheral tissue. Because methemoglobin has iron in its oxidized state, it is unable to bind to oxygen and participate in oxygen transport. Blood contains a very small amount of this molecule. Carboxyhemoglobin is another abnormal form of hemoglobin; it involves the binding of heme to carbon monoxide instead of oxygen. Because the bond with carbon monoxide is 210 times stronger than oxygen, it displaces oxygen and inhibits oxygen's binding capacity.

The percentage of oxyhemoglobin to total hemoglobin provides an indication of how well the blood has been oxygenated by the lungs. This is termed the *percent oxyhemoglobin saturation*. In the systemic arteries, at a partial pressure of 100 mm Hg, the percent hemoglobin is 97%, indicating that 97% of hemoglobin molecules in blood are bound to oxygen. The remaining 3% reflects deoxyhemoglobin, methemoglobin, and carboxyhemoglobin concentrations. The gold standard for measuring oxyhemoglobin saturation is through an analysis of arterial blood gases. However, pulse oximeter can also be used to obtain this number.

The oxygen-carrying capacity of the body is determined by the concentration of hemoglobin. Normal levels of hemoglobin are between 12 and 16 g/dL for women and 13 and 18 g/dL for men.[17] A below-normal level of hemoglobin occurs with anemia and compromises the ability to carry oxygen. Conversely, an increase in hemoglobin concentrations, a condition called *polycythemia*, increases oxygen-carrying capacity within the system.

Oxyhemoglobin Dissociation Curve

The oxyhemoglobin dissociation curve (Fig. 2-10) describes the relation between the amount of O_2 bound to hemoglobin (Hb), clinically referred to as the percentage of saturation of hemoglobin, and the partial pressure of O_2 (Po_2) with

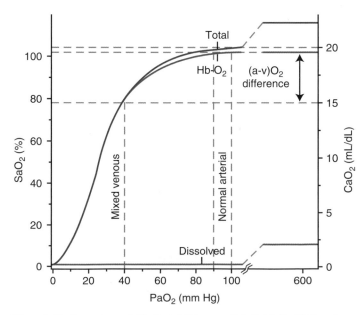

Figure 2-10 The oxyhemoglobin dissociation curve. Note that in the "flat" portion of the curve (80 mm Hg and above), a change in the partial pressure of arterial oxygen (PaO_2) of as much as 20 mm Hg does not appreciably alter the hemoglobin saturation. However, in the "steep" portion of the curve (below 60 mm Hg), relatively small changes in saturation result in large changes in the PaO_2. pH, the logarithm of the reciprocal of hydrogen ion concentration; *DPG*, diphosphoglycerate.

which the Hb is in equilibrium.[18–20] Under ideal conditions (blood pH = 7.4, body temperature = 37° C, Hb = 147 g · L−1), less than 10% of the O_2 dissociates from the Hb as Po_2 falls to 40 mm Hg from 100 to 60 mm Hg. However, nearly 60% of the O_2 is dissociated from the Hb as Po_2 falls another 40 mm Hg from 60 to 20 mm Hg. Decreasing the pH (increasing acidemia) of the blood from the normal value of 7.40 to 7.30 shifts the hemoglobin dissociation curve downward and to the right an average of 7% to 8%; in contrast, alkalemia shifts the curve to the left. Increasing the concentration of CO_2 in the tissue capillary beds displaces oxygen from the hemoglobin, delivering the O_2 to the tissues at a higher Po_2 than would otherwise occur. In conditions of prolonged hypoxemia (lasting longer than a few hours), the amount of 2,3-diphosphoglycerate in the blood is increased, resulting in a rightward shift in the hemoglobin dissociation curve. 2,3-Bisphosphoglycerate is present in human red blood cells and binds with greater affinity to deoxygenated hemoglobin than it does to oxygenated hemoglobin. In bonding to partially deoxygenated hemoglobin, it allosterically upregulates the release of the remaining oxygen molecules bound to the hemoglobin, thus enhancing the ability of red blood cells to release oxygen near tissues that need it most. Furthermore, increasing the temperature of the tissue, as happens normally in exercising muscle, also results in a shift of the hemoglobin dissociation curve to the right. The result of these rightward shifts is a decreased hemoglobin affinity for oxygen. Although a rightward shift in the hemoglobin dissociation curve can be beneficial, the reader is cautioned that the range of variability normally tolerated by the body is relatively narrow: rapid fluctuations in pH or core temperature are not at all well tolerated.

Carbon Dioxide Transport

Carbon dioxide released from metabolically active cells is carried by blood in one of three ways:

- Dissolved in plasma
- Bound to the protein component of hemoglobin (carbaminohemoglobin)
- As bicarbonate ion

Dissolved carbon dioxide.

Carbon dioxide released from tissue may get dissolved in blood plasma and transported through the system. A very small percentage of carbon dioxide, approximately only 7% to 10%, is transported in this manner.

Carbaminohemoglobin.

Carbon dioxide can also be transported by binding to the hemoglobin molecule in blood. The carbon dioxide molecule binds to the protein chains rather than the heme component of the hemoglobin molecule. The complex formed from the binding of carbon dioxide and hemoglobin is termed *carbaminohemoglobin*. About one-fifth of the total blood carbon dioxide is carried in this manner.

Bicarbonate ions and the chloride and reverse chloride shifts.

The majority of carbon dioxide combines with water to form a compound called *carbonic acid*. This reaction is facilitated through the action of the carbonic anhydrase enzyme under conditions of high partial pressure of carbon dioxide

at the level of the tissue.[2,7] This enzyme is confined to the red blood cell, thereby allowing most of the carbonic acid to be produced within the red blood cell. A small amount of carbonic acid is also produced spontaneously within the plasma of blood.

$$CO_2 + H_2O - \text{carbonic anhydrase} \rightarrow H_2CO_3$$

Carbonic acid that is built up within the red blood cell dissociates into positively charged hydrogen ions (protons) and negatively charged bicarbonate ions.

$$H_2CO_3 \rightarrow H^+ + HCO_3^-$$

The hydrogen ions released from carbonic acid combine with deoxyhemoglobin molecules within red blood cells. As a result, fewer hydrogen ions move out of red blood cells, causing the negatively charged bicarbonate ions to leak out of the blood cell into plasma. The trapping of hydrogen ions within the red blood cell results in a net positive charge within the blood cell and a compensatory shift of negative chloride ions into the red blood cell as bicarbonate moves out. This exchange of anions as blood travels through tissue capillaries is termed the *chloride shift* (Fig. 2-11).

It is important to appreciate that deoxyhemoglobin bonds more strongly to hydrogen ions than to oxyhemoglobin. In light of this, the unloading of oxygen to peripheral tissue is increased (the Bohr effect) as more hydrogen ions are released from carbonic acid to produce a greater amount of deoxyhemoglobin for the hydrogen ions to bind to. In summary, increased carbon dioxide production increases oxygen unloading into the tissue, which, in turn, improves carbon dioxide transport out of the tissue.

At the level of the lung, deoxyhemoglobin is converted to oxyhemoglobin. As mentioned earlier, oxyhemoglobin has a weaker affinity for hydrogen ions. With the partial pressure of oxygen being high at the level of the lung, free hydrogen ions are released from hemoglobin within the red blood cell. The free hydrogen ions attract bicarbonate ions from the plasma and join to form carbonic acid.

$$H^+ + HCO_3^- \rightarrow H_2CO_3$$

Under conditions of low partial pressures of carbon dioxide within the lung, carbonic anhydrase facilitates the breakdown of carbonic acid into carbon dioxide and water. The carbon dioxide is then released from the lungs through the process of expiration.

$$H_2CO_3 - \text{carbonic anhydrase} \rightarrow CO_2 + H_2O$$

A reverse chloride shift occurs at the level of the lungs to facilitate the entry of bicarbonate into the red blood cell. As bicarbonate ion leaves the plasma to enter the blood cell, chloride ions shift out of the red blood cell and enter the plasma. These processes are vital in maintaining acid–base regulation and normal pH of blood.

Acid–Base Balance

Metabolically produced acids are largely eliminated from the body via the lungs in the form of CO_2 because the major blood acid, carbonic acid (H_2CO_3), is volatile; that is, it can chemically vary between a liquid and gaseous state. The

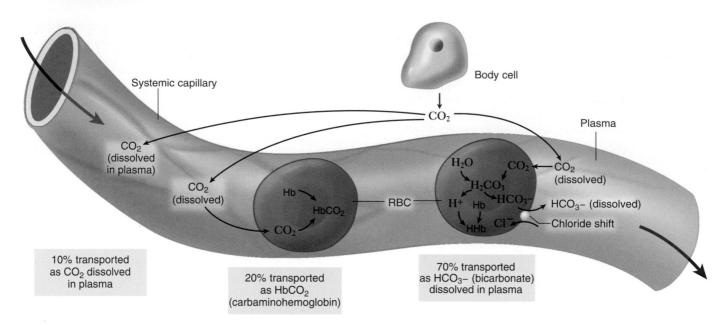

Figure 2-11 Transport of carbon dioxide and the chloride shift.

other blood acids (dietary acids, lactic acids, and ketoacids) are regulated by the kidneys and the liver. The measurement of arterial oxygen or carbon dioxide tension and hydrogen ion concentration for assessment of acid–base balance and oxygenation status are commonly accomplished by means of laboratory analysis of arterial blood gases (ABGs). Generally, an ABG report contains the pH, the $PaCO_2$, the PaO_2, and the HCO_3-, and base excess (BE) values for the sample analyzed. Chapter 10 provides a detailed discussion of acid–base balance and arterial blood gases.

The Cardiovascular System

The primary function of the cardiovascular (circulatory) system is the transportation and distribution of essential substances to the tissues of the body and the removal of the byproducts of cellular metabolism (Fig. 2-12). The heart provides the principal force that pushes blood through the vessels of the pulmonary and systemic circuits. In the case of the systemic circuit, the forward movement of blood is also facilitated by the recoil of the arterial walls during diastole, skeletal muscle compression of veins during exercise, and negative thoracic pressure during inspiration. The pulmonary circuit receives the entire output of the right ventricle with each cardiac cycle.

The Cardiac Cycle

The period from the beginning of one heartbeat to the beginning of the next is called the *cardiac cycle*. Figs. 2-13 and 2-14 depict selected events during the cardiac cycle. Beginning with an action potential in the sinoatrial (SA) node, a depolarization wave is spread through both atria to the atrioventricular (AV) node and then, through the His–Purkinje complex, into the ventricles. However, because of the nature of the specialized conduction system, the impulse is delayed for about 0.1 second in the upper two-thirds of the AV node. This allows the atria to contract (a result of

excitation–contraction coupling) and pump an additional volume of blood into the ventricles—an atrial "kick."[21] The ventricles provide the primary force to move blood through the vascular system.

The cardiac cycle may be further divided into two periods: systole and diastole. Systole is the period of ventricular contraction; diastole is the period of ventricular relaxation. Fig. 2-14 illustrates left-sided pressure and volume, electrocardiogram (ECG), and phonocardiographic events associated with the cardiac cycle. Closure of the tricuspid and mitral valves generates the first heart sound (S_1), signaling the onset of ventricular systole, and is shown on the phonocardiographic tracing just after the peak of the R wave on the ECG tracing. In early ventricular systole, the ventricular volume remains unchanged despite a rapid rise in ventricular pressure. This isovolumic contraction occurs until the aortic valve opens, at which time the ventricular ejection phase begins. The retrograde bulging of the mitral valve into the left atrium is responsible for the rise in atrial pressure seen during the isovolumic ventricular contraction, the c wave. Ventricular ejection continues until the aortic valve closes, terminating systole and generating the second heart sound (S_2). Immediately following aortic valve closure, there is a phase of isovolumic relaxation that continues until the mitral valve opens when ventricular pressure falls below atrial pressure. The rise in atrial pressure indicated by the v wave of the atrial pressure tracing is probably brought about by the relative

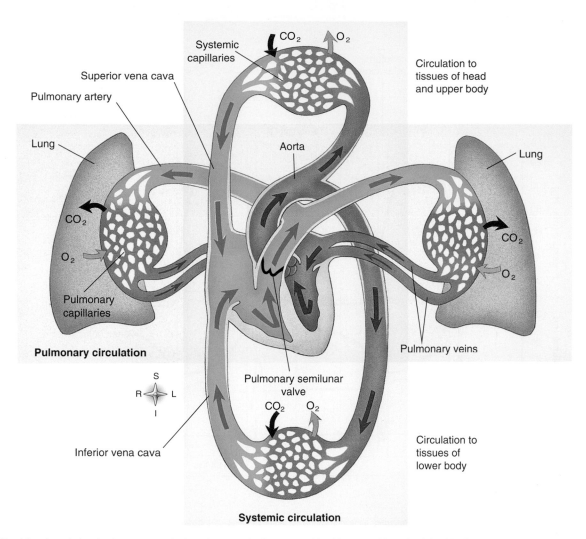

Figure 2-12 Blood flow through the circulatory system. In the pulmonary circulatory route, blood is pumped from the right side of the heart to the gas-exchange tissues of the lungs. In the systemic circulation, blood is pumped from the left side of the heart to all other tissues of the body. (From Thibodeau GA: *The Human Body in Health & Disease,* ed 4, St. Louis, 2006, Mosby.)

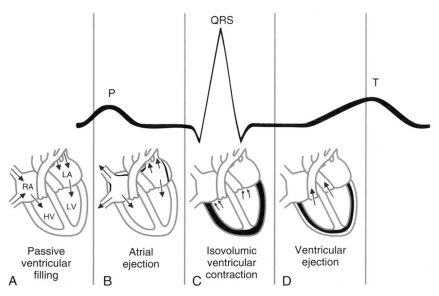

Figure 2-13 The mechanical events of the cardiac cycle shown in relation to the electrical events of the electrocardiogram. In late diastole, just before the P wave, the ventricles fill passively **(A).** At about the time that the P wave ends, the atria contract to eject up to 20% of the end-diastolic ventricular volume **(B).** A period of isovolumic ventricular contraction begins very shortly after the onset of the QRS complex **(C).** Ventricular ejection coincides with the early portion of the ST segment **(D).**

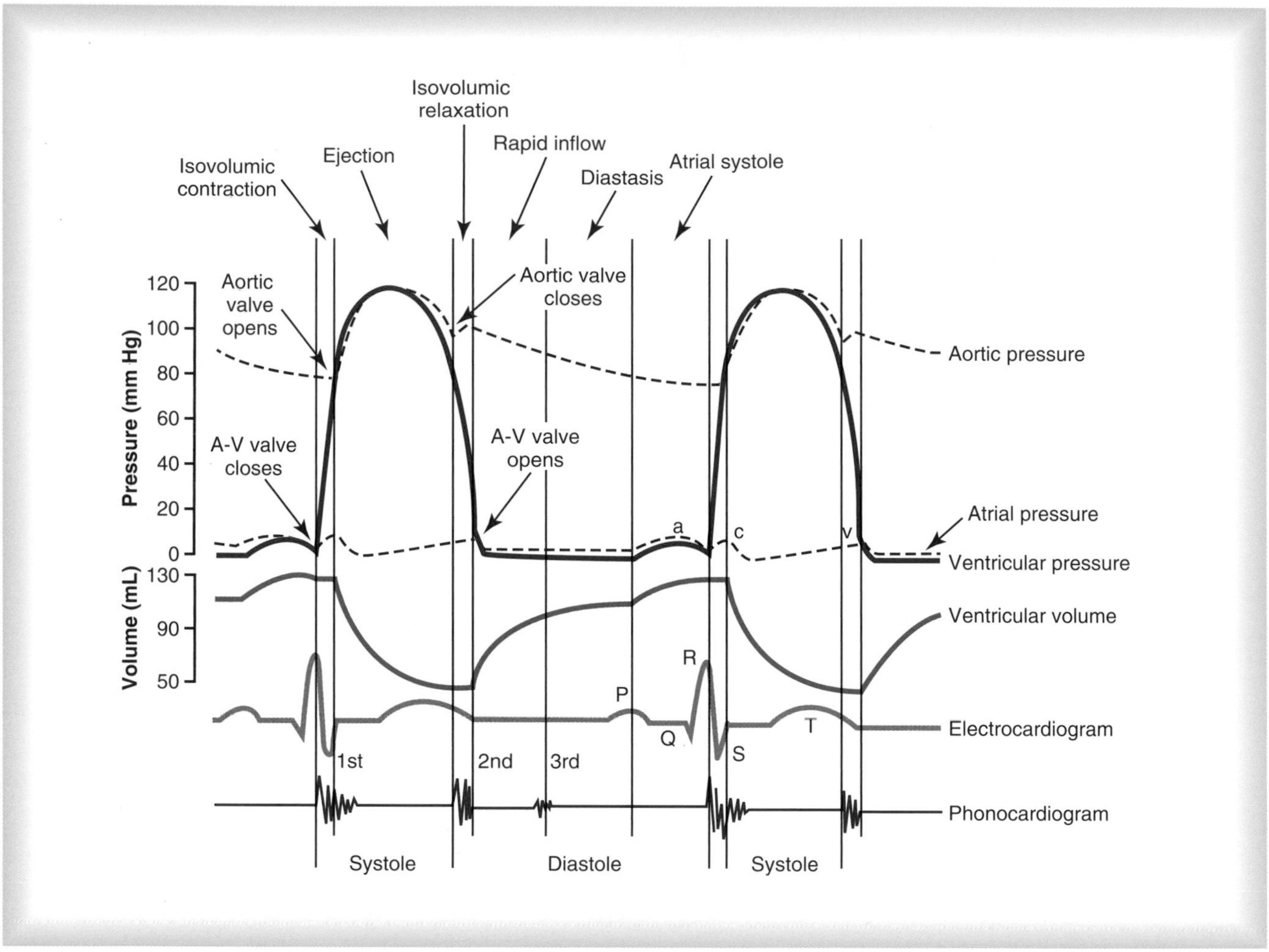

Figure 2-14 Events of the cardiac cycle for left ventricular function, showing changes in left atrial pressure, left ventricular pressure, aortic pressure, ventricular volume, the electrocardiogram, and the phonocardiogram. (From Guyton AC, Hall JE: *Textbook of Medical Physiology*, ed 11, St. Louis, 2006, Saunders.)

negative pressure resulting from ventricular relaxation. Once the mitral valve opens, ventricular volume begins rising as the ventricle passively fills during the rapid-filling phase. Immediately following the rapid-filling phase is the slow-filling phase, also called *diastasis*, which continues until atrial systole. Atrial systole is indicated on the atrial pressure tracing as a wave. These same events are essentially mirrored on the right side of the heart.

Physiology of Cardiac Output

The previous section outlines the sequence of events to allow the heart to function as an efficient pump, with the end product being an ejection of blood out of the heart. An adequate volume of blood must be ejected out of the heart to sustain life and activity. The cardiac output reflects the volume of blood ejected out of the left ventricle into the systemic vasculature per minute. It is a function of the number of heartbeats per minute (heart rate) and the volume of blood ejected per beat (stroke volume). On average, the cardiac output at rest is between 4 and 6 L/min to allow for sufficient tissue perfusion.

Cardiac Output = Heart Rate × Stroke Volume

It is also interesting to note that the average total blood volume is approximately 5.5 L.[7] This indicates that the ventricle

pumps an amount of blood equivalent to the total blood volume each minute. Therefore it takes approximately 1 minute for a given volume of blood (a drop of blood) to complete the systemic and pulmonary circuits. With exercise, an increase in cardiac output is warranted to meet the metabolic needs of the working muscles. To allow for this increase in cardiac output, an increase in blood volume must also exist. The following section reviews factors that regulate heart rate and stroke volume to accomplish an increase in blood volume and cardiac output.

Regulation of Heart Rate

As mentioned in Chapter 1, the heart continues to beat automatically between 60 and 100 beats per minute (bpm) as long as myocardial cells are alive as a consequence of spontaneous depolarization of the pacemaker cells in the SA node. Sympathetic and parasympathetic nerve fibers to the heart are activated to alter this intrinsic pacing rate of the SA node.[23] Epinephrine from the adrenal medulla of the adrenal gland and norepinephrine from the sympathetic axons open channels of the pacemaker cells of the SA node and increase the rate of depolarizations, resulting in an increase in heart rate.[1,5,7] Conversely, parasympathetic influence is achieved through the release of acetylcholine released by vagus nerve endings that bind to acetylcholine receptors, slowing down the rate of action potential production at the level of the SA node, thereby depressing heart rate.[1,5,7] It is important to understand that the actual pacing rate of the SA node is because of the net effect of these antagonistic influences. Mechanisms that alter the cardiac rate are said to have a chronotropic effect. Influences that increase heart rate are said to have a positive chronotropic effect, whereas those that decrease heart rate are said to produce negative chronotropic effects.

Autonomic nervous system influences not only affect the firing of the SA node, but also affect sympathetic endings (β-adrenergic receptors) in the myocardial wall of the atria and ventricles.[2,5] Sympathetic stimulation vasodilates coronary arteries to increase blood flow to the heart and increases myocardial contraction. On the other hand, parasympathetic influence vasoconstricts coronary arteries, reducing blood flow to the myocardium and depressing myocardial contractility.[2,5] Mechanisms that affect the contractility of the myocardium are said to have an ionotropic effect, those that increase contractility have a positive ionotropic effect, and those that reduce contractility have a negative ionotropic effect.

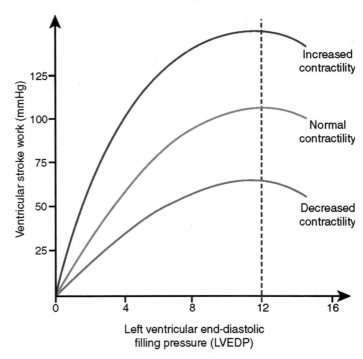

Figure 2-15 Contractility. (From Irwin S, Tecklin SJ: *Cardiopulmonary Physical Therapy: A Guide to Practice*, ed 4, St. Louis, 2005, Mosby.)

Clinical tip

A common goal in the pharmacologic management of patients with heart failure is to provide medications that cause a positive ionotropic effect to increase the pumping ability of the failing heart. These medications include phosphodiesterase inhibitors and dobutamine that allow the heart to pump stronger and increase cardiac output.

A bout of aerobic exercise causes a linear increase in heart rate with increasing intensity as a result of decreased vagus nerve inhibition and increased sympathetic nerve stimulation. In addition, the slow resting heart rate, or bradycardic, responses seen in endurance-trained athletes continues to be controversial, but is often thought to occur as a consequence of enhanced parasympathetic input to the heart.

Patients on β blockers have a blunted heart rate response during exercise, as β receptors on the myocardial wall are unable to respond to sympathetic stimulation and appropriately increase heart rate. In light of this, it is effective to use a subjective assessment of intensity (Borg rate of perceived exertion), as objective measures of intensity examined through heart rate responses will be inaccurate.

Regulation of Stroke Volume

The stroke volume, or volume of blood ejected out of the heart per beat, is affected by three variables:

- Preload
- Contractility
- Afterload

Preload

The preload is a reflection of the volume of blood returning to the heart. It is often correlated with the end-diastolic volume (EDV), which is the maximum amount of blood that can be in the ventricles immediately before contraction. In normal cardiovascular physiology, the preload is directly proportional to the stroke volume. In other words, as more blood returns to the heart, a greater volume of blood leaves the heart with every contraction. Two physiologists, Otto Frank and Ernst Starling, demonstrated an intrinsic property of heart muscle to increase stroke volume based on the precontractile myocardial cell length. Within physiologic limits, the strength of ventricular contraction resulting in increased stroke volume varies proportionally to its precontraction length.[6,12] This length is influenced by the volume of blood in the ventricles before contraction. This is termed the *Frank–Starling mechanism* and in summary explains how a greater volume of blood is ejected out of the ventricles when a greater volume of blood is returned to the heart (Fig. 2-15). Clinically the term *preload*, directly influenced by the EDV, refers to the amount of stretch, or load, on the myocardial wall before contraction (precontraction).

It is interesting to note that in patients with congestive heart failure and a resultant failing heart, an increase in the EDV does not produce an increase in the preload and subsequent increase in stroke volume through the Frank–Starling mechanism. In fact, an increase in the preload puts additional stress on the failing heart. Therefore a variety of treatments are geared at reducing the preload or stretch on the myocardial wall. One such intervention appropriate in physical therapy practice is appropriate positioning to help adjust the preload in patients with left-sided heart failure. These patients will often not tolerate a supine or recumbent position, when the effects of gravity are minimized and a greater volume of blood returns to the heart. This increased volume puts greater load or stretch on a heart, causing blood to back up into the lungs and exacerbate signs and symptoms. Conversely, these patients tolerate the upright position better, as the effects of gravity are maximized, allowing less blood to return to the heart and relatively less stress on the failing heart.

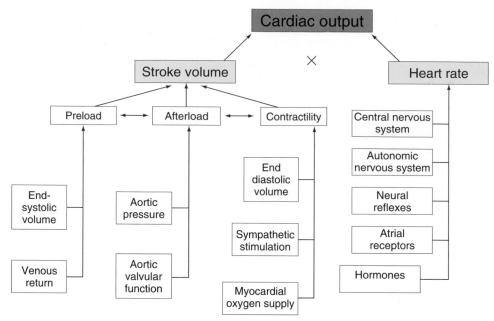

Figure 2-16 Factors affecting cardiac performance. Cardiac output, which is the amount of blood (in liters) ejected by the heart per minute, depends on heart rate (beats per minute) and stroke volume (milliliters of blood ejected during ventricular systole). (From McCance KL, Huether SE, Brashers VL, et al, editors: *Pathophysiology: The Biologic Basis for Disease in Adults and Children*, ed 6, St. Louis, 2010, Mosby.)

Contractility

Myocardial contractility is influenced by intrinsic and extrinsic factors. The intrinsic control of contraction strength is a result of the degree of myocardial stretch caused by changes in the EDV.[12,13] This is discussed more comprehensively in the preceding section. In addition, force–frequency relationships cause an increase in myocardial contractility when heart rate increases. Physiologically, at higher heart rates (>120 bpm), an increased availability of calcium ions allows for excitation–contraction coupling and a resultant stronger contraction.[13]

The extrinsic control of contractility depends on the activity of the sympathoadrenal system (Fig. 2-16). Epinephrine from the adrenal medulla and norepinephrine from the sympathetic nerve endings produce a positive ionotropic effect, or increase myocardial contractility, by promoting an influx of calcium available to the sarcomeres of the myocardial cells. Conversely, a reduction in sympathetic stimulation and reduction in heart rate results in reduced myocardial contractility.

Afterload

Blood flows from areas of high pressure to areas of low pressure. Therefore to enable blood to be ejected out of the ventricle into the aorta, the pressure generated within the ventricle must exceed the pressure within the systemic vasculature.[24] The pressure within the arterial system during the diastolic phase of the cardiac cycle, while the heart is filling, is a function of the total peripheral resistance. An increase in the total peripheral resistance increases the pressure within the systemic vasculature. The afterload is a reflection of the pressure against which the heart has to contract to pump blood into the aorta. The total peripheral resistance presents a hindrance to the ejection of blood from the ventricles or represents an afterload on the ventricular wall after contraction has begun (Fig. 2-17). The afterload is inversely proportional to the stroke volume. Thus an increase in the afterload or total peripheral resistance reduces the amount of blood ejected with each contraction.

It is valuable to note that a reduced stroke volume from an increased afterload triggers compensatory mechanisms to maintain the cardiac output at a normal level of approximately 5.5 L/min. Initially, as blood has greater difficulty being ejected because of an increase in the afterload, a greater volume of blood builds within the ventricle, triggering the Frank–Starling mechanism and a resultant greater myocardial contraction to help increase the stroke volume. An inability of the heart to compensate in this way leads to congestive heart failure and a compensatory increase in the heart rate to maintain the cardiac output at a normal level of approximately 5.5 L/min.

Ejection Fraction

The ejection fraction is the best indicator of cardiac function and represents a ratio or percentage of the volume of blood ejected out of the ventricles relative to the volume of blood received by the ventricles before contraction.[10] In other words, the ventricles receive a certain volume of blood during the diastolic phase, then contract and surge out a certain volume of blood. The ejection fraction reflects the ratio of the volume of ejected relative to what was received before systole or contraction of the ventricles. This can be mathematically presented as systolic volume (SV)/EDV. The normal ejection fraction is 60% to 70%. This means that for every 100 mL of blood poured into the ventricles during relaxation, 60 to 70 mL of blood is ejected per contraction. The volume of blood that remains in the ventricle following contracting is termed the *end-systolic volume* (ESV) and is approximately 30% of the EDV. A certain volume of blood must remain within the ventricles at the end of the contraction to maintain a certain degree of stretch within muscle fibers of the myocardial cells.[25]

In patients with systolic heart failure, the ejection fraction is compromised as evidenced by a ratio less than 40%. This means that for every 100 mL of blood brought into the ventricles, less than 40 mL of blood is ejected per contraction caused by a failing heart. Thus blood that cannot be ejected backs up

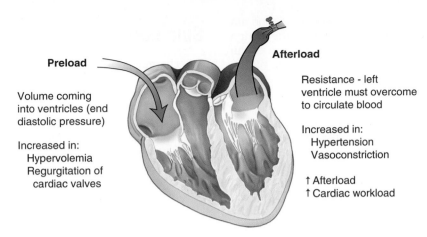

Preload

Volume coming
into ventricles (end
diastolic pressure)

Increased in:
Hypervolemia
Regurgitation of
cardiac valves

Afterload

Resistance - left
ventricle must overcome
to circulate blood

Increased in:
Hypertension
Vasoconstriction

↑ Afterload
↑ Cardiac workload

Figure 2-17 Preload and afterload. (From Irwin S, Tecklin SJ: *Cardiopulmonary Physical Therapy: A Guide to Practice,* ed 4, St. Louis, 2005, Mosby.)

into the ventricle and causes an array of complications. These consequences are more comprehensively discussed in subsequent chapters.

Venous Return

Venous return represents the return of blood to the right side of the heart via the veins. Two factors dictate the rate at which the right atrium fills with venous blood. These include the total blood volume and the pressure within the venous vasculature. Blood returned to the heart is primarily returned because of venous pressure. The mean venous pressure through the venous vasculature is approximately 2 mm Hg and is very different from mean arterial pressure, which is 90 to 100 mm Hg. This pressure is highest in the distal venules (approximately 10 mm Hg) and lowest at the junction of the vena cava with the right atrium (0 mm Hg). This pressure difference is the driving force of blood back to the heart. In addition, return is aided by the muscle pump activity, whereby the squeezing of peripheral muscles milk veins and assist with venous return. Also, sympathetic nerve fibers stimulate smooth muscle cell contraction in veins. Finally, pressure differences between the thoracic and abdominal cavities promote flow back to the heart. This phenomenon may be facilitated by active deep diaphragmatic inspiratory maneuvers. During contraction of the diaphragm, the central tendon contracts and pulls the two hemidiaphragms caudally. This creates an increase in the abdominal pressure and a partial vacuum in the thoracic cavity, driving blood from the abdominal cavity into the thoracic cavity.

It is also noteworthy that veins have very thin walls and are less muscular compared with arteries. This increases their compliance, and they can distend much more with any given amount of pressure. In light of this, veins have an ability to hold large volumes of blood and are often referred to as *capacitance vessels*, being similar to electrical capacitors that store electrical charges. Approximately two-thirds of total blood volume is stored within the venous vasculature.

It is often thought that the Trendelenburg position (elevation of the pelvis and lower extremities above the horizontal plane in the supine position) is effective for assisting with venous return in patients who are dehydrated or hypovolemic. The Trendelenburg position is not likely to augment cardiac output because of the high capacitance of veins.[26] The high capacitance of veins acts as a volume reservoir and counteracts any changes in the pressure gradient between peripheral and central veins. The venous system is more likely to transmit pressure when the veins are overloaded and less distensible. Therefore the Trendelenburg position is more likely to assist with venous return when the patient has excess volume and not during episodes of volume depletion. Thus using the Trendelenburg position with patients in hypovolemia is not recommended.

Coronary Blood Flow

The coronary arteries, discussed in Chapter 1, have a multitude of capillaries that help to perfuse myocardial tissue. It is interesting to note that the capillary density in myocardial tissue ranges from 2500 to 4000 capillaries per cubic millimeter of myocardial tissue, in contrast to skeletal muscle tissue where the capillary density is only 300 to 400 capillaries per cubic millimeter of muscle tissue.[27] The heart is a muscle that survives through constant aerobic respiration, both at rest and during heavy exercise. Thus it is imperative that adequate amounts of blood and oxygen be constantly perfused to myocardial tissue.

During systole, or contraction of the myocardium, coronary arteries are squeezed, reducing perfusion of blood. Consequently, coronary perfusion to the myocardium occurs more during the diastolic or relaxation phase of each cardiac cycle. To provide a continuous supply of oxygen to myocardial cells despite the temporary reduction in the flow of blood during systole, the myocardium contains a large amount of molecules called *myoglobin*. These structures are similar to the hemoglobin found in red blood cells and have the ability to store oxygen during diastole and release it during systole to myocardial cells.

Coronary blood flow is regulated by autonomic nervous system influence. The fight-or-flight response triggers the sympathetic hormone epinephrine that affects the β-adrenergic receptors on the coronary arteries, producing vasodilatation.[28] Therefore to fight or flight during a stressful state, a surge of blood is perfused to the myocardium because of vasodilation to excite myocardial tissue and increase cardiac output.

Blood Flow to Muscles During Exercise

As the body transitions from rest to exercise, blood flow patterns change markedly as a consequence of actions of the sympathetic nervous system.[10] Systemic vessels contain both α and β receptors that cause peripheral vasoconstriction and vasodilation, respectively. Through the action of the sympathetic nervous system, blood can be redirected from certain organs and shunted to working muscles to provide oxygen and energy and sustain activity. The shift in blood flow to muscle tissue is accomplished primarily by reducing blood to the kidneys, intestines, liver, and stomach.

During exercise, when the active muscles experience a need for additional blood, norepinephrine released by sympathetic nerve fibers stimulate the α-adrenergic receptors along the blood vessels of the digestive organs and kidneys. Stimulation of these receptors raises vascular resistance through vasoconstriction of the vessels, thereby diverting blood to skeletal muscles. At the level of the working muscles, epinephrine released by the adrenal medulla stimulates the β-adrenergic receptors within the blood vessel of the muscle to produce vasodilation and increase blood flow to the active muscles.[10]

During exercise, alterations in autonomic nervous system stimulation also influence coronary blood flow by directly affecting heart rate and force of contraction—the two primary determinants of the myocardium's metabolic rate. The rate pressure product, or double product, is a clinically useful tool to estimate the myocardial oxygen demand and is calculated by multiplying heart rate by systolic blood pressure.

Clinical tip

During aerobic exercise, heart rate and systolic blood pressure are the two main factors determining the workload on the heart. If these factors increase, the heart has to work harder and will require more oxygen and nutrients to keep going, requiring greater myocardial blood flow.

Aging and Cardiovascular Physiology

Normal aging alters functioning of the cardiovascular system. In addition, chronic illnesses and comorbidities, seen more in the geriatric population, further affect functioning of the system. This section addresses normal cardiac system changes that occur with aging. It is important to note, however, that because exercise has positive physiologic effects on aging, the changes mentioned may not be evidenced in all older individuals.

With increasing age, left ventricular wall thickness increases as a consequence of increased collagen and enhanced size of myocardial cells.[6] Increased vascular thickness and vascular intimal thickness are additional changes noted in older individuals. The diastolic or filling properties of the heart are negatively influenced, with reduced rate of ventricular filling and prolonged period of isovolumic myocardial relaxation, which is the time between aortic valve closure and the opening of the mitral valve.[6]

Maximal oxygen uptake (VO_2max) and cardiac output also reduce with increasing age. Reduced exercise performance and increased body weight collectively contribute to reductions in the relative oxygen consumption. Additionally, central and peripheral factors, including decreased maximum heart rate, reduced stroke volume, and compromised arteriovenous oxygen uptake, have been documented as factors contributing toward the decline in the VO_2max.[24] Finally, cardiac output during exercise reduces with increasing age as a result of low exercise heart rate and stroke volume values.

Summary

This chapter reviews the basic physiology of the cardiovascular and pulmonary systems and its clinical relevance for the practitioner. The physiologic principles of ventilation, respiration, and transport of gases provide the clinician with an understanding of the mechanisms involved in getting oxygen to the peripheral tissue and removal of waste products generated through metabolic processes. In addition, the physiologic principles involved within each cardiac cycle, both electrical and mechanical, that enable the delivery of oxygen to vital organs to sustain life and activity are discussed. Finally, factors influencing cardiac output, blood flow to peripheral tissue, and venous return provide a basis for understanding possible pathophysiologic processes that can occur with disease.

References

1. West JB: Respiratory Physiology. In *The Essentials*, ed 7, Baltimore, 2004, Lippincott Williams & Wilkins.
2. Beachy W: Respiratory Care Anatomy and Physiology. In *Foundations of Clinical Practice*, ed 2, St. Louis, 2008, Mosby.
3. Kendrick AH: Comparison of methods of measuring static lung volumes, *Monaldi Arch Chest Dis* 51(5):431–439, 1996.
4. Baydur A, Sassoon CS, Carlson M: Measurement of lung mechanics at different lung volumes and esophageal levels in normal subjects: Effects of posture change, *Lung* 174:139–151, 1996.
5. Fox S: *Human Physiology*, ed 11, Boston, 2009, McGraw-Hill.
6. Frownfelter D, Dean E: *Cardiovascular and Pulmonary Physical Therapy: Evidence and Practice*, ed 4, St. Louis, 2006, Mosby.
7. Guyton AC, Hall JE: *Textbook of Medical Physiology*, ed 11, Philadelphia, 2006, Saunders.
8. Kim V, Benditt JO, Wise RA, et al.: Oxygen therapy in chronic obstructive pulmonary disease, *Proc Am Thorac Soc* 5(4):513–518, 2008.
9. Cahalin LP: Heart failure, *Phys Ther* 76:516–533, 1996.
10. Wilmore JH, Costill DL: *Physiology of Sport and Exercise*, ed 2, Champaign, IL, 2000, Human Kinetics.
11. Gould BE: *Pathophysiology for the Health Professions*, ed 3, St. Louis, 2007, Saunders.
12. Irwin S, Tecklin J: *Cardiopulmonary Physical Therapy: A Guide to Practice*, ed 4, St. Louis, 2005, Mosby.
13. DeTurk W, Cahalin L: *Cardiovascular and Pulmonary Physical Therapy: An Evidence-Based Approach*, New York, 2004, McGraw-Hill.
14. Lacaze-Masmonteil T: Pulmonary surfactant proteins, *Crit Care Med* 21:S376–S379, 1993.
15. Johansson J, Curstedt T: Molecular structure and interactions of pulmonary surfactant components, *Eur J Biochem* 244(3):675–693, 1993.
16. Heuther S, McCance KL: *Understanding Pathophysiology*, ed 3, St. Louis, 2004, Mosby.
17. Goodman C, Fuller K: *Pathology: Implications for the Physical Therapist*, ed 3, St. Louis, 2009, Saunders.
18. Goodfellow LM: Application of pulse oximetry and the oxyhemoglobin dissociation curve in respiratory management, *Crit Care Nurs Q* 20(2):22–27, 1997.
19. Sims J: Making sense of pulse oximetry and oxygen dissociation curve, *Nurs Times* 92(1):34–35, 1996.
20. Dickson SL: Understanding the oxyhemoglobin dissociation curve, *Crit Care Nurse* 15(5):54–58, 1995.
21. Berne RM, Levy MN: *Cardiovascular Physiology*, ed 8, Philadelphia, 2000, Mosby.
22. Cheitlin MD: *Clinical Cardiology*, ed 7, Stamford, CT, 2004, Appleton & Lange.

23. Dubin D: *Rapid Interpretation of EKGs: A Programmed Course*, ed 6, Tampa, FL, 2006, Cover Publishing.

24. Ehrman JK, Gordon PM, Visich PS, et al.: *Clinical Exercise Physiology*, Champaign, IL, 2003, Human Kinetics.

25. Ganong WF: *Review of Medical Physiology*, ed 21, New York, 2003, McGraw-Hill.

26. Marino P: *The ICU Book*, ed 2, Philadelphia, 1998, Lippincott Williams and Wilkins.

27. Moore K, Dalley A: *Clinically Oriented Anatomy*, ed 5, Baltimore, 2006, Lippincott, Williams and Wilkins.

28. Paz J, West M: *Acute Care Handbook for Physical Therapists*, ed 3, St. Louis, 2009, Saunders.

3

Ischemic cardiovascular conditions and other vascular pathologies

Ann Fick and Ellen Hillegass

The current estimate is that at least 83 million Americans have one or more forms of cardiovascular disease (CVD).[1] Cardiovascular disease is, in reality, many diseases. The American Heart Association (AHA) considers ischemic (coronary) heart disease, hypertension (HTN), heart failure, and cerebrovascular disease (stroke) to be the major cardiovascular diseases. Of the leading causes of death in the United States in 2010, heart disease continued to rank first. Heart disease was responsible for 31.9% of all deaths in 2010, which represents a 16.7% decline in the mortality rate from 2000, with CVD responsible for 54.5% of total deaths.[1]

This chapter presents a detailed description of the anatomy and physiology of normal myocardial perfusion, a discussion of the pathologic changes that occur in coronary arteries as the result of coronary artery disease (CAD), and common cardiovascular diseases that are linked to the same process called *atherosclerosis*, including HTN, cerebrovascular disease, peripheral arterial disease (PAD), and other vascular disorders such as vascular aneurysms. The risk factors associated with the development of atherosclerosis are presented along with the major patterns of clinical presentation for CAD—chronic stable angina and acute coronary syndrome (ACS) (unstable angina, sudden cardiac death, and acute myocardial infarction [MI]).

The clinical presentation of the patient with CAD, the clinical signs and symptoms caused when the myocardium becomes ischemic, was first described by Heberden[2] in his lecture "Disorders of the Breast" in 1772:

There is a disorder of the breast, marked with strong and peculiar symptoms considerable for the kind of danger belonging to it, and not extremely rare, of which I do not recollect any mention among medical authors. The seat of it, and sense of strangling and anxiety, with which it is attended, may make it not improperly be called angina pectoris. Those, who are afflicted with it, are seized while they are walking and most particularly when they walk soon after eating, with a painful and most disagreeable sensation in the breast, which seems as if it would take their life away, if it were to increase or to continue; the moment they stand still, all this uneasiness vanishes.

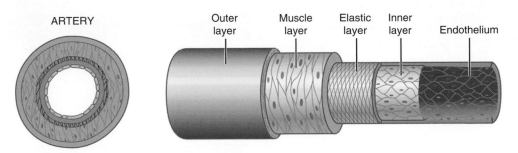

Figure 3-1 Artery wall structure. (Modified from Chabner DE: The language of medicine, ed 8, St Louis, 2007, Saunders.)

The prevalence of CAD and its surprising presence in seemingly healthy young men was not fully appreciated until 1953, when Enos and colleagues[3] published the results of the autopsies they performed on soldiers killed in the Korean conflict. The investigation found that 77.3% of the 300 soldiers examined (mean age: 22.1 years) had observable blockages of their coronary arteries.[4] In ten of the men, complete obstruction of one or more coronary arteries was found. As a direct result of the work of Enos and coworkers,[3] the medical community now distinguishes CAD (the presence of an obstruction that limits coronary blood flow but does not significantly inhibit heart muscle function) from coronary heart disease (CHD)—the presence of an obstruction that causes permanent damage to heart muscle fibers downstream, thus inhibiting heart muscle function.

Enos's report[3] was followed by the now famous Framingham Heart Study in which 5209 apparently healthy men and women between the ages of 30 and 62 years were followed for 20 years.[5] During that period, the subjects were seen for biennial examinations, which consisted of questionnaires on activity and smoking history, blood chemistry studies, blood pressure measurement, and a resting 12-lead electrocardiogram (ECG). Although no one specific cause of CAD could be identified in the Framingham cohort, several major and minor risk factors for its development were discovered and are discussed later in this chapter.

> **Clinical tip**
>
> The Framingham Heart Study provided landmark epidemiologic research that has led to the public and professional acceptance of the role of risk factors in the development and progression of CVD.[5]

Anatomy of the Coronary Arteries

Although the anatomy of the coronary arteries has been well understood for several years, to fully understand what is known about the coronary atherosclerotic process, a presentation of the normal triple-layered structure of arteries is necessary.[6]

Outer Layer

The outer layer of an artery (adventitia) consists chiefly of collagenous fibers, mostly fibroblasts, and provides the basic support structure for the artery (Fig. 3-1). This portion of the artery also houses the vessels that furnish the middle layer of the artery with its blood supply—the *vasa vasorum*.

Middle Layer

The middle layer (media) of all arteries (of which the coronary arteries are considered medium-size) consists of multiple layers of smooth muscle cells separated from the inner and outer layers by a prominent elastic membrane, or lamina. Through alterations in vasomotor tone, as demands for changes in blood flow to the myocardium are perceived, this muscular layer is responsible for making adjustments to the luminal diameter. These smooth muscle cells are also capable of synthesizing collagen, elastin, and glycosaminoglycans, especially when they react to different physical and chemical stimuli.

Inner Layer

The inner layer (intima) consists of an endothelial layer, the basement membrane, and variable amounts of isolated smooth muscle cells, as well as collagen and elastin fibers. The boundary of the intima and media is marked by the internal elastic lamina.

The two inner layers of the artery wall have received the most attention with regard to the development of the processes that lead to myocardial ischemia. The arterial endothelium is selectively permeable to macromolecules of the size of a low-density lipoprotein (LDL). The concentration of LDL in the lymph of the arterial wall has been found to be approximately one-tenth of that in the bloodstream.[7] Although many plasma proteins can enter the artery wall in this concentration, lipoproteins and fibrinogen are particularly likely to accumulate in the intima.[8]

Myocardial Perfusion

Before discussing the particulars of myocardial perfusion, it is important to review two basic rules of fluid dynamics. First, all fluids flow according to a pressure gradient, that is, from an area of higher pressure to an area of lower pressure. Second, all fluids follow the path of least resistance. Consequently, if an obstruction is encountered, fluid tends to follow the less-resistant path, thereby reducing the fluid volume across the obstruction and decreasing the pressure that would drive the fluid farther down the path beyond the obstruction.

As with all muscle beds, myocardial perfusion occurs primarily during periods of muscle relaxation, in this case, during diastole.[9,10] Fig. 3-2 shows the relationship between mean aortic pressure and blood flow in the coronary arteries. Blood

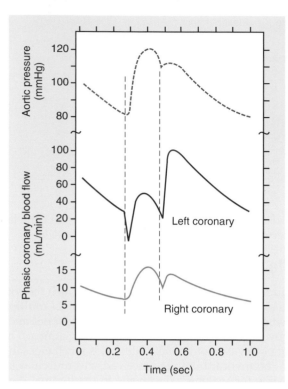

Figure 3-2 The relationship between blood pressure in the aorta (top) and blood flow in the left (middle) and right (bottom) coronary arteries. The first vertical dotted line is the beginning of systole, and the second dotted line is the beginning of diastole. (Modified from Boucek R, Morales A, Romanelli R, et al: *Coronary Artery Disease: Pathologic and Clinical Assessment*, Baltimore, 1984, Williams & Wilkins.)

flow increases retrogradely into both the right and left coronary arteries at the onset of systole (first vertical dotted line). When the aortic valve is closed, aortic diastolic pressure is transmitted through the dilated Valsalva sinuses to the openings of the coronary arteries themselves. Throughout diastole, the sinuses act as miniature reservoirs, facilitating maintenance of relatively uniform coronary inflow. The pressure generated by the right ventricle during systole is in the range of 15 to 25 mm Hg, whereas the left ventricle produces pressures of 120 mm Hg or higher. Consequently, the occlusive pressure on the right coronary artery terminal vessel is less than that on the left vessel during systole, so there is less difference in blood flow in the right coronary artery between systole and diastole.

Just as with any other arteries, the coronary arteries distend when blood is forced back into them by the contracting muscle. Inasmuch as the pressure within the coronary arteries is less than that in the aorta, the coronary arteries themselves become reservoirs for the storage of blood. The resultant engorgement provides the initial "pressure head" that drives blood into the myocardium once intramyocardial pressure drops following systole (see Chapter 2).

Clinical tip

The coronary arteries receive their blood supply during diastole. One mechanism to optimize the filling of the coronary arteries in individuals with disease is to place patients on β-blocking medications that lower the resting and exercise heart rates and increase diastolic filling time.

BOX 3-1 Myocardial blood flow relationship

F = DBP + VMT − R − LVEDP

F = flow of blood to the myocardium

DBP = diastolic blood pressure

VMT = vasomotor tone (additive if the vessel is in a dilated state and subtractive if constricted)

R = the resistance to flow offered by an obstructive lesion

LVEDP = left ventricular end-diastolic pressure

An especially important difference between the coronary vascular bed and most others is the presence of anastomotic connections that lack intervening capillary beds (known as *collateral vessels*). In human hearts, the distribution and extent of collateral vessels are quite variable.[11] Under normal conditions, such vessels are generally less than 40 μm in diameter and appear to have little or no functional role. However, when myocardial perfusion is compromised by obstructions that affect major vessels, these collateral vessels enlarge over several weeks and blood flow through them increases.[12-14] Given the time to make this adaptation, perfusion via collateral vessels may equal or exceed perfusion via the obstructed vessel.

Major Determinants of Myocardial Blood Flow

- Diastolic blood pressure (DBP) is the primary driving force moving blood into the myocardial tissue.
- Vasomotor tone (VMT) plays a major role in determining the volume of blood passed along to the tissue by regulating the caliber of the artery. Vasomotor tone is usually uniform throughout the coronary vascular tree. It aids or opposes DBP.
- Resistance to flow (R) is most commonly caused by atherosclerosis. A significant increase in the size and number of collateral vessels decreases total resistance to flow by providing an alternative route for the blood to take around an obstruction.
- Left ventricular end-diastolic pressure (LVEDP) is the pressure within the ventricle at end diastole; it causes an occlusive force on the capillary beds of the muscle closest to the pumping chamber, the endocardium.
- Myocardial blood flow relationship (Box 3-1).

Atherosclerosis

Atherosclerosis is a disease that causes progressive hardening and narrowing of the coronary, cerebral, and peripheral arteries. The development of atherosclerosis is a complex process dependent on the interaction of several risk factors and the sensitivity of the individual to these factors. Atherosclerotic plaques are composed of lipid and thrombus; the relative concentration of each varies widely from individual to individual (Fig. 3-3). In an effort to clarify this process, atherosclerosis is presented here as two processes—"atherosis" and "sclerosis"—that occur within the intima and endothelium of arterial walls. Undoubtedly, one of these components is more prominent than the other in each person who develops this disease. However, in very rare cases (homozygous familial hypercholesterolemia), atherosis is the only cause of the obstructive lesion.

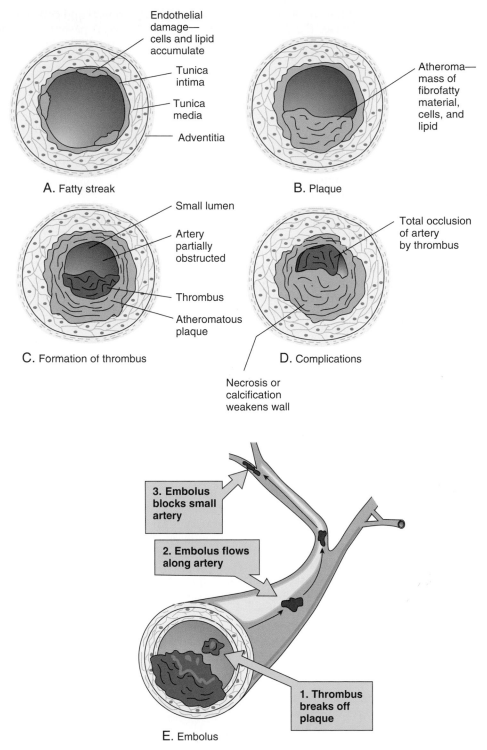

Figure 3-3 A-E, Development of an atheroma leading to arterial occlusion. (From Gould BE: *Pathophysiology for the Health Professions,* ed 4, St. Louis, 2011, Saunders.)

Pathophysiology

Atherosis

The first detectable lesion of atherosclerosis is the often-discussed fatty streak, which consists of lipid-laden macrophages and smooth muscle cells. Fatty streaks have been found in the arteries of patients as young as 10 years of age at the sites where major lesions appear later in life (see Fig. 3-3, *A*).[15,16]

The development and progression of the fatty streak in humans can be inferred from the findings of animal studies. In such studies, fatty streaks have been found in the lining of the aorta within 12 days of starting a high-fat, high-cholesterol diet. Clusters of monocytes have been found in junctional areas, between endothelial cells, where they accumulate lipid and are known as *foam cells.*[16,17] The subendothelial accumulation of these macrophages constitutes the beginning stage of fatty streak development. After several months, accumulations of lipid-laden macrophages grow so large that the endothelium is stretched and begins to separate over them (see Fig. 3-3, *B*). Such endothelial separation exposes the intima-based lesion and the underlying connective tissue to the circulation. Consequently, platelets aggregate and thrombus forms at these locations, a hallmark characteristic of the "sclerotic" phase of atherosclerosis (see Fig. 3-3, *C*).

Sclerosis

The sclerotic components of the lesions of atherosclerosis are responsible for a reduction of blood vessel compliance. Atherosclerotic intimal lesions that produce symptoms or end-organ damage (ischemia or infarction in the organs fed by the vessel involved) invariably have a major fibrous component. Increased lesion collagen and destruction of medial elastin, in addition to changes in the composition of these fibrous proteins, are important mechanisms underlying sclerosis in atherosclerosis.[18,19] Pure atherosis (lipid deposition alone), such as that in fatty streaks, does not produce end-organ damage (except with homozygous familial hypercholesterolemia), but may contribute to sclerosis. The exposure of subendothelial structures to the raw material of thrombus formation and the subsequent effect of such exposure on endogenous factors such as endothelium-derived relaxation factor contribute to the process of sclerosis.

One of the long-standing theories of the development of the atherosclerotic lesion is that of encrustation, that is, the formation of an organized "fibrous cap" of thrombi over advanced plaques that have developed on the endothelial lining.[6,20,21] Although this theory has never adequately accounted for the exact origin of the lesions, it has always been considered an important part of the process because of findings of extensive thrombus formation on microscopic examination of these plaques. A "response-to-injury" hypothesis has been postulated in an effort to define the initial stages of development of the atherosclerotic plaque (see Fig. 3-3).[22,23]

Although the response-to-injury hypothesis does not identify the agent or process responsible for it, investigations of vasospasm have provided some clues to the origin.[24–28] Platelet-derived growth factor (PDGF) contributes to lesion formation in two ways. First, as the name implies, PDGF stimulates the replication of connective tissue cells in the areas in which it is released. Second, PDGF is a chemoattractant; when released from tissues at the site of endothelial injury, it attracts smooth muscle cells so that they migrate from the media into the intima.[29–31]

When examining patients who are diagnosed with atherosclerosis in one organ, one should keep in mind that atherosclerosis occurs throughout the body in large and small arteries based upon the disease process. Therefore patients may have undiagnosed disease in other arteries because of a lack of presenting symptoms.

Vasospasm

At the beginning of this century, Sir William Osler was the first to suggest that a basic abnormality existed in the smooth muscle of coronary arteries that were affected by atherosclerosis when he reported to the Royal College of Physicians: "We have, I think, evidence that sclerotic arteries are especially prone to spasm."[32] For the next 50 years, coronary vasospasm was considered only a minor factor in the myocardial blood flow equation. Prinzmetal and colleagues[33] first identified the connection between vasospasm and what they called "variant angina." Variant angina differs from "typical angina," as first described by Heberden,[2] in that it is associated with ST-segment elevation instead of depression, occurs at rest (typically in the early morning) instead of during a predictable level of activity, and is not associated with any preceding increase in myocardial oxygen demand. This syndrome, which became known as *Prinzmetal angina*, was similar to typical angina in that it was promptly relieved with nitroglycerin and other vasodilators. Subsequent investigators found that this syndrome was considerably more widespread than had been previously believed, and by 1976, the "proved hypothesis" of a vasospastic nonlesion cause for angina was widely accepted.[34] Hyperreactivity of the coronary smooth muscle is thought to be a key factor in Prinzmetal angina.[35]

It has long been known that hyperplasia of intimal smooth muscle cells is a hallmark of advanced atherosclerosis.[22,23,36] It should not be surprising, therefore, that coronary arteries so afflicted would be prone to spasm. Experiments have shown that if the endothelium of the coronary artery is damaged, the intimal smooth muscle constricts instead of relaxing when stimulated.[37,38] A reduction in the release of endothelium-derived relaxing factors, that is, nitric oxide (NO), is thought to be the primary cause of this endothelial vasodilator dysfunction.[39]

Risk Factors

The Framingham study[5] was the first to test relationships between genetic and behavioral factors and their contribution to the development of coronary atherosclerosis and CHD in a long-term, large-scale epidemiologic trial. As a result of the original Framingham study and subsequently many other studies, the AHA has identified several risk factors for coronary heart disease; some of these factors can be changed, although others cannot (Box 3-2).[1] Vita and colleagues[40] suggested that in addition to accelerating the disease process once it is established, risk factors may themselves constitute the "injury" in the response-to-injury hypothesis of Ross and Glomset.[22,23] Although the presence or absence of significant

---

BOX 3-2 **Risk factors of heart and cardiovascular disease**

- Smoking
- Physical inactivity
- Obesity
- Suboptimal diet
- Hypertension
- Elevated serum total cholesterol
    - Elevated low-density lipoprotein (LDL)
    - Decreased high-density lipoprotein (HDL)
- Diabetes
- Family history
- Age
- Gender
    - Male risk is higher until females reach menopause; then risk is equal
- Stress

CAD cannot be determined by any simple arithmetic formula, there is considerable evidence to support the contention that the greater the number of risk factors present, the greater the likelihood that CAD, and ultimately CHD, will be present.[41–45] In addition to being risk factors of CAD, these are the risk factors of the other vascular diseases that are discussed later in this chapter (carotid and vertebral disease, PAD).

Seven Health Metrics for Ideal Cardiovascular Health

The AHA now identifies seven health metrics for ideal cardiovascular health in adults and children for reducing CAD and CVD. Four of the metrics embrace health behaviors, including no cigarette smoking, appropriate physical activity, a healthy diet, and normal body weight. The remaining three involve managing health factors, especially blood pressure, cholesterol, and fasting blood glucose.[46] Other nonmodifiable risk factors are heredity, male sex, and increased age. Each of these risk factors not only has an additive effect on the ability of the other factors to contribute to the development of CAD and to subsequent CHD, but also exerts a multiplicative effect. Consequently, although each risk factor is discussed individually, it is critical to remember that these factors exist individually only in the isolation of the scientist's laboratory.

Cigarette Smoking

Approximately 15% of all deaths related to heart disease are a result of cigarette smoking.[1,47] Cigarette smoking has been associated with increased risk of CVD since 1958.[48] Although no one component of cigarette smoke has been identified as the causative agent for this association, a number of studies have shown how cigarette smoking has a deleterious effect on other known factors involved in the development of atherosclerosis.[49–52] As few as four cigarettes a day increases a smoker's risk of developing CAD and CHD above that of a nonsmoker or an ex-smoker.[53,54] In comparison to nonsmokers, smokers have been shown to manifest leukocytosis, lower serum high-density lipoprotein (HDL) levels, elevated fibrinogen and plasma catecholamine levels, and increased blood pressure.[55,56] That similar alterations in the risk factor profiles of the preadolescent children of smoking parents have also been observed suggests that cigarette smoking increases the risk of developing CHD in both the smoker and the nonsmoking family members.[57,58]

Physical Activity

The role of exercise in the management of CHD has been acknowledged since Morris[59] reported a lower incidence of MI in conductors (who were physically active) of British double-decker buses, compared with drivers. Physical inactivity remains a significant risk factor for developing CHD and is comparable to that observed for cigarette smoking.[1] The Centers for Disease Control and Prevention reported that an insufficient amount of exercise is the most prevalent risk factor for CHD, and approximately 60% of adults in the United States do not perform the minimum recommended amount of physical activity.[1,60–62] In addition, the prevalence of sedentary lifestyle in the United States was higher among women compared with men, and higher among diabetics versus nondiabetics.[63]

There is more than ample evidence that regular aerobic exercise has a beneficial impact on many CHD risk factors.[64–69] The effects of regular aerobic exercise training on lipids and lipoproteins have been reviewed in several metaanalyses, yet controversy exists as to the amount of change that occurs in lipids as a result of exercise training. Kelley performed a metaanalysis on aerobic exercise and lipid changes and found that changes were equivalent to improvements of 2% for total cholesterol (TC) and HDL cholesterol (HDL-C), 3% of LDL cholesterol (LDL-C), and 9% for triglycerides (TG).[70] Carroll and Dudfield reported that regular aerobic exercise was effective in reducing TG (−18.7 mg/dL, −12%) and increasing HDL-C (1.6 mg/dL, +4.1%) in overweight and obese, sedentary adults with dyslipidemia.[71] Katzel and coworkers[72] showed that aerobic exercise coupled with weight training can yield reductions in plasma TG of 17% and LDL-C of 8%, in addition to increasing HDL-C by 11% (3.7 mg/dL). Although the amount of change may vary depending on the type of activity, evidence exists to conclude that activity does improve the lipid profile, whether it is resistive, aerobic, or both.[73]

Some of the lesser-known benefits of long-term endurance training are an increase in fibrinolysis and red blood cell deformability, as well as a decrease in platelet aggregability,[74–79] which may be beneficial in preventing initial or subsequent coronary ischemic events. It has been shown that exercise of adequate intensity, duration, and frequency is beneficial in preventing cardiovascular disease and increasing longevity in the healthy population.[69,76,80–84] The AHA has defined a goal of 150 min/week of moderate or 75 min/week of vigorous intense exercise as a main component necessary for ideal cardiovascular health.[46]

> **Clinical tip**
>
> The major risk factors for CHD are also major risk factors for carotid artery disease and PAD. The professional should also assess these other systems when assessing the patient for CHD, and should consider the possibility of underlying disease in other systems if these risk factors are present.

Body Weight

It is estimated that 68% of the population is either overweight or obese.[1] Several studies have associated obesity (body mass index [BMI] ≥ 30 kg/m^2) with the development of CHD.[85–87] This relationship appears to be more significant if the excess body fat is concentrated in the abdomen (central obesity) as opposed to being more evenly distributed throughout the body.[88,89] The AHA now considers obesity and being overweight as a main risk factor for CVD, with a goal for ideal cardiovascular health of less than 25 kg/m^2.[46]

Diet

Proper nutrition can play a significant role in decreasing the risk factors of HTN, hyperlipidemia, obesity, and glucose levels. Therefore the impact of dietary habits is thought to be quite underestimated in the development of CHD and CVD. The AHA recommends a healthy diet of at least 4½ cups of fruits and vegetables per day, 2 servings of fish per week, and 3 servings of whole grains per day. In addition, they recommend limiting sugar-sweetened drinks to 36 oz/week or less and sodium to 1500 mg/day or less.[1]

Blood Pressure

According the AHA, 77.9 million Americans, including nearly a third of all black adults and more than half of all adults older than age 60 years, have HTN, or high blood pressure.[1] Hypertension, both systolic (≥140 mm Hg) and diastolic (≥90 mm Hg), is believed to be an independent risk factor for the development of CAD and peripheral and cerebral vascular disease. So far, efforts to lower the morbidity and mortality rates associated with HTN have proved better at reducing stroke than heart attack.[1] Such findings have led some investigators to believe that high blood pressure and coronary vascular disease merely coexist instead of influencing one another in a causal relationship.[90] Nonetheless, the epidemiologic evidence still overwhelmingly points to HTN as a significant risk factor for the development of CAD.[1,91,92]

Cholesterol

Since the first published results of the Framingham study, the direct link between abnormal levels of cholesterol and the development of CHD has been well established.[93,94] Several forms of cholesterol have been shown to play a role in atherogenesis: very-low-density lipoprotein (VLDL), intermediate-density lipoprotein (IDL), LDL, and lipoprotein a (LpA).[95–97] Direct dietary intake of cholesterol is not the principal influence on the level of cholesterol in the blood; instead, intake of saturated fat influences the lipoproteins.[98–102] The cholesterol-to-saturated fat index (CSI) has proved to be a valuable clinical education tool because it clearly shows the discrepancy between dietary and serum levels of cholesterol.[103–105]

From the CSI formula (CSI = [1.01 × g saturated fat] + [0.05 × mg cholesterol]), it is clear that the contribution of saturated fat in any particular food item is about 20 times more atherogenic than its cholesterol content.

Other studies have documented the importance of HDL as an independent predictor of CHD risk.[106–108] A value of less than 40 mg/dL for men and less than 50 mg/dL for women is considered low.[1] Although the exact mechanism by which increased levels of HDL provide protection from coronary disease is poorly understood, several theories have been proposed. The concept of "reverse cholesterol transport"—bringing free cholesterol from the tissues back to the liver for safe storage—is most often cited.[109–116] The best predictor of risk for developing cholesterol-related blockages in an artery is the ratio of total cholesterol to HDL (CHOL/HDL); a ratio of greater than 4.5 increases an individual's risk of developing atherosclerosis.[117–119] Elevated triglycerides have also become a marker for the development of coronary atherosclerosis (>150 mg/dL), particularly when they are associated with low levels of HDL (<35 mg/dL).[120–122] In 2004 the National Cholesterol Education Program (NCEP) published treatment goals and intervention strategies for cholesterol testing and management and endorsed the use of the Framingham Risk Score (FRS) for identifying 10-year CHD risk.[123] The 2013 American College of Cardiology/AHA Task Force on Practice Guidelines also supported the use of high-intensity and moderate-intensity statin therapy for prevention of atherosclerosis. However, the panel stated more research is needed before supporting any currently proposed LDL and HDL target treatment levels.[124]

Fasting Blood Glucose

Nonenzymatic glycosylation, or the chemical attachment of glucose to proteins without the involvement of enzymes, is known to affect fibrinogen, collagen, antithrombin III, HDL, and LDL, all of which are involved in the evolution of CAD.[125–127] The attachment of glucose to these molecules renders them less sensitive to the enzymes and other substances with which they interact. For example, antithrombin III activity, which normally inhibits excessive blood coagulation, is decreased when it undergoes glycosylation, and fibrinogen is less likely to perform its function of degrading fibrin when so affected. In both these cases, thrombus formation is enhanced. This process may even be the principal cause of basement membrane thickening, long known to be a major tissue change associated with prolonged diabetes (see Chapter 7).

The Adult Treatment Panel (ATP) III guidelines identified diabetes as a high-risk condition based upon the evidence demonstrating patients with diabetes have a relatively high 10-year risk for developing CVD.[123] The Heart Protective Study (HPS) studied individuals who had both diabetes and CVD and discovered that these individuals were at very high risk for future cardiovascular events, warranting lipid-lowering therapy.[128] According to the AHA, diabetes is now a main risk factor, and an untreated fasting blood glucose level of lower than 100 mg/dL is suggested for prevention of CVD.[1,46]

Other Risk Factors

The contributing risk factors are not independently significant in predicting the likelihood of an individual's developing CHD. As their name implies, however, they do play a role in its establishment and growth.

Family History

Family history of CHD, defined as its presence in a parent or sibling, has been shown to be a minor risk factor for the development of CAD.[129–132] With the exception of the familial hypercholesterolemias, no genetic link has been established for CHD; like obesity, the atherogenic contribution of family history is not entirely genetic. Fortunately, the modification of risk factors in subjects with a strong family history of premature coronary disease provides a reduction in overall risk of developing subsequent disease.[133,134] Premature or early coronary disease is defined as men younger than age 50 years and women younger than age 60 years, but the AHA defines family history as significant if either parent (genetic linked parents) had a diagnosis of heart disease (first event of MI, angina, coronary artery bypass graft [CABG], or percutaneous transluminal coronary angioplasty [PTCA]) at an age younger than 60 years. Although the Framingham Score does not take into account family history, most experts report a premature or early family history of heart disease doubles one's risk for CVD.[135,136]

Although scientific literature has not established a genetic link with HDL cholesterol specifically, there appear to be findings of lower HDL and higher total CHOL/HDL ratios in offspring of individuals with CHD. Another genetic theory involves a possible inheritance of platelet stickiness in individuals with CHD. The current theory is to recommend aspirin use on a long-term basis in offspring with a strong family history of CHD, as well as to monitor C-reactive protein levels (an antiinflammatory marker) in individuals with a positive family history.[135–138]

Age

Increased age is known to be a risk factor for CHD.[139] The average age of an initial MI for men is 64.7 and 72.2 for women.[140] Whether older age is an independent pathologic process or simply a consequence of prolonged exposure to the risk factors is less clear. Studies show that interventions on other risk factors have proved to be beneficial in older subsets of patients and have resulted in the reduction of clinical end points, for example, MI and symptoms.[141,142] Also, both patients and subjects without known disease in the young-old and middle-old age groups (ages 67 to 76 years) have responded to the same extent as young subjects to attempts at risk factor reduction.[143–145]

Although biochemical changes are known to occur as people age—for example, decreased nerve conduction velocity and decreased aerobic enzyme activity—the functional significance of these changes appears to be negligible if they are not complicated by preexisting disease.[146,147]

Gender

It is a common perception that premenopausal women are "immune" from CHD. Men are much more likely than women to experience an MI before age 55 years,[107,148–150] and the overall onset of clinically significant CHD in women lags 10 years behind that in men.[150,151]

Although it is true that, in general, women experience lower CHD morbidity and mortality rates than men do, heart disease is the leading cause of death in both men and women.[1,152] Once an MI occurs, women of all age groups have a higher mortality rate than men. Slightly more women have unrecognized or "silent" MIs than men (34% vs. 27%), but interestingly, the initial clinical event in women is most often angina, whereas in men it is an acute MI. Women who have diabetes are more susceptible to developing CHD than are men.[153–155] Females who develop preeclampsia during pregnancy are also identified at increased risk of CVD, as they are more likely to develop HTN and cerebrovascular disease.[156] Women who also develop placental problems during pregnancy and who have traditional cardiovascular risk factors, including pre-pregnancy HTN, diabetes mellitus, obesity, dyslipidemia, or metabolic syndrome, are also defined as at elevated risk for CVD.[156]

In terms of age group, the largest "gain" in either sex during which the greatest increase in CHD occurs is in women ages 55 to 64 years.[157–159] Because the gap between CHD incidence in men and women closes in the years following menopause, it has been argued that menopause plays some nonspecific role in regulating this disease process. Therefore estrogen replacement was thought to be cardioprotective.[160–164] However, research has not confirmed this belief. The AHA guidelines for hormone replacement report that hormone therapy and selective estrogen-receptor modulators (SERMs) should not be used for the prevention of CHD.[165]

Stress

Although the pathogenesis may not have been defined, Friedman and Rosenman[166] related the sense of time urgency and easily aroused hostility to a sevenfold increase in prevalence of CHD—what they termed *type A behavior*. Therefore the personality characteristics of hostility and anger may be more descriptive than the traditional term "type A behavior." The identification of what has been termed type A behavior as an independent risk factor for CHD is still being debated.[167–169] The exact mechanism by which this predominantly psychological trait increases the risk for the tissue changes of CHD is believed to be related to platelet activation. This contribution to the sclerotic component of CHD is known to be related to increases in levels of catecholamine and platelet-secreted proteins, which have been found in subjects undergoing emotional stress.[170,171] It is known also that alterations in this type A behavior can reduce morbidity and mortality rates for post-MI patients.[115] However, further research is essential to determine how stress influences CHD.

> ### Clinical tip
>
> Psychosocial distress is also associated with increased mortality and morbidity rates after MI. In addition, social isolation and depression are associated with a poor prognosis after MI. These findings should emphasize the importance of identifying this risk before rehabilitation to ensure it is addressed in the total rehabilitation of the patient.

Emerging Risk Factors

Additional risk factors for atherosclerotic disease that may or may not have a role in thrombus development or initiation of atherosclerosis include the following:[172–175]

- Lp(a)
- LDL subclasses
- Oxidized LDL
- Homocysteine
- Hematologic factors (primarily fibrinogen, factor VII, and tissue plasminogen activator [tPA])
- Inflammatory markers such as C-reactive protein (CRP) and lipoprotein-associated phospholipase A_2 (Lp-PLA_2)

Each of these risk factors is discussed in greater detail in Chapter 8 in the clinical laboratory section. Lipoprotein(a) appears to have an atherogenic and prothrombic effect that interferes with plasminogen and tPA binding to fibrin. Lipoprotein(a) levels are thought to be genetic in origin and were found in 50% of the offspring of patients with CAD in the Framingham study.[172] Increased Lp(a) levels are associated with a threefold increase in the risk of a primary CAD event.[172] In addition to Lp(a), the presence of an elevated amount of small dense LDL particle subtype (phenotype B) is associated with an elevated risk for CAD (threefold increased risk).[172,173] Small dense LDL is also associated with elevated triglyceride levels.

Homocysteine, a type of amino acid found in the blood, has been linked to an increased risk of development of CVD when the levels in the blood are elevated.[174,175] However, the use of screening homocysteine levels to direct treatment remains debatable.[176]

Elevated levels of inflammatory markers are also seen in individuals with CVD. Elevated CRP levels are associated with CHD and sudden cardiac death, and high Lp-PLA_2 levels are linked to MI and stroke.[177,178] Therefore if an individual has high levels of these inflammatory markers, aggressive CVD risk modification may be beneficial.

Clinical Course

The clinical presentation of the patient with CHD typically occurs in one of four ways:

- Sudden cardiac death
- Chronic stable angina
- Acute coronary syndrome (ACS), an umbrella term used to define acute myocardial ischemia that is further divided into three components:
  - Unstable angina
  - ST-segment elevation myocardial infarction (STEMI)
  - Non-STEMI
- Cardiac muscle dysfunction (see Chapter 4)

Sudden Cardiac Death

In 40% to 50% of patients with CHD, sudden cardiac death (SCD—death within 1 hour of onset of symptoms) is the initial presenting syndrome.[179,180] Studies also show coronary atherosclerosis was found in most of the victims.[180] Ventricular tachycardia and ventricular fibrillation, leading to cessation of cardiac output, are the usual causes of death. Box 3-3 lists the risk factors for SCD. For these patients, prompt delivery of bystander cardiopulmonary resuscitation with an automatic external defibrillator (AED) and entry into the emergency medical system within 10 minutes is their only chance of survival.[1,181]

Angina

The majority of patients with CHD first seek medical attention because of angina (an Old English term meaning "strangling") pectoris. This sensation, most commonly described as a substernal pressure, can occur anywhere from the epigastric area to the jaw and is described as squeezing, tightness, or crushing (Fig. 3-4). It is now known to be caused by an imbalance in supply and demand of myocardial oxygen. Table 3-1 lists the types of chest discomfort.

Chronic Stable Angina

Chronic stable angina, as its name implies, usually has a well-established level of onset and is the result of not enough blood supply to meet the metabolic demand (Fig. 3-5). Patients are able to predict reliably those activities that provoke their discomfort; this condition is usually associated with a set level of myocardial oxygen demand. As mentioned earlier, myocardial oxygen demand is closely related to heart rate and systolic blood pressure (SBP). By multiplying these values, the so-called *double product* or *rate pressure product* (RPP), an index that is useful in correlating functional activities with myocardial capabilities, can be obtained. Wall stress, the third determinant of the myocardial oxygen consumption (MVO_2) rate, can be accurately measured only with invasive monitoring and is therefore not usually available to the patient performing routine activities.

Patients with stable angina are usually able to bring their symptoms under control by reducing slightly the intensity of the exercise they are performing or by taking sublingual nitroglycerin. Patients have some variability in their tolerance for activity—that is, they have "good days and bad days"—which is probably related to variations in coronary vascular tone, but overall, stable angina is a predictable syndrome.

BOX 3-3　**Risk factors associated with sudden death**

Undiagnosed CHD population	Diagnosed CHD population
Age	Decreased left ventricular ejection fraction (LVEF) (<35%)
Systolic blood pressure (elevated)	
Left ventricular hypertrophy	
Intraventricular block on ECG	
Nonspecific ECG abnormalities	
Serum cholesterol (elevated)	
Heart rate (elevated resting HR)	
Vital capacity (low, especially a factor in females)	
Cigarettes consumed daily	
Relative weight	

The ventricular fibrillation (VF) sudden cardiac arrest survival rate is only 2% to 5% if defibrillation is provided more than 12 minutes after collapse.[1] Early cardiopulmonary resuscitation (CPR) and rapid defibrillation, combined with early advanced care, can produce high long-term survival rates for witnessed cardiac arrest. In some cities with public access to defibrillation or "community AED programs," when bystanders provide immediate CPR and the first shock is delivered within 3 to 5 minutes, the reported survival rates from VF sudden cardiac arrest are as high as 48% to 74%.[1] *CHD,* Coronary artery disease; *ECG,* electrocardiogram; *HR,* heart rate.

Acute Coronary Syndrome

Chest discomfort continuing for greater than 20 minutes is the most common symptom in individuals with ACS. Acute coronary syndrome is used to describe individuals diagnosed with either unstable angina or acute myocardial infarction (AMI).

The definition of acute/evolving/recent MI has been redefined in recent years. Since 2007, AMI has been defined as a clinical event resulting in myocardial necrosis due to ischemia. In 2012 a third universal definition of AMI was adopted to include criteria of a rise/drop of troponin *plus* evidence of symptoms of ischemia, ECG changes (pathologic Q wave, ST-segment changes, and/or new left bundle branch block), or new cardiac muscle damage/wall motion abnormalities seen on imaging.[182–184] Acute myocardial infarction is divided into STEMI and non-STEMI. When individuals arrive in the emergency department, medical interventions are chosen based on the presence or absence of ST-segment elevation on ECG and elevated serum cardiac biomarkers such as troponin I or troponin T.[185]

Unstable angina can be defined as the presence of signs or symptoms of an inadequate blood supply to the myocardium in the absence of the demands that usually provoke such an imbalance (usually at rest, often waking an individual in the middle of the night). The patient who presents with unstable angina or has chronic stable angina that develops an unstable pattern (see later discussion) requires quick recognition and referral for treatment. Although the physical therapist is not responsible for making the diagnosis of unstable angina, he or she may be the person who first detects its presence while following a patient in a cardiac rehabilitation program. It is therefore important for such professionals to have a basic understanding of the mechanisms of unstable angina and know how to detect it.

Patients who have unstable angina are known to have increased morbidity and mortality rates compared with those who have stable angina, even though the absolute amount of coronary atherosclerosis in both groups is not significantly

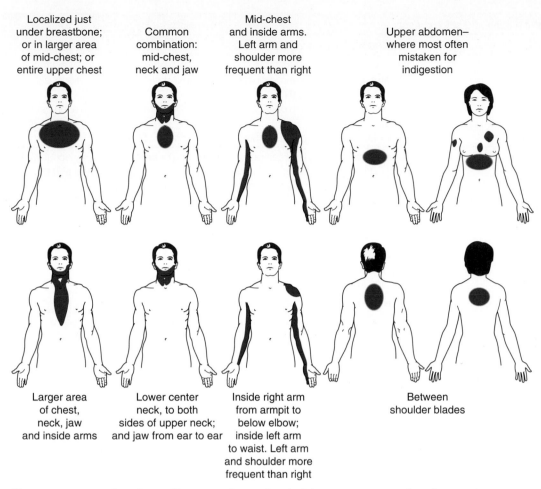

Localized just under breastbone; or in larger area of mid-chest; or entire upper chest

Common combination: mid-chest, neck and jaw

Mid-chest and inside arms. Left arm and shoulder more frequent than right

Upper abdomen— where most often mistaken for indigestion

Larger area of chest, neck, jaw and inside arms

Lower center neck, to both sides of upper neck; and jaw from ear to ear

Inside right arm from armpit to below elbow; inside left arm to waist. Left arm and shoulder more frequent than right

Between shoulder blades

Most common warning signs of heart attack

- Uncomfortable pressure, fullness, squeezing or pain in the center of the chest (prolonged)
- Pain that spreads to the throat, neck, back, jaw, shoulders, or arms
- Chest discomfort with lightheadedness, dizziness, sweating, pallor, nausea, or shortness of breath
- Prolonged symptoms unrelieved by antacids, nitroglycerin, or rest

Atypical, less common warning signs (especially women)

- Unusual chest pain (quality, location, e.g., burning, heaviness; left chest), stomach or abdominal pain
- Continuous midthoracic or interscapular pain
- Continuous neck or shoulder pain
- Isolated right biceps pain
- Pain relieved by antacids; pain unrelieved by rest or nitroglycerin
- Nausea and vomiting; flu-like manifestation without chest pain/discomfort
- Unexplained intense anxiety, weakness, or fatigue
- Breathlessness, dizziness

Figure 3-4 Early warning signs of a heart attack. Multiple segmental nerve innervation shown in accounts for the varied pain patterns possible. A woman can experience any of the various patterns described but is more likely to develop atypical symptoms of pain as depicted here. (From Goodman CC: *Pathology: Implications for the Physical Therapists,* ed 3, St. Louis, 2009, Saunders.)

different.[186,187] The major physiologic difference between unstable and chronic stable angina is the absence of an increase in myocardial oxygen demand to provoke the syndrome. Chierchia and colleagues proved that imbalances in myocardial blood flow could be related to a primary reduction in oxygen supply without an increase in demand.[188] They were able to show that a fall in cardiac vein oxygen saturation always preceded the electrocardiographic or hemodynamic indicators of ischemia in 137 patients who experienced angina while at rest.

Factors That Contribute to Unstable Angina

According to Cannon and Braunwald, several factors are implicated as contributors to unstable angina and non-STEMI.

The most common cause is atherosclerotic plaque rupture in an already partially blocked artery. Other processes include dynamic obstruction (coronary vasoconstriction), inflammation, and extrinsic factors causing myocardial ischemia (e.g., anemia, tachycardia).[185]

The atherosclerotic plaque is known to undergo physical changes when a patient is experiencing unstable angina (Fig. 3-6). There are distinct differences in the morphology of atherosclerotic lesions of persons who are experiencing unstable angina compared with that of persons who have stable angina.[189,190] Technology allows direct visual inspection of coronary atherosclerotic lesions, thus permitting differentiation of plaques by their appearance.

Table 3-1 Types of angina and other chest pain

Types	Descriptors
Classic stable angina	Described as tightness, pressure, indigestion anywhere above waist (substernum, neck, left arm, right arm, cervical, between shoulder blades) that develops with exertional activity and diminishes with rest or nitroglycerin (NTG). Women typically complain of nausea, indigestion, discomfort between shoulder blades, or excessive fatigue. Individuals with diabetes often complain of shortness of breath.
Unstable angina (UA)	Chest discomfort that is accelerating in frequency or severity and may occur while at rest but does not result in myocardial necrosis. The discomfort may be more severe and prolonged than typical angina pain or may be the first time a person has angina pain.
Prinzmetal angina	Chest discomfort associated with ST-segment elevation instead of depression, occurs at rest (typically in the early morning) instead of during a predictable level of activity, and is not associated with any preceding increase in myocardial oxygen demand.
Pericarditis	Pain at rest, may worsen with activity, but is not relieved with rest or NTG. Responds to antiinflammatory medications. Common in post-CABG patients.
Chest wall pain (musculoskeletal)	Pain/discomfort that is increased with palpation over chest wall.
Pulmonary/pleuritic (pleurisy, pneumothorax, pneumonia)	Discomfort/pain, often sharp in nature that changes with breathing. Upon auscultation may hear pleural friction rub, decreased breath sounds, or other adventitious sounds. Check for tracheal shift and fever.
Bronchospasm	Exertionally related or induced by cold, extreme difficulty breathing, relieved with bronchodilator or stopping of activity.
Vascular (pulmonary embolism, aortic dissection)	Sudden onset of pain, constant. Pleuritic pain with shortness of breath often seen in pulmonary embolism and "unrelenting" in aortic dissection.
Gastrointestinal (esophageal reflux, peptic ulcer, gallbladder disease)	Prolonged epigastric discomfort usually related to food intake and/or relieved by antacid.

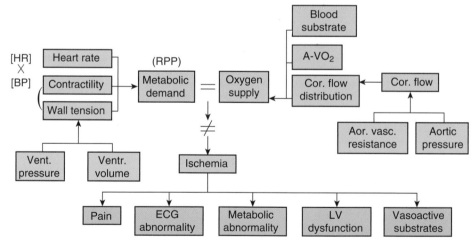

Figure 3-5 Factors that affect the supply of blood to the heart and factors that affect the demand or workload on the heart muscle. Ischemia results when there is an imbalance in supply and demand, and an individual will often perceive symptoms of angina.

Coronary plaque can be a dynamic process; therefore the stability of the disease can be altered quickly. Several clinical clues to the development of unstable angina should alert the health professional to notify a patient's physician:
- Angina at rest often lasting more than 20 minutes
- Occurrence of the patient's typical angina at a significantly lower level of activity than usual
- Deterioration of a previously stable pattern, for example, discomfort occurring several times a day compared with several times a week

- Evidence of loss of previously present myocardial reserve, such as a drop in blood pressure or increase in heart rate with levels of activity previously well tolerated

Unstable angina should be distinguished from Prinzmetal or variant angina (see Table 3-1). Both are likely to occur in the first few hours of rising, but variant discomfort is usually not as severe and is often seen in younger patients. Patients with variant angina are able to perform high levels of work later in the day without discomfort, but patients with unstable angina are unable

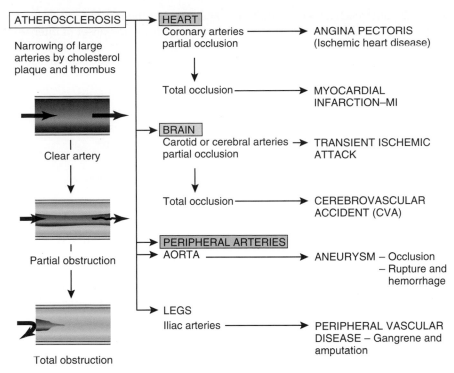

Figure 3-6 Possible consequences of atherosclerosis. (From Gould BE: *Pathophysiology for the Health Professions*, ed 4, St. Louis, 2011, Saunders.)

to increase their cardiac output significantly without provoking further discomfort, even if their earlier pain has waned.

Up to this point, consideration has been given only to primary prevention schemes. Health care professionals must not lose sight of the fact that although the number of Americans dying from heart disease is decreasing, the number of those living with heart disease is increasing. Primary health care providers must realize that risk factor modification interventions that have proven to be effective for the primary prevention of CAD and CHD are also applicable to secondary prevention and should be incorporated into the plan of care (see Chapter 18).

Other Acute Coronary Syndrome: STEMI and Non-STEMI

Acute coronary syndrome refers to symptoms that signify AMI and/or infarction as a result of insufficient supply to the heart muscle. Individuals with symptoms of insufficient blood supply to the myocardium will be given an ECG to look for STEMI or other ECG changes indicative of ischemia or infarction (non-STEMI or unstable angina). A STEMI develops a Q wave on the ECG in the subsequent 24 to 48 hours, and these previously were defined as Q wave or transmural (full- or near-full-thickness) infarctions. The percentage of ACSs with ST elevation on ECG has been reported to range from 29% to 47%.[1] A STEMI with transmural injury occurs distal to a totally occluded coronary artery that has become occluded secondary to a thrombus that occluded an area of plaque or ruptured plaque. However, other factors may affect the extent of injury, including whether or not collateral flow exists in the area, and whether or not vasospasm also occurred to complete the blockage of the area with plaque and thrombus. A non-STEMI does not develop a Q wave on the ECG and has been referred to as a *non–Q-wave infarction* or *subendocardial* (nontransmural, or affecting only the subendocardial

region) *infarction*. Studies using magnetic resonance imaging (MRI) actually show that the development of a Q wave on the ECG is caused by the size of the infarct and not the depth of the mural involvement (see Fig. 3-3, *D* and *E*).[191]

Progression of atherosclerosis may be gradual or sudden. In the case of a sudden change in plaque, the plaque may disrupt and promote platelet aggregation, thrombus generation, and thrombus formation. The thrombus may temporarily disrupt blood flow by becoming lodged in a plaque-laden area of a coronary artery. When this occurs, the thrombus interrupts the supply of oxygen to the myocardium and may cause myocardial necrosis. If the blood flow interruption is greater than 20 minutes, the patient may experience symptoms of unstable angina with myocardial ischemia and demonstrate reversible changes in the myocardial tissue. When elevation of a cardiac biomarker such as troponin I or T is present, this is considered to be a non-STEMI. Non-STEMIs often occur when coronary arteries are not completely blocked but have severely narrowed diameters and are at risk of becoming completely blocked (Fig. 3-7).[185] Identification of the location of the injury/infarction is made on the 12-lead ECG based upon the leads that demonstrate the ST elevation (for STEMIs) or ST depression or T-wave changes (in non-STEMIs) (Table 3-2).

If arterial reperfusion of the myocardium occurs within 20 minutes of MI, necrosis can be prevented. Beyond this phase, the extent of damage varies depending on factors such as the total time of coronary artery occlusion, possible collateral blood flow, and myocardial oxygen requirements (see Fig. 3-8 and Fig. 3-9 for more information). After reperfusion, where areas have become necrotic, mitochondria may develop deposits of calcium phosphate. Reperfusion of infarcted myocardium also promotes removal of intracellular proteins, resulting in early exaggerated values of cardiac markers such as troponin T and I. Table 3-3 describes changes that occur in the first few hours to weeks.[192]

Pathologic processes other than atherosclerosis can result in MI. These processes include coronary arterial disorder due to:

- Embolization
- Arteritis (e.g., Kawasaki syndrome)
- Trauma
- Congenital anomalies
- Metabolic disease (e.g., amyloidosis)
- Hematologic disorders
- Myocardial oxygen supply–demand imbalance
- Other (e.g., vasospasm)

Cocaine abuse has become one of the more frequent causes of vasospastic-induced MI in patients with and without CAD.[124]

Medical Management of Acute Coronary Syndrome

Prompt recognition is crucial for successful acute management of ACS. The primary concern for management of ACS is to reperfuse the area of the heart not receiving enough blood and oxygen, as well as to control for cardiac pain, limit any amount of necrosis, and prevent complications. Early reperfusion is accomplished with fibrinolysis (thrombolytic agents)

and PTCA if the individual receives emergent care within 60 to 90 minutes of the onset of intense chest pain (the earlier the reperfusion, the less the necrosis and the better the prognosis). The other general treatment measures include:[192]

- Aspirin
- Anticoagulant therapy
- Control of cardiac pain
  - Use of nitrates
  - Use of morphine
  - Use of β blockers
- Improve oxygenation
  - Use of oxygen
- Limitation of infarct size
  - Early reperfusion—consider need for percutaneous coronary intervention (PCI)
- Treatment of arrhythmias if needed for hemodynamic stability
- Control of other complications
  - Treatment of left ventricular dysfunction
  - Treatment for heart block with temporary or permanent pacemaker

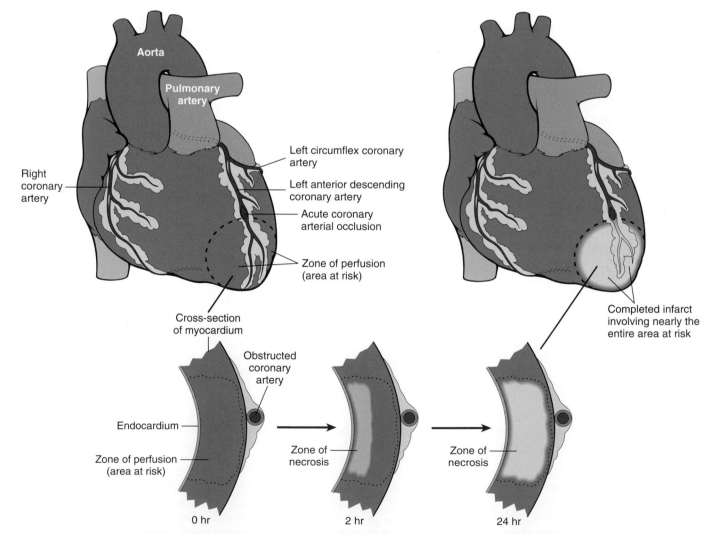

Figure 3-7 Progression of myocardial necrosis after coronary artery occlusion. Necrosis begins in a small zone of the myocardium beneath the endocardial surface in the center of the ischemic zone. The area that depends on the occluded vessel for perfusion is the "at-risk" myocardium (shaded). Note that a very narrow zone of myocardium immediately beneath the endocardium is spared from necrosis because it can be oxygenated by diffusion from the ventricle. (From Kumar V, Abbas AK, Fausto N, et al, editors: *Robbins and Cotran Pathologic Basis of Disease*, ed 8, St. Louis, 2010, Saunders.)

Table 3-2 Coronary anatomy and location of infarction

Anatomy	Location of Infarct	ECG Changes	Common Complications
Right coronary artery	Inferior	II, III, aVF	Risk of atrioventricular block and/or arrhythmias 50% have right ventricular infarct
Left main	Anterior and lateral	V1-V6, I, aVL	Pump dysfunction or failure
Left anterior descending (LAD)	Anterior	V1-V4	Pump dysfunction or failure
Circumflex	Lateral	V5, V6, aVL, I	None specific

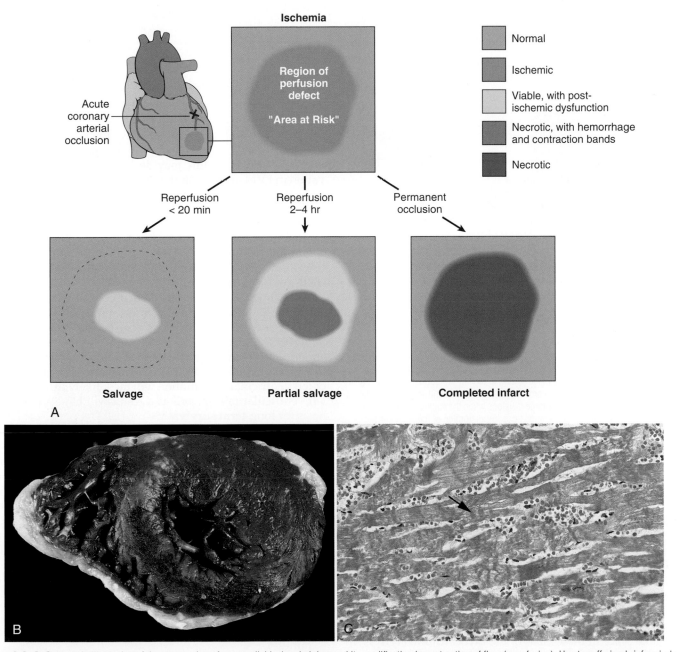

Figure 3-8 **A,** Schematic illustration of the progression of myocardial ischemic injury and its modification by restoration of flow (reperfusion). Hearts suffering brief periods of ischemia of longer than 20 minutes followed by reperfusion do not develop necrosis (reversible injury). Brief ischemia followed by reperfusion results in stunning. If coronary occlusion is extended beyond 20 minutes' duration, a wavefront of necrosis progresses from subendocardium to subepicardium over time. Reperfusion before 3 to 6 hours of ischemia salvages ischemic but viable tissue. This salvaged tissue may also demonstrate stunning. Reperfusion beyond 6 hours does not appreciably reduce myocardial infarct size. **B,** Large, densely hemorrhagic, anterior wall acute myocardial infarction from patient with left anterior descending artery thrombus treated with streptokinase intracoronary thrombolysis (triphenyl tetrazolium chloride-stained heart slice). (Specimen oriented with posterior wall at top.) **C,** Myocardial necrosis with hemorrhage and contraction bands, visible as dark bands spanning some myofibers *(arrow).* This is the characteristic appearance of markedly ischemic myocardium that has been reperfused. (From Kumar V, Abbas AK, Fausto N, et al, editors: *Robbins and Cotran Pathologic Basis of Disease,* ed 8, St. Louis, 2010, Saunders.)

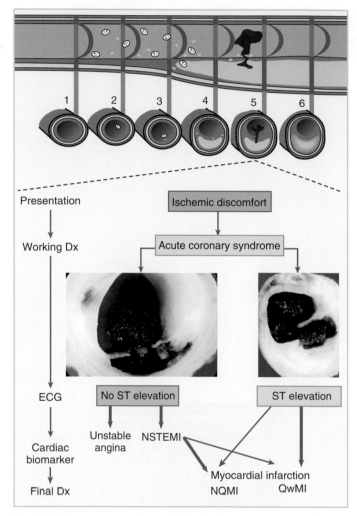

Figure 3-9 Acute coronary syndromes. The longitudinal section of an artery depicts the "timeline" of atherogenesis from (1) a normal artery, to (2) lesion initiation and accumulation of extracellular lipid in the intima, to (3) the evolution to the fibrofatty stage, to (4) lesion progression with procoagulant expression and weakening of the fibrous cap. An acute coronary syndrome develops when the vulnerable or high-risk plaque undergoes disruption of the fibrous cap (5); disruption of the plaque is the stimulus for thrombogenesis. Thrombus resorption may be followed by collagen accumulation and smooth muscle cell growth (6). *CK-MB*, MB isoenzyme of creatine kinase; *Dx*, diagnosis; *NQMI*, non–Q-wave myocardial infarction; *QwMI*, Q-wave myocardial infarction.   (Top portion: Modified from Libby P: Current concepts of the pathogenesis of the acute coronary syndromes, *Circulation* 104(3):365-72, 2001. Photos: From Davies MJ: The pathophysiology of acute coronary syndromes, *Hart* 83(3):361-6, 2000. IN Libby P, Bonow RO, Mann DL, et al: Braunwald's heart disease: A textbook of cardiovascular medicine, ed 8, Philadelphia, 2008, Saunders.)

Complications with STEMI and Non-STEMI

When epicardial coronary arterial occlusion occurs, the area of the myocardium it supplies loses its capability to perform contractile work (see Fig. 3-9). According to Antman and Morrow[192], a sequence of four abnormal contraction patterns then take place in these areas of the myocardium: (1) dyssynchrony—uncoordinated contraction with adjacent segments; (2) hypokinesis—reduction in the strength of contraction; (3) akinesis—no contraction; and (4) dyskinesis—abnormal movement during contraction.[124,193,194] Hyperkinesis, or overactivity of the noninfarcted areas, is thought to be due to increased sympathetic nervous system activity and the Frank–Starling mechanism. If more than 15% of the left ventricle is

Table 3-3	Progression of STEMI
Timeline	**Pathophysiologic Changes**
First hours	Myocardial injury is potentially reversible for about the first 20 min after onset
	Progressive loss of viable tissue from 20 min up to 6–12 hrs post onset
	Zones of necrosis identified as early as 2–3 hrs post-MI
First days	Affected myocardium is pale and swollen
	18–36 hrs post-MI erythrocytes are trapped
	48 hrs post-MI neutrophils infiltrate
First weeks	8–10 days post-MI thickness of infracted cardiac wall ↓
	Mononuclear cells remove necrotic muscle
	From 3 wks to 3–4 mons infracted area converts to shrunken thin firm scar

involved, stroke volume may decline with a subsequent elevation in LVEDP and volume. A lower stroke volume leads to a lower aortic pressure and subsequently a reduction in coronary perfusion pressure. Ultimately, this may intensify myocardial ischemia and thereby initiate a vicious circle. When greater than 25% of the left ventricle is involved, signs and symptoms of heart failure are seen. Death is often associated in individuals who have over 40% involvement of the left ventricle myocardium.[124]

As healing ensues, improvement in contractility takes place. An increase in end-diastolic volume and decrease in diastolic pressure toward normal levels also occurs. The size of the infarct is associated with the degree of systolic and diastolic abnormality seen. Regardless of the amount of time since the infarct happened, individuals with 20% to 25% abnormality of left ventricular wall motion will most likely exhibit signs of left ventricular failure, and as a result will have a poor prognosis for long-term survival.[124]

Other common complications that occur with STEMIs include persistent angina and arrhythmias due to persistent ischemia possibly in other coronary arteries. Table 3-4 has a full list of complications that may occur in other organs with STEMI. Knowing the complications the individual might have or has demonstrated as a result of the STEMI will affect hospital course and prognosis. Criteria for a complicated post-MI hospital course was defined by McNeer and coworkers and includes the following (complications should have occurred within first 24 to 48 hours):[195]

- Ventricular tachycardia and fibrillation
- Atrial flutter or fibrillation
- Second- or third-degree atrioventricular (AV) block
- Persistent sinus tachycardia (above 100 beats per minute)
- Persistent systolic hypotension (below 90 mm Hg)
- Pulmonary edema
- Cardiogenic shock
- Persistent angina or extension of infarction

Patients who were characterized as "uncomplicated" had significantly lower morbidity and mortality rates following

Table 3-4 Postmyocardial infarction complications

System/Hormones	Complications
Pulmonary	Problems with gas exchange, ventilation, and perfusion Interstitial edema/pulmonary edema Hypoxemia, ↓ vital capacity
Circulation	↓ Affinity of hemoglobin for O_2 Platelets: hyperaggregable, ↑ aggregation, release vasoactive substances
Endocrine	Impaired glucose tolerance Hyperglycemia/insulin resistance Excessive secretion of catecholamines
Renin-angiotensin-aldosterone (RAS) system	Activation of RAS with ↑ angiotensin II production May get vasoconstriction, impaired fibrinolysis, ↑ Na retention
Natriuretic peptides	Released early, peak at 16 hrs Elevated levels 6 hrs after onset of symptoms have ↑ in mortality
Adrenal cortex	Rise in cortisol (correlates with infarct size and mortality) Rise in aldosterone, ketosteroids, and hydroxycorticosteroids
Renal	Prerenal azotemia and acute renal failure can occur as a result of ↓ CO

Data from Libby P, Bonow RO, Mann DL, et al: *Braunwald's Heart Disease: A Textbook of Cardiovascular Medicine*, ed 8, Philadelphia, 2007, Saunders.

BOX 3-4 **Secondary prevention methods to reduce the risk factors of CHD and CVD**

- Maintaining a normal blood pressure
- Smoking cessation
- Maintaining normal total cholesterol, lowering LDLs and raising HDLs
- Maintaining normal blood glucose levels and glycosylated hemoglobin (Hb A_{1c})
- Maintaining normal BMI and weight
- Eating a healthy diet
- Performing 150 min/wk of moderate or 75 min/wk vigorous intense exercise
- Reducing stress, anger, and hostility

their initial cardiac events. A prolonged or complicated hospital course affected an individual's activity progression due to the effects of inactivity or bed rest.

Ventricular Remodeling

With STEMI there is a change in shape, size, and thickness of the myocardium as a result of both infarcted and noninfarcted areas. This is called *ventricular remodeling* and includes areas of ventricular dilation and ventricular hypertrophy. Factors that affect remodeling include:

- Size of infarct
- Ventricular load (increased pressure or increased volume will increase the load)
- Patency of the artery that was infarcted.

When there is an increased infarction size, an increased ventricular load, or poor blood supply to the area infarcted, there will be decreased remodeling, possibly increased infarction expansion, and higher risk of complications and increased mortality. With a decrease in infarction size, decreased ventricular load, or increase in blood supply to the infarcted area, there will be an increase in scar formation and improved remodeling.[124]

Prognosis

An individual's prognosis post-MI is related to the complications, infarction size, presence of disease in other coronary arteries, and, most importantly, left ventricular function.[196] Therefore although mortality rates have continued to decrease over the years, monitoring an individual post-MI is extremely important, especially in individuals with complicated post-MI.

Natural History of Coronary Disease

Although many population and longitudinal studies have been carried out that document the relative importance of single factors or combinations of risk factors, still little is known about the natural history of CHD as it applies to an individual patient.[197,198] Knowledge of risk factors has allowed the establishment of a model from which relative risk can be approximated, but such tools decrease in value for those who are at either end of the normal distribution of the population. The only "guarantee" that can be offered to the patient with known CHD is that if the factors that caused the disease to be present in the first place remain unchanged, it will progress.

There is some evidence that the progression of atherosclerotic CHD is not inevitable and, in fact, that it is reversible.[19,199–201] The safety and effectiveness of the use of aspirin for individuals with ischemic heart disease has been reported in more than 50 randomized trials. The range recommended for the prevention of a secondary event, based on strong clinical evidence, is 75 to 325 mg per day.[202,203] Other guidelines recommend prescribing only 75 to 100 mg per day because the evidence for higher doses providing extra protection against MI is lacking and higher doses may cause more gastrointestinal bleeding. In addition, the strict control of diabetes appears to decrease atherosclerotic changes in endothelial and intimal elastin, contributing to beneficial decreases in vessel wall compliance.

Since the Cholesterol Lowering in Atherosclerosis Study,[204,205] the importance of treating patients pharmacologically to lower cholesterol levels and lessen the risk of developing atherosclerosis is well accepted. There is also clear evidence that aggressive lifestyle modification can elicit significant results without the use of medication (Box 3-4).[1,201] Perhaps physical therapists should seize the opportunity to incorporate secondary prevention measures for CVD into their clinical practices. Chapter 18 provides a full discussion of secondary prevention as an intervention. The establishment of secondary prevention clinics in England resulted in reduced hospital admissions for participants.[206]

Hypertension

Hypertension (HTN) is diagnosed when DBP equals or exceeds 90 mm Hg or when SBP is consistently higher than 140 mm Hg, with values of 130 to 139/85 to 89 mm Hg being considered high normal (prehypertension), as shown in Table 3-5.[207] Labile HTN refers to blood pressure that fluctuates between hypertensive and normal values; however, this variability in blood pressure is thought by some to be much more normal than previously thought.[208] Usually, individuals with HTN have elevated levels of both systolic and diastolic blood pressures; however, isolated systolic hypertension (ISH), which occurs when SBP exceeds 140 mm Hg but DBP remains within the normal range, becomes increasingly more common in the elderly.[209,210] Approximately 90% to 95% of individuals with HTN have no discernible cause for their disease and are said to have primary or essential HTN. The remainder have secondary HTN resulting from another identifiable medical problem, such as renovascular or endocrine disease.

Despite much research, the etiology of essential HTN continues to be unknown. Both genetic and environmental factors, such as dietary sodium excess, stress, obesity, and alcohol consumption, have been implicated. Regardless of the underlying cause(s), the result is a failure of one or more of the control mechanisms that are responsible for lowering blood pressure when it becomes elevated.

The major determinants of arterial blood pressure are cardiac output and total peripheral resistance. If either one or both of these factors becomes elevated, blood pressure will rise. However, both cardiac output and total peripheral resistance are determined by a number of other factors (Fig. 3-10). Cardiac output is the product of heart rate and stroke volume; yet, each of those factors has several determinants, as described in Chapter 2. Similarly, total peripheral resistance (TPR) is affected by several variables, including the caliber of the arteriolar bed, the viscosity of the blood, the elasticity of the arterial walls, and sympathetic influence and activity.

Consequently, there are many physiologic pathways where abnormal function can result in high blood pressure, and many of these share a number of common features, as shown in Fig. 3-10. Furthermore, it is probable that the mechanisms that are responsible for initiating HTN differ from those that serve to maintain it. For example, there is evidence that many individuals with labile or early mild HTN have increased cardiac output, probably related to enhanced activity of the sympathetic nervous system and apparently normal peripheral resistance.[211,212] However, later when HTN becomes established, the classic findings of elevated TPR and normal or decreased cardiac output are found.[212]

Category		Systolic (mm Hg)	Diastolic (mm Hg)
Normal		<120	<80
High normal/prehypertension		120–139	80–89
Hypertension	Stage 1	140–159	90–99
	Stage 2	>159	>99

Table 3-5 Blood pressure levels for adults*

*These values are for adults ages 18 years and older who are not taking antihypertensive medications and are not acutely ill.
From Rosendorff C, Black HR, Cannon CP, et al: Treatment of hypertension in the prevention and management of ischemic heart disease: a scientific statement from the American Heart Association Council for High Blood Pressure Research and the Councils on Clinical Cardiology and Epidemiology and Prevention [published correction appears in *Circulation* 116(5):e121, 2007]. *Circulation* 115(21):2762, 2007.

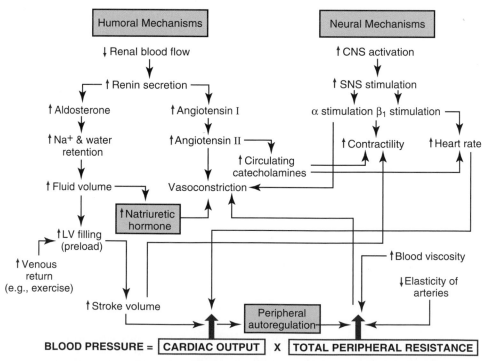

Figure 3-10 Factors contributing to elevated blood pressure. Because blood pressure is a product of cardiac output and peripheral resistance, any influence that increases either of these factors results in a rise in blood pressure. The enclosed boxes identify some of the proposed mechanisms involved in the pathogenesis of essential hypertension. Note the number of interrelationships among the different mechanisms. *CNS*, Central nervous system; *LV*, left ventricle; *SNS*, sympathetic nervous system; ↑, increased; ↓, decreased.

The consequences of HTN are directly related to the level of blood pressure, even within the accepted normal range. Actuarial data reveal that persons with diastolic blood pressures of greater than 88 to 92 mm Hg have a 32% to 36% higher mortality rate over 20 years of follow-up than those with diastolic pressures less than 80 mm Hg.[213] Higher SBP levels at any given level of DBP also are associated with an increased morbidity rate in both men and women.[210,214–216] The most common complications of HTN include atherosclerotic heart disease (AHSD), congestive heart failure, cerebrovascular accidents, renal failure, dissecting aneurysm, peripheral vascular disease, and retinopathy (Fig. 3-11).

Hypertensive Heart Disease

Regardless of its etiology and pathophysiologic mechanisms, HTN produces a pressure overload on the left ventricle, which is compensated for by left ventricular hypertrophy (LVH).[217] Initially, normal systolic left ventricle function is maintained by the hypertrophied left ventricle. However, diastolic dysfunction with impairment of left ventricle relaxation develops early in the course of essential HTN (Box 3-5).[218–221,222] The combination of LVH and diastolic dysfunction leads to reduced left ventricle compliance (i.e., a stiffer left ventricle), which creates a greater load on the left atrium and resultant left atrial enlargement. In addition, LVH alters the equilibrium between the oxygen supply and demand of the myocardium. Coronary reserve is reduced in patients with HTN and LVH, even in the absence of any coronary artery stenosis.[219,223,224] Thus

there is a predisposition toward myocardial ischemia, atrial fibrillation, and ventricular dysrhythmias. Superimposed is the role of HTN as a major risk factor for ASHD, as previously discussed. This interaction makes it difficult to differentiate between the ischemic effects of ASHD and hypertensive heart disease.

If adequate left ventricle filling volume is not achieved, either because of reduced filling times associated with higher heart rates or arrhythmias in which active atrial contraction is missing (e.g., atrial fibrillation, nodal rhythm, frequent premature ventricular beats), stroke volume will diminish. Thus symptoms of inadequate cardiac output, such as lightheadedness or dizziness, dyspnea, and impaired exercise tolerance, can result from diastolic dysfunction rather than impaired systolic function.[225,226] However, as HTN becomes more severe or prolonged, impairment of systolic function may also develop, appearing as subnormal left ventricle functional reserve initially during exercise and later at rest.[227–230]

Although normal cardiac output may be maintained for some time at the expense of pulmonary congestion, the ultimate consequence of progressive LVH is the development of left ventricular failure, as shown in Fig. 3-12. A number of factors, such as further elevation of blood pressure, increased

BOX 3-5 Systolic vs. diastolic dysfunction

Systolic Dysfunction	Diastolic Dysfunction
An impairment in ventricular contraction, resulting in decrease in stroke volume and decrease in ejection fraction (<40%). An increase in end systolic volume will also occur. Now called heart failure with reduced ejection fraction or HFREF.	Changes in ventricular diastolic properties that lead to an impairment in ventricular filling (reduction in ventricular compliance) and an impairment in ventricular relaxation. A consequence of diastolic dysfunction is the rise in end diastolic pressure. Now called heart failure with preserved ejection fraction or HFPEF.

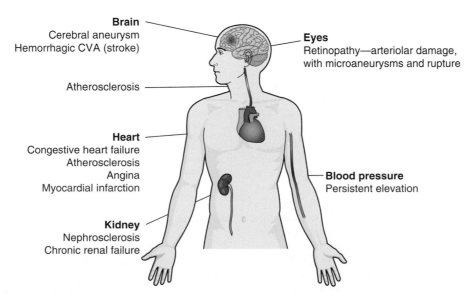

Brain
Cerebral aneurysm
Hemorrhagic CVA (stroke)

Eyes
Retinopathy—arteriolar damage, with microaneurysms and rupture

Atherosclerosis

Heart
Congestive heart failure
Atherosclerosis
Angina
Myocardial infarction

Blood pressure
Persistent elevation

Kidney
Nephrosclerosis
Chronic renal failure

Figure 3-11 Effects of uncontrolled hypertension.

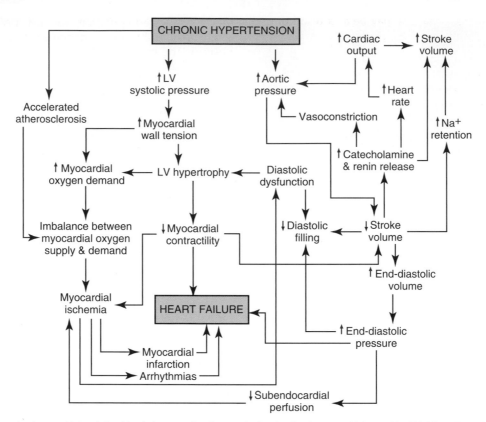

Figure 3-12 Some of the mechanisms and interrelationships in hypertension that may lead to the development of left ventricle (LV) failure. Repeating cycles tend to aggravate the problem. ↑, Increased; ↓, decreased.

venous return, or impaired contractile function, may precipitate decompensation and overt left ventricle failure.

Treatment of Hypertension

The goals of antihypertensive therapy are to normalize BP both at rest and during exertion and to reverse LVH and the myocardial dysfunction it creates.[1,231-234] Pharmacologic therapy is the most commonly prescribed intervention in the management of HTN. However, the latest medical guidelines recommend beginning with lifestyle modifications in most patients diagnosed with HTN (Table 3-6).[207] The most effective modifications have proved to be weight reduction, sodium restriction, moderation of alcohol intake, and regular aerobic exercise.[235,236] Although these interventions may not eliminate the need for antihypertensive medications in most patients, they often permit a lower dosage of medications to be used, thus reducing the potential for adverse side effects. In addition, because HTN tends to cluster with other coronary risk factors, such as dyslipidemia, insulin resistance, glucose intolerance, and obesity,[210] some of the interventions, such as aerobic exercise and weight reduction, by virtue of their effect on more than one factor, may significantly reduce the risk of CVD and death.

The medications used to treat HTN fall into the following major categories: diuretics, β-adrenergic blockers, α-adrenergic blockers, vasodilators, centrally acting adrenergic antagonists, calcium-channel blockers, angiotensin II receptor blockers, and angiotensin-converting enzyme (ACE) inhibitors.[237-241] Many of these drugs have additional cardiovascular effects and side effects and may be used to treat other clinical problems. Chapter 14 has more complete information on these drugs.

Table 3-6 Treatment guidelines for hypertension		
Category	**Blood Pressure** Range	Treatment
Prehypertension	120–139 systolic 80–89 diastolic	Lifestyle modification
Stage 1 hypertension	140–159 systolic 90–99 diastolic	Thiazide diuretics May consider angiotensin-converting enzyme (ACE) inhibitor, angiotensin II receptor blockers, β Blocker, calcium-channel blocker
Stage 2 hypertension	>159 systolic >99 diastolic	Two-drug combination Thiazide and ACE or other

Modified from Rosendorff C, Black HR, Cannon CP, et al: Treatment of hypertension in the prevention and management of ischemic heart disease: a scientific statement from the American Heart Association Council for High Blood Pressure Research and the Councils on Clinical Cardiology and Epidemiology and Prevention [published correction appears in *Circulation* 116(5):e121, 2007], *Circulation* 115(21):2762, 2007.

Hypertension and Exercise

Research involving hypertensive individuals has revealed that exercise capacity is reduced by 15% to 30%, even in those who are asymptomatic, compared with age- and fitness-matched control subjects.[228,242,243] Stroke volume increases subnormally and peak heart rate is lower; therefore cardiac output is decreased. There is some evidence that these changes may be as a result of diastolic dysfunction and impaired coronary flow reserve.[223,224,228] In addition, exercise time and anaerobic threshold are reduced.

Treatment of HTN with medications may modify the physiologic responses to exercise. Antihypertensive medications lower resting blood pressure, but many do not maintain the same degree of effectiveness during exertion, especially with isometric activities.[227,244–246] Thus patients on antihypertensive medications may have acceptable blood pressure levels at rest but display exaggerated responses to exercise. Furthermore, some of the drugs have side effects that are affected by or have an effect upon exercise. Of particular concern is the hypokalemia that can be induced by diuretic therapy using the thiazides and loop diuretics. When combined with the systemic demands of exercise, hypokalemia can precipitate dangerous arrhythmias, skeletal muscle fatigue and cramps, weakness, and occasionally other problems. The potassium-sparing diuretics and β blockers are associated with a greater risk of hyperkalemia, which can also cause arrhythmias.

A great deal of research has been directed at assessing the efficacy of exercise training for the treatment of HTN. Although the data are not consistent, the general consensus is that reductions of up to 10 mm Hg in both systolic and diastolic blood pressure can be achieved through exercise training in the hypertensive population. These reductions are significant enough to allow some patients to avoid or discontinue drug treatment and many others to reduce their drug dosages.[244,247–251] In addition, exercise training has been demonstrated to cause a significant regression of LVH.[252]

Clinical tip

The problem with exercise training as a treatment for HTN is the high percentage of dropouts from exercise programs or noncompliance. The effects of exercise training on blood pressure are maintained only as long as the individual remains compliant with the exercise program.

Implications for Physical Therapy Intervention

One in three adults in the United States has HTN. Approximately one-fourth of individuals with HTN are unaware that they have it.[207] Therefore the percentage of patients referred to physical therapy who may have recognized or unrecognized HTN is very high. Patients with any of the following diagnoses are particularly likely to have HTN: stroke, diabetes, CAD, aortic aneurysm, PAD, obesity, renal failure, and alcoholism. In addition, patients with chronic pain syndromes and those in high-stress occupations, such as air traffic controllers, firefighters, and middle-level and upper-level managers, may be at higher risk for HTN.

With the growing trend toward independent practice, physical therapy may represent the mode of entry into the medical care system for a number of adults. This fact, combined with the prevalence of HTN, supports the need for inclusion of blood pressure monitoring during the physical therapy evaluation and treatment of all adults older than age 35 years. In addition to the valuable information this might provide for both the client and the physician, the positive professional image created could improve acceptance by the medical community of the physical therapy position as an independent health care provider. Furthermore, when a client with diagnosed HTN is seen for physical therapy, the clinician should question the client about prescribed treatments, determine the level of compliance, and reinforce the importance of strict adherence. If the client complains of unpleasant side effects of a particular medication, the client should be encouraged to discuss the side effects with the physician so that a different medication can be prescribed. With so many antihypertensive agents available, most patients can receive comfortable and effective treatment.

Because blood pressure values vary considerably during the day, it is beneficial to include monitoring during two to three different treatment sessions. Also, inasmuch as blood pressure can be normal or borderline at rest but become excessively elevated during exertion, it is important to monitor blood pressure during exercise as well as at rest.

Clinical tip

Proper technique for monitoring of blood pressure is important. Proper cuff size is essential to accuracy: A cuff that is too small will produce a reading that is falsely elevated, and one that is too large will yield a reading that is erroneously low. The arm should be relaxed and supported at the level of the heart. If the arm is lower than the heart or if the arm muscles are not relaxed, the blood pressure readings, both systolic and diastolic, will be erroneously high.

If resting BP is uncontrolled and severe (SBP ≥180 mm Hg and DBP ≥110 mm Hg), patients must have medical clearance and prescribed medication for HTN before advising them on the appropriate exercise regimen. Furthermore, any evidence of target organ damage secondary to HTN, such as retinopathy, renal disease, or LVH, necessitates that blood pressure be controlled both at rest and during exercise before physical therapy intervention. If the resting blood pressure before exercise testing is excessively high (SBP >200 mm Hg or DBP >110 mm Hg), physician clearance must be obtained. Exercise testing should be terminated if blood pressure becomes excessively high (SBP >250 mm Hg or DBP >115 mm Hg).[237] The risk of myocardial ischemia during exercise is enhanced in individuals with HTN, especially those with evidence of LVH, and angina may occur. Furthermore, if left ventricle function is impaired, LV end-diastolic volume and pressure, and therefore intrapulmonary pressures, will rise during exercise, resulting in shortness of breath (Box 3-6).

Clinical tip

Orthostatic hypotension is defined as a systolic pressure drop of more than 20 mm Hg or a diastolic drop of more than 10 mm Hg when assuming an upright position, which often renders the individual symptomatic (dizzy, lightheaded, or cognitive changes). It is not the same as a hypotensive blood pressure response to activity.

BOX 3-6 Guidelines for exercise in individuals with hypertension

- Exercise testing
  - If resting BP >200 mm Hg systolic, >100 mm Hg diastolic: obtain physician clearance
  - Discontinue exercise if >250 mm Hg systolic, >115 mm Hg diastolic
- Exercise training
  - If resting BP is uncontrolled and severe, ≥180 mm Hg systolic, ≥110 mm Hg diastolic: medical clearance needed.
- Consider side effects of medications
- Particularly watch for hypotension with:
  - Change of position
  - Postexercise
  - Long-term standing
  - Warm environments
- Avoid breath hold and Valsalva, especially with resistive exercises
- Low weights, high repetitions in deconditioned/high risk; 60% to 80% one repetition maximum others
- Endurance training at moderate intensity

Data from American College of Sports Medicine: *Guidelines for Exercise Testing and Prescription,* ed 9, Baltimore, Williams & Wilkins, 2014.

Cerebrovascular Disease

Approximately 795,000 individuals experience a new or recurrent cerebrovascular accident (stroke) in the United States each year. It is estimated that 87% of these events result from ischemia and the remaining from a hemorrhage.[1] Stroke is the leading cause of disability and the fourth leading cause of death after CAD, cancer, and chronic lung disease in the United States.[1] Fig. 3-13 shows the actual anatomy of the vascular supply to the brain, demonstrating two internal carotid arteries and two vertebral arteries that come together at the base of the skull to form the circle of Willis. There is a vast amount of individual variability in the circle of Willis, and some individuals do not even have a complete circle.

A cerebrovascular event is defined as a transient ischemic attack (TIA) if symptoms resolve completely within 24 hours, and as a stroke if deficit results after 24 hours. Patients with a TIA have a higher chance of stroke within 90 days, with many of these occurring within the first 2 days.[253] Individuals who have involvement of a carotid artery may experience hemispheric symptoms such as contralateral hemiparesis, contralateral sensory loss, aphasia, and/or a visual field deficit. Individuals who have vertebrobasilar or circle of Willis arterial involvement may have nonhemispheric symptoms, which include ataxia, dysarthria, diplopia, vertigo, syncope, and/or cranial nerve involvement.

Many of the risk factors for stroke are the same as those of cardiac and peripheral vascular disease, yet stroke presents with a variety of different conditions and pathophysiologic processes. The treatment interventions for stroke are too numerous to present in this chapter, but the interventions for stroke prevention as outlined by the American Stroke Association/American Heart Association are presented in the following sections.[1,254–258]

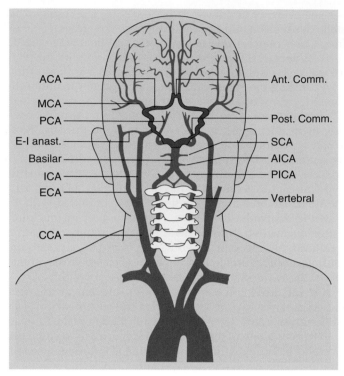

Figure 3-13 Extracranial and intracranial arterial supply to the brain. Vessels forming the circle of Willis are highlighted. *ACA,* Anterior cerebral artery; *AICA,* anterior inferior cerebellar artery; *Ant. Comm.,* anterior communicating artery; *CCA,* common carotid artery; *ECA,* external carotid artery; *E-I anast.,* extracranial–intracranial anastomosis; *ICA,* internal carotid artery; *MCA,* middle cerebral artery; *PCA,* posterior cerebral artery; *PICA,* posterior inferior cerebellar artery; *Post. Comm.,* posterior communicating artery; *SCA,* superior cerebellar artery. (Modified from Lord K: *Surgery of the occlusive cerebrovascular disease,* St. Louis, 1986, Mosby. In Goodman CC: *Pathology: Implications for the Physical Therapist,* ed 3, St. Louis, 2009, Saunders.)

Treatment for Stroke Prevention: Primary and Secondary Prevention

According to the American Stroke Association, primary and secondary prevention includes risk factor reduction and medical management. Medical management includes platelet antiaggregants (primarily aspirin), anticoagulants, lipid-lowering medications, glycemic control, antihypertensive medications, and appropriate interventional methods.[254,255,258] The benefit of the use of aspirin outweighs the risk of bleeding in all individuals who are at moderate to high risk of stroke based upon risk factors, especially women. Women who were defined as having a moderate to high risk of stroke demonstrated a 17% reduction in risk with the inclusion of aspirin in their daily regimen as defined in the Women's Health Study.[259] Aspirin in combination with sustained-release dipyridamole was found to reduce risk of a second stroke by 37%.[255,260] Anticoagulation (warfarin/Coumadin) has been used for years to reduce the risk of a first event of embolism due to conditions like mechanical heart valves, atrial fibrillation, and cardiomyopathy; however, the Warfarin-Aspirin Recurrent Stroke Study (WARSS) found a slight advantage with the use of aspirin compared with warfarin for prevention of a second stroke because of the risk of bleeding complications with warfarin and the need for additional monitoring.[261]

The role of statins is well documented in the management of patients with CAD and is also well documented in the primary prevention of stroke. The HPS was the first large study to document the use of statins for secondary prevention of stroke.[128] Individuals with a prior history of stroke showed a 20% reduction in frequency of major vascular events (MI, stroke, revascularization procedure, or vascular death) with the use of statins.

Finally, the American Stroke Association and the *Seventh Report of the Joint National Committee on Prevention, Detection, Evaluation, and Treatment of High Blood Pressure* (JNC 7) agree that the reduction in blood pressure is far more important than the actual medications used to achieve the reduction and that with a reduction in blood pressure, risk for stroke is reduced between 28% and 35%.[207,254] Therefore a combination of aspirin, lipid-lowering medication, glycemic control, and antihypertensive medication may be the optimal regimen for primary and secondary prevention of stroke in addition to risk factor modification. Chapter 11 discusses other treatments for those with documented carotid disease in greater detail.

Implications for Physical Therapy Intervention

Because of the incidence of atherosclerotic disease in this patient population, patients with a diagnosis of carotid or vertebral disease should have their blood pressure monitored at rest and with all new activities, should be educated about primary or secondary prevention of stroke (medical management as outlined earlier), and should be taught the symptoms of instability (signs of TIAs) and the need for immediate medical treatment should these symptoms appear. The earlier a patient receives emergency medical management for an impending stroke, the lower the risk of permanent brain injury.

Peripheral Arterial Disease

Peripheral arterial disease, or more specifically atherosclerotic occlusive disease (AOD), involves atheromatous plaque obstruction of the large- or medium-size arteries supplying blood to one or more of the extremities (usually lower). Atherosclerotic occlusive disease is a result of the same atherosclerotic process previously described and causes symptoms when the atheroma becomes so enlarged that it interferes with blood flow to the distal tissues, it ruptures and extrudes its contents into the bloodstream or obstructs the arterial lumen, or it encroaches on the media, causing weakness of that layer and aneurysmal dilation of the arterial wall. The hemodynamic significance of the disease depends on the location and number of lesions in an artery, the rapidity with which the atherosclerotic process progresses, and the presence and extent of any collateral arterial system. When blood flow is not adequate to meet the demand of the peripheral tissues (i.e., during activity), the patient may experience symptoms of ischemia, such as intermittent claudication of a lower extremity. As the disease progresses, the patient experiences more severe symptoms, such as rest pain and skin changes. Complete obstruction to flow will cause tissue necrosis and possibly loss of the limb (Fig. 3-14).

Individuals with lower extremity PAD should be assumed to have ASHD, which is the main cause of higher morbidity and mortality rates in these individuals.[262] Studies report up to 60% to 80% of those with PAD have significant coronary atherosclerosis in at least one coronary artery.[263] Individuals with asymptomatic disease appear to have the same increased risk of cardiovascular events and death found in those with symptoms of claudication.[264] Further information on PAD and medical diagnostic testing and interventions can be found in the American College of Cardiology Foundation and American Heart Association's Guidelines for the management of patients with PAD, updated in 2011.[265]

Exercise and Peripheral Arterial Disease

Individuals with PAD are unable to produce the normal increases in peripheral blood flow essential for enhanced oxygen supply to exercising muscles. If the oxygen supply is inadequate to meet the increasing demand of the exercising muscles, ischemia develops and leads to the production of lactic acid. When excessive lactic acid accumulates in the muscle, pain is experienced (this symptom is known as *intermittent claudication*); when it reaches the central circulation, respiration is further stimulated and patients may experience shortness of breath (Table 3-7).

Patients with intermittent claudication have moderate to severe impairment in walking ability that usually comes on with a particular amount of activity and is relieved with rest. Their peak exercise capacity during graded treadmill exercise is severely limited, allowing for only light to very-light activities;[266–268] the energy requirements of many leisure and work-related activities usually exceed their capacity. Metabolic measurements during exercise testing reveal that maximal oxygen consumption and anaerobic threshold are reduced in patients with AOD.[266,268] Yet, even though the anaerobic threshold may be so low that it cannot be detected, evidence of systemic lactic acidosis may be minimal because of the reduced muscle perfusion.

Several studies have documented the efficacy of exercise training in the management of patients with AOD. Increases in both pain-free and maximal walking tolerance on level ground and during constant-load treadmill exercise achieved during exercise testing have been reported.[269–277] A recent Cochrane Review found patients healthy enough to participate in exercise programs can improve the time and distance of walking, with results lasting for approximately 2 years.[278] Studies even have concluded that greater symptomatic relief and functional improvement in patients with mild to moderate claudication not requiring immediate therapeutic interventions is achieved through supervised exercise therapy rather than PTCA.[270,279] Some studies have demonstrated the benefit of exercise for patients with rest pain.[280] Several mechanisms have been postulated to account for these improvements: increased walking efficiency, increased peripheral blood flow through changes in the collateral circulation, reduced blood viscosity, regression of atherosclerotic disease, raising of the pain threshold, and improvements in skeletal muscle metabolism. There is evidence that periods of brief repetitive walking can successfully improve oxygenation in the feet of limbs with more severe arterial obstruction.[281]

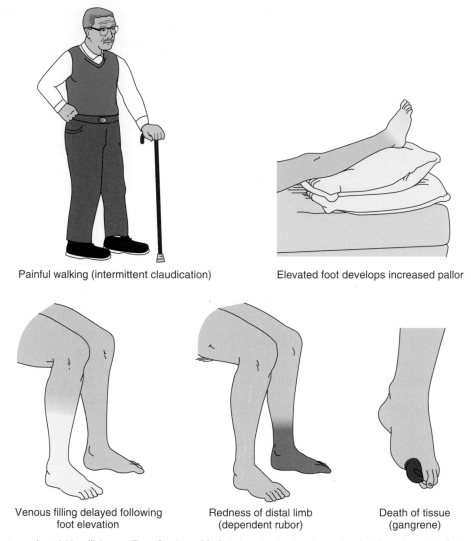

Painful walking (intermittent claudication)

Elevated foot develops increased pallor

Venous filling delayed following foot elevation

Redness of distal limb (dependent rubor)

Death of tissue (gangrene)

Figure 3-14 Signs and symptoms of arterial insufficiency. (From Goodman CC: *Pathology: Implications for the Physical Therapists,* ed 3, St. Louis, 2009, Saunders.)

Table 3-7 Subjective gradation of claudication discomfort	
Grade	**Pain Description**
I	Initial discomfort (established, but minimal)
II	Moderate discomfort but attention can be diverted
III	Intense pain (attention cannot be diverted)
IV	Excruciating and unbearable pain

From American College of Sports Medicine: *Guidelines for Exercise Testing and Prescription*, ed 3, Baltimore, 2009, Williams & Wilkins.

Implications for Physical Therapy Intervention

Because of the high prevalence of ASHD in patients with PAD, all patients should be monitored during physical therapy evaluation and initial treatment, including the monitoring of heart rate and blood pressure. Such monitoring is especially needed when working with patients who have undergone amputation, which implies severe disease. Notably, patients with PAD may exhibit precipitous rises in blood pressure during exercise due to their atherosclerosis and diminished vascular bed.

Physical therapists can also use SBP measurements to predict the severity of PAD by performing an ankle–brachial index (ABI). Systolic blood pressures should be higher in the lower extremities; if the upper extremity SBPs are higher than the lower extremity SBPs, one should suspect PAD. If an ABI (SBP of ankle/SBP of arm) is 0.90 or less, it is considered abnormal (see Chapters 8 and 22). Physical therapists should also look for other signs of PAD in the extremity, including dry, shiny skin; hair loss; thick toenails; muscle atrophy; impaired sensation; and decreased pulses.

Intermittent claudication is considered a classic symptom during activity. Claudication in the calf is associated with stenosis of the femoral and/or popliteal artery, whereas thigh, hip, or buttock claudication is usually caused by aortoiliac arterial disease. However, studies state that less than half of individuals with PAD express any type of leg symptoms, and many others describe other various leg symptoms, whereas only 10% actually report classic claudication.[1,237,282] Still, including a subjective gradation of pain for expressing claudication discomfort, as described in Table 3-8, can be useful during exercise.[237,282] Patients should exercise to levels of maximal tolerable pain—that is,

Table 3-8 Two-level DVT wells score	
Clinical Feature	**Points**
Active cancer (treatment ongoing, within 6 months, or palliative)	1
Paralysis, paresis, or recent plaster immobilization of the lower extremities	1
Recently bedridden for 3 days or more, or major surgery within 12 weeks requiring general or regional anesthesia	1
Localized tenderness along the distribution of the deep venous system	1
Entire leg swollen	1
Calf swelling at least 3 cm larger than asymptomatic side	1
Pitting edema confined to the symptomatic leg	1
Collateral superficial veins (nonvaricose)	1
Previously documented DVT	1
Alternative diagnosis at least as likely as DVT	-2
Clinical probability simplified score	
DVT "likely"	2 points or more
DVT "unlikely"	Fewer than 2 points

BOX 3-7 **Exercise recommendations for individuals with peripheral arterial disease**
Perform exercise in intervals as short as 1 to 5 minutes, alternating with rest periods.
Increase the length of exercise intervals and decrease the length of rest periods.
Most convenient and functional mode is walking.
Non–weight-bearing activities may allow for longer duration and higher intensities, but progressive walking should be encouraged.
Longer warm-up time required in colder environments because of peripheral vasoconstriction.
Sensory examination should be performed before providing an exercise prescription because of the possibility of peripheral neuropathy.
Footwear and foot hygiene should be emphasized.

to grade III discomfort—in order to obtain optimal symptomatic benefit over time, possibly through enhanced collateral circulation or increased muscular efficiency.[237,281,283] And, in order to achieve as much benefit as possible, an individual should consider a supervised exercise program. A recent Cochrane Review reported that people in supervised exercise programs improved their distance of walking significantly more (up to 180 meters) than those in unsupervised exercise programs.[284] Box 3-7 provides additional exercise recommendations.

Other Vascular Disorders

Venous Disease

Venous disease comprises the major categories of venous problems, including venous insufficiency, venous stasis ulcers, and venous thromboembolism (VTE). Prevalence of venous insufficiency varies depending on the age and ethnic population studied; however, mild forms have been reported in more than 40% of individuals. In more serious venous disease, it is estimated that 300,000 to 600,000 Americans are affected yearly by VTE, resulting in approximately 60,000 to 100,000 deaths despite advances in medical care.[285,286] Venous stasis ulcers affects half a million people. These venous conditions are thought to be underdiagnosed and often preventable.

Venous Insufficiency

Approximately 65% to 70% of the blood is housed in the veins at one time, thus the term *capacitance vessels* for veins. Veins have the job of being the body's "clean-up crew," carrying carbon dioxide and other cellular waste back to the heart and liver. The walls of veins are thinner and less rigid with a larger lumen diameter than arteries. They are equipped with one-way valves that, when open, function to move blood back toward the heart and liver and, when closed, prevent blood from flowing backward. If damage occurs to the valves, the blood pools and flows backward, causing the veins to become enlarged and weak. Tension can then build up, leading to venous HTN, obstruction of venous flow, and overall failure of the pump.

Muscle action is also essential to help the valves move venous blood toward the heart. When inadequate muscle action, incompetent venous valves, or venous obstruction occurs, venous insufficiency can result.

Risk factors for venous insufficiency include, but are not limited to, advancing age, genetics, obesity, prolonged standing, sedentary lifestyle, smoking, and female hormones. Symptoms may include complaints of dull ache, heaviness, swelling, itching, tingling, or cramping in the extremity (typically in the leg).

Types of venous insufficiency range from mild forms of spider veins (telangiectasias) and varicose veins to chronic venous insufficiency. Spider veins are dilated veins in the dermal layer of the skin (Fig. 3-15). Varicose veins are superficial subcutaneous veins appearing knotted, swollen, and/or twisted.

Chronic venous insufficiency leads to skin changes caused by a "chronic release of inflammatory mediators,"[287] swelling, and wounds. Dermatitis and hemosiderin staining are typically visible skin changes caused by venous insufficiency. Hemosiderin staining is thought to happen when red blood cells "leak" into the tissues secondary to venous HTN. These red blood cells later break down, leaving behind a rusty brown skin color due to iron contained in the blood (Fig. 3-16). Venous wounds can also develop. These wounds are typically described as beefy red in color, with moderate to severe exudate and irregular borders, and are usually seen in the lower one-third of the leg.

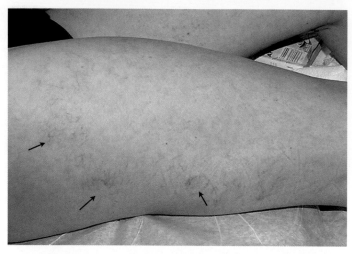

Figure 3-15 Spider veins. (From Travers R, Hsu J: Skin in the spotlight: Cosmetic treatments, *Sexuality, Reproduction and Menopause* Volume 4, Issue 2, October 2006, Pages 80–85.)

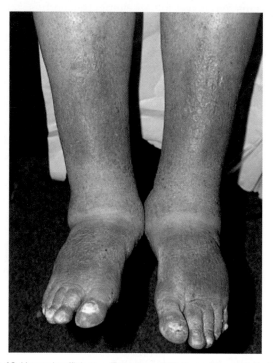

Figure 3-16 Venous insufficiency. (From James WD, Berger TG, and Elston DM: Andrews' Diseases of the Skin: *Clinical Dermatology*, ed 10, St. Louis, 2006, Elsevier.)

Venous Thromboembolic Disease

Venous thromboembolism includes both deep venous thrombosis (DVT) and pulmonary embolism (PE). Deep vein thrombosis usually refers to the development of a clot in a deep vein of the lower extremity or pelvis, with a smaller percentage occurring in the arm (Fig. 3-17). A PE is a clot that reaches the lungs. In both cases, the thrombosis obstructs blood flow in the affected area.[286]

Major risk factors for the development of VTE are thought to arise from one or more of three main categories described as *Virchow's triad*; hypercoagulability, venous stasis, and endothelial injury.[288] A hypercoagulable state encompasses any situation where there is an increased propensity of developing blood clots, such as with cancer, hormonal replacement, and inherited clotting disorders such as factor V Leiden mutation.[289] Venous stasis is a condition in which blood flow is slowed or congested such as what happens with prolonged bed rest, travel, and paralysis. Endothelial injury, or injury to the inner lining of the vein, can occur from surgery, trauma, or insertion of a central venous catheter.

Pain, ipsilateral swelling, a palpable cord, and redness are signs of a DVT. The Wells Decision Tool can assist the therapist in assessing the probability of a DVT (see Chapters 8 and 16). Medical testing, including D dimer, a Doppler assessment, compression ultrasonography, or MRI, can be used to confirm the presence of lower extremity or upper extremity DVT.

Signs and symptoms of a PE are shortness of breath, decreased SpO$_2$, pleuritic chest pain, cough, and tachycardia. However, one systematic review found one-third of patients with a DVT to have had an asymptomatic, or "silent," PE.[290] Therefore it is crucial to assess for these warning signs, especially when patients have a history of a proximal DVT (above the knee), previous PE, or other significant risk factors. Medical testing consisting of ventilation/perfusion scan or computed tomography (CT) pulmonary angiogram can be used for medical diagnosis of a PE.

Implications for Physical Therapy

Through effective screening, examination, and interventions, physical therapists can be instrumental in prevention and further development of complications from venous disease experienced in patients. When obtaining the patient's history, the risk factors and signs/symptoms for venous

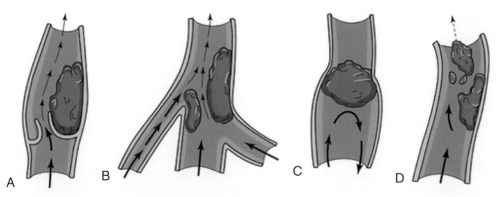

Figure 3-17 Development of deep venous thrombosis with arrows indicating direction of blood flow. **A,** Thrombus in valve pocket of a deep vein with blood flowing beside thrombus. **B,** Thrombi tend to form at bifurcations of deep veins with some slowing of blood flow. **C,** Complete occlusion of vein by thrombus forcing backflow of blood. **D,** Embolus that has broken off from a thrombus and is floating in bloodstream could migrate to lungs and cause pulmonary embolism. (From Monahan FD, Sands JK, Neighbors M: *Phipps' Medical-Surgical Nursing*, ed 8, St. Louis, 2007, Mosby.)

insufficiency and VTE are important to consider (utilization of the Wells Prediction Model for VTE is important and found in Chapters 8 and 16; see Table 3-8).[291] When examining the lower extremity for a DVT, the therapist must distinguish a DVT from other medical problems that can mimic a DVT, such as a baker's cyst or muscle injury. And throughout the session, it is essential to assess vital signs as well as for signs and symptoms of a PE.

Interventions for venous insufficiency comprise exercise, elevation of the extremity, avoiding long periods of sitting or standing, compression, and aggressive wound management, along with education to prevent further progression of the disorder.

Mechanical compression, early mobility, and anticoagulation are vital for the prevention and further progression of venous thromboembolic disease.[292] Anticoagulation, such as heparin, low-molecular-weight heparin, or a new oral anticoagulant is a key treatment for individuals at risk for or diagnosed with a DVT. These medications work by blocking proteins needed for clot formation, which in turn slows and/or prevents this process. The clot gradually dissolves and is reabsorbed by the body as healing occurs. This process can take weeks to months (see Chapter 14 for further information about anticoagulation used in VTE).[293] It has been found that anticoagulation therapy is best continued for 3 to 6 months to avoid recurrence or progression of VTE. In these individuals, especially if balance is impaired, fall prevention education is vital for those taking anticoagulation medication because of an increased risk of complications related to bleeding.[292]

Research supports early ambulation as soon as possible.[294] Patients who have a documented lower extremity DVT and have reached therapeutic levels of the prescribed anticoagulant should be mobilized out of bed and encouraged to ambulate to prevent venous stasis, as well as deconditioning, a lengthened hospital stay, and other adverse effects of bed rest.[292] A common concern of mobilizing a patient with a lower extremity DVT is that the clot will dislodge and embolize to the lungs, causing a potentially fatal PE. However, mobilization has been shown to lead to no greater risk of PE than bed rest for those with a diagnosed DVT who have been treated with anticoagulants.[294]

In the metaanalysis by Aissaoui in 2009, the authors concluded there is no increased risk of PE/DVT with early ambulation after anticoagulation.[294] Similar findings were reported in a systematic review reporting strong prospective evidence that early walking did not increase the risk of PE in the days after diagnosis of DVT and initiation of anticoagulation therapy.[295] Early mobilization of lower extremity DVT patients has also demonstrated a potentially reduced risk of extension of proximal DVT and reduced long-term symptoms of postthrombotic syndrome (PTS).[295]

Ambulation postdocumented lower extremity DVT after initiation of an anticoagulant has been reported to be safe as soon as an individual has reached the therapeutic dosing of the anticoagulant. Different anticoagulants have different times to therapeutic levels, but in general, heparin will be prescribed for individuals with renal dysfunction and a creatinine clearance of less than 30 mL/min, and it achieves a therapeutic level within 12 to 24 hours; low-molecular-weight heparins usually achieve therapeutic levels within 3 to 5 hours, and the new oral anticoagulants achieve therapeutic levels within 2 to 3 hours.[296–301] The time frames allow earlier mobility based upon the time to achieve a level in the blood to dissolve any larger clots floating in the blood or that break off from the original clot that would cause problem with the lungs.[296–301] These time frames are based upon the documented therapeutic levels and give some guidance for mobility, yet all physical therapists should still be watching for signs/symptoms of PE in all patients with a documented lower extremity DVT. Physical therapists should continue to assess for DVT/PE in these individuals since they will often be prescribed anticoagulant medications for 3 to 6 months or more. Individuals with a proximal lower extremity DVT or a PE may require different anticoagulation or time before mobilization, as these are more unstable clots.

Mechanical compression, in addition, is important to utilize for prevention of DVT as well as postthrombotic syndrome.[292,301,302] A Cochrane Systematic Review showed evidence that graduated compression stockings worn by hospitalized surgical patients were effective in reducing the risk of DVT.[302] Another systematic review found compression stockings decreased the incidence of DVT in airline passengers.[303]

Postthrombotic syndrome is the most frequent complication of lower extremity DVT and develops in up to 50% of these patients even when appropriate anticoagulant therapy is used; therefore physical therapists should evaluate all patients who have a diagnosis of lower extremity DVT for PTS.[304–306] A clot remaining in the vein of the LE can obstruct blood flow, leading to venous hypertension. Additionally, damage to the vein itself occurs and leads to inflammation and tissue damage within the vein, which may compromise return of blood flow. As a result, PTS symptoms may develop, including chronic, aching pain; edema; limb heaviness; and leg ulcers.[304]

In summary, anticoagulation, ambulation, and even mechanical compression have been shown to decrease the incidence of progression of DVT, as well as development of PTS.

Renal Artery Disease

Renal artery stenosis (RAS) results from atherosclerosis of the renal artery and is associated with increased cardiovascular events and mortality. The prevalence of RAS is approximately 20% to 30% in the high-risk population.[307] Renal artery stenosis is a progressive disease that is associated with loss of renal mass, progressing to renal insufficiency, refractory HTN, and renal failure. Approximately 20% of individuals older than 50 years of age who begin renal dialysis have atherosclerotic RAS as the cause of their renal failure. Renal dialysis patients with RAS have a 56% 2-year survival rate, 18% 5-year survival, and 5% 10-year survival.[308] Clearly, the early diagnosis of RAS and the prevention of end-stage renal disease (ESRD) are important goals.

Aortic Aneurysm

The aorta is the largest artery in the body and is divided anatomically into the thoracic and abdominal aorta. An aneurysm of the aorta is a pathologic permanent dilation of the aortic wall that is at least 50% greater than the

Table 3-9 Risk factors of aneurysms

Risk Factors	Complications
Smoking (current or past)	Fivefold increase vs. nonsmokers
Age	Most occur in individuals >60 years of age
Gender	5–10× higher incidence in men than in women Women with aneurysm have a higher risk of rupture
Family history	First-degree relative has an increased risk
Hypertension	
Hyperlipidemia	
Atherosclerosis	

Data from Braverman A, Thompson R, Sanchez L: Diseases of the aorta. In Braunwald E, editor: *Heart Disease: A Textbook of Cardiovascular Medicine*, ed 9, Philadelphia, 2012, Saunders.

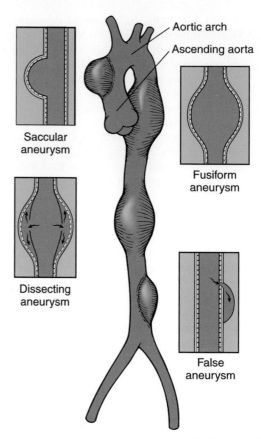

Figure 3-18 Abdominal aortic aneurysm. (From Frazier M: *Essentials of Human Diseases and Conditions*, ed 6, St. Louis, 2016, Saunders.)

expected normal diameter (>3 cm is considered aneurysmal in adults). Aneurysms are typically described in terms of their location, size, morphologic appearance, and origin. An aortic aneurysm is usually uniform in shape, although some form a sac or outpouching of a portion of the aorta (Table 3-9). The large majority of abdominal aortic aneurysms (AAAs) arise below the renal arteries and are known as *infrarenal aneurysms*. Only a small minority, known as *suprarenal aneurysms*, arise between the level of the diaphragm and the renal arteries.[309]

A thrombus may form as a result of stagnate blood flow along the wall of the aneurysmal section. This thrombus has the potential to break off and impede circulation of the distal arteries. However, rupture is the major risk of AAAs and is usually fatal. Rupture into the retroperitoneum is most common. When there is rupture into the peritoneal cavity, uncontrolled hemorrhage and rapid circulatory collapse occur. Because most AAAs expand over time at an average increase of 0.3 to 0.5 cm per year, the risk of rupture tends to increase with time. A sudden increase in enlargement can also predict the possibility of aneurysm rupture, especially for AAAs 5.5 cm or greater in diameter (Fig. 3-18).[309]

Implications for Physical Therapy

Although individuals with AAAs often have no symptoms, the most common signs/symptoms include:

- Pulsating tumor or mass in abdominal area (although often not reliable)
- Bruit heard over swollen area in abdomen
- Abdominal, back, or flank pain
- Leg pain/claudication pain
- Numbness in the lower extremities
- Excessive fatigue, especially with walking
- Poor distal pulses, especially the dorsalis pedis
- Low back pain with elevated pressure that may indicate renal artery aneurysm

During the initial assessment, the therapist should identify risk factors for aneurysm, especially age (>60 years) and

immediate family history (see Table 3-9). According to Braverman et al, moderate activity in individuals with small AAAs has not been shown to influence the risk of rupture; therefore regular exercise should be promoted.[309]

Summary

- Coronary heart disease is the most common disease in the industrialized world.
- The presence of CHD in a given individual is dependent on the presence of any of the following risk factors for the disease and the susceptibility of the individual to those factors:
  - Cigarette smoking
  - Hypertension
  - Elevated cholesterol levels
  - Physical inactivity
  - Diabetes
  - Obesity
  - Poor dietary habits
  - Family history
  - Age
  - Gender
  - Stress
- The risk factors of CAD are the same risk factors of PAD, carotid and vertebral vascular disease, and other vascular diseases. Therefore individuals with any of these diseases should be examined for all other diseases.

- The plaques that obstruct the coronary arteries are a combination of atheroma and thrombus, and they begin to form early in life, probably in the second decade.
- The majority of the risk factors for CAD are modifiable.
- Through control of these risk factors, the progress of CAD can be arrested and in some cases reversed.
- Patients with diabetes have a relatively high 10-year risk for developing CVD.
- Premature or early coronary disease is defined as men older than age 50 years and women older than age 60 years, but the AHA defines family history as significant if either parent (genetic linked parents) had a diagnosis of heart disease (first event of MI, angina, CABG, or PTCA) at an age earlier than 60 years.
- Psychosocial distress is also associated with increased mortality and morbidity rates after MI. In addition, social isolation and depression are associated with a poor prognosis after MI.
- Individuals with elevated CRP and Lp-PLA$_2$ levels might benefit from more aggressive long-term dietary, lifestyle, and coronary risk factor modification than would be the standard of care in a primary prevention population.
- In 40% to 50% of patients with CHD, SCD (death within 1 hour of onset of symptoms) is the initial presenting syndrome.
- The term *acute coronary syndrome* is used to describe patients who present with either unstable angina or AMI, which includes STEMI and non-STEMI.
- A third universal definition of AMI has been adopted to include criteria of a rise or drop of troponin *plus* evidence of symptoms of ischemia, ECG changes (pathologic Q wave, ST-segment changes, and/or new left bundle branch block), or new cardiac muscle damage or wall motion abnormalities seen on imaging.
- If arterial reperfusion of the myocardium occurs within 20 minutes of myocardial ischemia, necrosis can be prevented. Beyond this phase, the extent of damage varies depending on factors such as the total time of coronary artery occlusion, possible collateral blood flow, and myocardial oxygen requirements.
- An individual's prognosis post-MI is related to the complications, infarction size, presence of disease in other coronary arteries, and, most importantly, left ventricle function.
- Standards of physical therapy practice should include the assessment of resting and activity vital signs during an initial examination as part of the systems review.
- Systolic dysfunction refers to an impairment of ventricular contraction, resulting in decrease in stroke volume and decrease in ejection fraction. Diastolic dysfunction refers to changes in ventricular diastolic properties that lead to an impairment in ventricular filling (reduction in ventricular compliance) and an impairment in ventricular relaxation.
- A cerebrovascular event is defined as a TIA if symptoms resolve completely within 24 hours, and as a stroke if deficit results after 24 hours.
- Medical management includes platelet antiaggregants (aspirin), anticoagulants, lipid-lowering medications, glycemic control, antihypertensive medications, and appropriate interventional methods.
- Studies report up to 60% to 80% of those with PAD have significant coronary atherosclerosis in at least one coronary artery.
- Renal artery stenosis results from atherosclerosis of the renal artery and is associated with increased cardiovascular events and mortality.
- An aneurysm of the aorta is a pathologic permanent dilation of the aortic wall that is higher than 50% of the expected normal diameter (>3 cm is considered aneurysmal in adults). Aneurysms are usually described in terms of their location, size, morphologic appearance, and origin.

Case study 3-1

Mr. H is a 38-year-old white male, who, at the age of 30 years, was experiencing angina with low levels of exertion and was found to have severe obstructions of his left anterior descending (LAD), first diagonal (DI), circumflex (CIRC), first obtuse marginal (OMI), and right coronary (RCA) arteries. He underwent five-vessel coronary artery bypass grafting, which relieved his angina. He now has a 2-year history of chronic stable angina, which in the past month has become more frequent, occurring with minimal exertion and occasionally while at rest. Mr. H was admitted to the hospital.

He underwent a repeat cardiac catheterization, which revealed total obstructions of his native proximal LAD, mid-CIRC, and RCA. His venous bypass grafts to his LAD and DI were also 100% occluded, whereas the grafts to his OMI and distal RCA were patent.

He has a 20 pack/year (number of packs per day multiplied by the number of years smoked) history of smoking, which he stopped at the time of his bypass surgery. He has a 12-year history of hypertension, which is controlled by medication. He is 67 inches tall and weighs 270 pounds, which is 50 pounds more than he weighed at the time of his bypass surgery. His current blood lipids are TC = 188 mg/dL, triglycerides = 147 mg/dL, HDL = 27 mg/dL, and CHOL/HDL = 6.96 mg/dL. He had been employed as an accountant, but stated that he had to quit his job because he was experiencing frequent angina during stressful situations at work. He has never engaged in an organized exercise program.

Study Questions
What is this patient's admitting diagnosis?
Why did this patient's angina return less than 5 years after bypass surgery?
Which risk factors did Mr. H modify after his bypass surgery?
Which risk factors did he not modify after his surgery?
What lifestyle changes should this patient make to keep his remaining grafts patent?

Case study 3-2

Mrs. F is a 65-year-old referred for gait training. Medical history includes PAD, hyperlipidemia, and 40 pack/year of smoking. After ambulating 150 feet, she complains of moderate discomfort in her right calf, which quickly subsides during rest.

Study Questions

What is this type of pain called?

What is the level of pain she is describing?

During a visual inspection of the patient's legs, what signs of PAD can be expected?

When the patient arrives the next day, she complains of chest discomfort.

Study Questions

What type of pain is most likely in her case?

What questions should be asked to help differentiate the type of chest discomfort she is experiencing?

What patient signs/symptoms should be closely observed?

What examination procedures can be performed to help determine the urgency of this matter?

References

1. Go A, Mozaffarian D, Roger V, et al.: Heart disease and stroke statistics—2014 update: A report from the American Heart Association Statistics Committee and Stroke Statistics Subcommittee, *Circulation* 129:e28–e292, 2014.

2. Heberden E: William Heberden the elder (1710–1801): aspects of his London practice, *Med Hist Jul* 30(3):303–321, 1986.

3. Enos W, Holmes R, Beyer J: Coronary disease among United States soldiers killed in action in Korea, *JAMA* 152(12):1090–1093, 1953.

4. Strong JP: Landmark perspective: Coronary atherosclerosis in soldiers. A clue to the natural history of atherosclerosis in the young, *JAMA* 256(20):2863–2866, 1986.

5. Kannel WB, Castelli WP, Gordon T, et al.: Serum cholesterol, lipoproteins, and the risk of coronary heart disease. The Framingham study, *Ann Intern Med* 74(1):1–12, 1971.

6. Libby P: The vascular biology of atherosclerosis. In Braunwald E, editor: *Heart Disease: A Textbook of Cardiovascular Medicine*, ed 9, Philadelphia, 2012, Saunders.

7. Reichl D: Lipoproteins of human peripheral lymph, *Eur Heart J* 11(Suppl E):230–236, 1990.

8. Haberland ME, Fless GM, Scanu AM, et al.: Malondialdehyde modification of lipoprotein(a) produces avid uptake by human monocyte-macrophages, *J Biol Chem 25*; 267(6):4143–4151, 1992.

9. Gorlin R: Coronary anatomy, *Major Probl Intern Med* 11:40–58, 1976.

10. Ambrose JA, Tannenbaum MA, Alexopoulos D, et al.: Angiographic progression of coronary artery disease and the development of myocardial infarction, *J Am Coll Cardiol* 12(1):56–62, 1988.

11. Fulton WFM: *Coronary Arteries: Arteriography, Microanatomy, and Pathogenesis of Obliterative Coronary Artery Disease*, Springfield, IL, 1965, Charles C Thomas.

12. Allwork SP: The applied anatomy of the arterial blood supply to the heart in man, *J Anat* 153:1–16, 1987.

13. Schaper W: The physiology of the collateral circulation in the normal and hypoxic myocardium, *Ergeb Physiol* 63:102–145, 1971.

14. Canty J: Coronary blood flow and myocardial ischemia. In Braunwald E, editor: *Heart Disease: A Textbook of Cardiovascular Medicine*, ed 9, Philadelphia, 2012, Saunders.

15. Tracy RE, Newman 3rd WP, Wattigney WA, et al.: Risk factors and atherosclerosis in youth autopsy findings of the Bogalusa Heart Study, *Am J Med Sci* 310(Suppl 1):S37–S41, 1995.

16. Stary HC: Evolution and progression of atherosclerotic lesions in coronary arteries of children and young adults, *Arteriosclerosis* 9(1 Suppl):I19–I32, 1989.

17. Srinivasan SR, Radhakrishnamurthy B, Vijayagopal P, et al.: Proteoglycans, lipoproteins, and atherosclerosis, *Adv Exp Med Biol* 285:373–381, 1991.

18. Hässig A, Wen-Xi L, Stampfli K: The pathogenesis and prevention of atherosclerosis, *Med Hypotheses* 47(5):409–412, 1996.

19. Blankenhorn DH, Kramsch DM: Reversal of atherosis and sclerosis. The two components of atherosclerosis, *Circulation* 79(1):1–7, 1989.

20. Campbell JH, Campbell GR: Cell biology of atherosclerosis, *J Hypertens Suppl* 12(10):S129–S132, 1994.

21. Kinlay S, Ganz P: Role of endothelial dysfunction in coronary artery disease and implications for therapy, *Am J Cardiol* 57:791–804, 1997.

22. Ross R, Glomset JA: The pathogenesis of atherosclerosis (second of two parts), *N Engl J Med* 295:420–425, 1976.

23. Ross R, Glomset JA: The pathogenesis of atherosclerosis (first of two parts), *N Engl J Med* 295:369–377, 1976.

24. DiCorleto PE: Cellular mechanisms of atherogenesis, *Am J Hypertens* 6:314S–318S, 1993.

25. Forstermann U, Mugge A, Alheid U, et al.: Selective attenuation of endothelium-mediated vasodilation in atherosclerotic human coronary arteries, *Circ Res* 62:185–190, 1988.

26. Ludmer PL, Selwyn AP, Shook TL, et al.: Paradoxical vasoconstriction induced by acetylcholine in atherosclerotic coronary arteries, *N Engl J Med* 315:1046–1051, 1986.

27. Marmur JD, Poon M, Rossikhina M, et al.: Induction of PDGF-responsive genes in vascular smooth muscle. Implications for the early response to vessel injury, *Circulation* 86:III53–III60, 1992.

28. Nilsson J, Volk-Jovinge S, Svensson J, et al.: Association between high levels of growth factors in plasma and progression of coronary atherosclerosis, *J Intern Med* 232:397–404, 1992.

29. Grotendorst GR, Chang T, Seppa HE, et al.: Platelet-derived growth factor is a chemoattractant for vascular smooth muscle cells, *J Cell Physiol* 113:261–266, 1982.

30. Krettek A, Fager G, Lindmark H, et al.: Effect of phenotype on the transcription of the genes for platelet-derived growth factor (PDGF) isoforms in human smooth muscle cells, monocyte-derived macrophages, and endothelial cells in vitro, *Arterioscler Thromb Vasc Biol* 17:2897–2903, 1997.

31. Marumo T, Schini-Kerth VB, Fisslthaler B, et al.: Platelet-derived growth factor-stimulated superoxide anion production modulates activation of transcription factor NF-kappa B and expression of monocyte chemoattractant protein 1 in human aortic smooth muscle cells, *Circulation* 96:2361–2367, 1997.

32. Osler W: Second Lumleian lecture on angina pectoris, *Lancet March* 26:839–844, 1910.

33. Prinzmetal M, Ekemecki A, Kennamer R, et al.: Angina pectoris. 1. A variant form of angina pectoris, *Am J Med* 27:375–388, 1959.

34. Meller J, Pichard A, Dack S: Coronary arterial spasm in Prinzmetal's angina: A proved hypothesis, *Am J Cardiol* 37:938–940, 1976.

35. Kaski J, Crea F, Meran D, et al.: Local coronary supersensitivity to diverse vasoconstrictive stimuli in patients with variant angina, *Circulation* 74(6):1255, 1986.

36. Haudenschild CC: Pathogenesis of atherosclerosis: State of the art, *Cardiovasc Drugs Ther* 4(Suppl 5):993–1004, 1990.

37. Yasue H, Matsuyama K, Matsuyama K, et al.: Responses of angiographically normal human coronary arteries to intracoronary injection of acetylcholine by age and segment. Possible role of early coronary atherosclerosis, *Circulation* 81:482–490, 1990.

38. Okumura K, Yasue H, Matsuyama K, et al.: Diffuse disorder of coronary artery vasomotility in patients with coronary spastic angina. Hyperreactivity to the constrictor effects of acetylcholine and the dilator effects of nitroglycerin, *J Am Coll Cardiol* 27:45–52, 1996.

39. Kitta Y, Obata JE, Nakamura T, et al.: Persistent impairment of endothelial vasomotor function has a negative impact on outcome in patients with coronary artery disease, *J Am Coll Cardiol* 53:323–330, 2009.

40. Vita JA, Treasure CB, Nabel EG, et al.: Coronary vasomotor response to acetylcholine relates to risk factors for coronary artery disease, *Circulation* 81:491–497, 1990.

41. Kannel WB: Some lessons in cardiovascular epidemiology from Framingham, *Am J Cardiol* 37:269–282, 1976.

42. Kannel WB: Contributions of the Framingham Study to the conquest of coronary artery disease, *Am J Cardiol* 62:1109–1112, 1988.

43. Mancia G: The need to manage risk factors of coronary heart disease, *Am Heart J* 115:240–242, 1988.

44. Battegay E, Gasche A, Zimmerli L, et al.: Risk factor control and perceptions of risk factors in patients with coronary heart disease, *Blood Press Suppl* 1:17–22, 1997.

45. Goble A, Jackson B, Phillips P, et al.: The family atherosclerosis risk intervention study (FARIS): Risk factor profiles of patients and their relatives following an acute cardiac event, *Aust N Z J Med* 27:568–577, 1997.

46. Lloyd-Jones D, Hong Y, Labarthe D, on behalf of the American Heart Association Strategic Planning Task Force and Statistics Committee, et al.: Defining and setting national goals for cardiovascular health promotion and disease reduction: the American Heart Association's strategic Impact Goal through 2020 and beyond, *Circulation* 121:586–613, 2010.

47. Chronic Disease Notes and Reports: In *National Center for Chronic Disease Prevention and Health Promotion, Centers for Disease Control and Prevention*, U.S. Department of Health and Human Services, 1997, pp 1–36.

48. Hammond EC, Horn D: Landmark article, March 15, 1958: Smoking and death rates—Report on forty-four months of follow-up of 187,783 men, *JAMA* 251:2840–2853, 1984.

49. Heitzer T, Yla-Herttuala S, Luoma J, et al.: Cigarette smoking potentiates endothelial dysfunction of forearm resistance vessels in patients with hypercholesterolemia. Role of oxidized LDL, *Circulation* 93:1346–1353, 1996.

50. Lin SJ: Risk factors, endothelial cell turnover and lipid transport in atherogenesis, *Zhonghua Yi Xue Za Zhi* 58(Taipei):309–316, 1996.

51. Vogel RA: Coronary risk factors, endothelial function, and atherosclerosis: A review, *Clin Cardiol* 20:426–432, 1997.

52. Veyssier Belot C: Tobacco smoking and cardiovascular risk, *Rev Med Interne* 18:702–708, 1997.

53. Rosengren A, Wilhelmsen L, Wedel H: Coronary heart disease, cancer and mortality in male middle-aged light smokers, *J Intern Med* 231:357–362, 1992.

54. Wilhelmsen L: Coronary heart disease: Epidemiology of smoking and intervention studies of smoking, *Am Heart J* 115:242–249, 1988.

55. Simon JA, Fong J, Bernert Jr JT, Browner WS: Relation of smoking and alcohol consumption to serum fatty acids, *Am J Epidemiol* 144:325–334, 1996.

56. van de Vijver LP, van Poppel G, van Houwelingen A, et al.: Trans-unsaturated fatty acids in plasma phospholipids and coronary heart disease: A case-control study, *Atherosclerosis* 126:155–161, 1996.

57. He Y, Lam TH, Li LS, et al.: The number of stenotic coronary arteries and passive smoking exposure from husband in lifelong non-smoking women in Xi'an, China, *Atherosclerosis* 127:229–238, 1996.

58. Moskowitz WB, Mosteller M, Schieken RM, et al.: Lipoprotein and oxygen transport alterations in passive smoking preadolescent children. The MCV Twin Study, *Circulation* 81:586–592, 1990.

59. Morris JN, Kagan A, Pattison DC, Gardner MJ: Incidence and prediction of ischaemic heart-disease in London busmen, *Lancet* 2:553–559, 1966.

60. Health risk factor surveys of commercial plan- and Medicaid-enrolled members of health-maintenance organizations: Michigan, 1995, *MMWR Morb Mortal Wkly Rep* 46:923–926, 1997.

61. Prevalence of physical inactivity during leisure time among overweight persons: Behavioral Risk Factor Surveillance System, 1994, *MMWR Morb Mortal Wkly Rep* 45:185–188, 1996.

62. Prevalence of sedentary lifestyle—behavioral risk factor surveillance system, United States, 1991, *MMWR Morb Mortal Wkly Rep* 42:576–579, 1993.

63. Cheng YJ, Gregg EW, Narayan KMV, et al.: Secular trend in sedentary lifestyle among US adults with and without diabetes 1997–2004, *Med Sci Sports Exerc* 38(5):S94, 2006.

64. Berg MH, Franz I, Keul J: Physical activity and lipoprotein metabolism: Epidemiological evidence and clinical trials, *Eur J Med Res* 2:259–264, 1997.

65. Fonong T, Toth MJ, Ades PA, et al.: Relationship between physical activity and HDL-cholesterol in healthy older men and women: A cross-sectional and exercise intervention study, *Atherosclerosis* 127:177–183, 1996.

66. Leon AS, Casal D, Jacobs Jr D: Effects of 2000 kcal per week of walking and stair climbing on physical fitness and risk factors for coronary heart disease, *J Cardiopulm Rehabil* 16:183–192, 1996.

67. Manninen V, Elo MO, Frick MH, et al.: Lipid alterations and decline in the incidence of coronary heart disease in the Helsinki Heart Study, *JAMA* 260:641–651, 1988.

68. Wood PD: Physical activity, diet, and health: Independent and interactive effects, *Med Sci Sports Exerc* 26:838–843, 1994.

69. Young DR, Haskell WL, Jatulis DE, Fortmann SP: Associations between changes in physical activity and risk factors for coronary heart disease in a community-based sample of men and women: The Stanford Five-City Project, *Am J Epidemiol* 138:205–216, 1993.

70. Kelley GA, Kelley KS: Vu Tran Z. Aerobic exercise, lipids and lipoproteins in overweight and obese adults: a meta-analysis of randomized controlled trials, *Int J Obes (Lond)* 29(8):881–893, 2005.

71. Carroll S, Dudfield M: What is the relationship between exercise and metabolic abnormalities? A review of the metabolic syndrome, *Sports Med* 34(6):371–418, 2004.

72. Katzel LI, Bleecker ER, Rogus EM, Goldberg AP: Sequential effects of aerobic exercise training and weight loss on risk factors for coronary disease in healthy, obese middle-aged and older men, *Metabolism* 46:1441–1447, 1997.

73. Katcher HI, Hill AM, Lanford JL, Yoo JS, Kris-Etherton PM: Lifestyle approaches and dietary strategies to lower LDL-cholesterol and triglycerides and raise HDL-cholesterol, *Endocrinol Metab Clin North Am* 38(1):45–78, 2009.

74. Huonker M, Halle M, Keul J: Structural and functional adaptations of the cardiovascular system by training, *Int J Sports Med* 17(Suppl 3):S164–S172, 1996.

75. Kvernmo HD, Osterud B: The effect of physical conditioning suggests adaptation in procoagulant and fibrinolytic potential, *Thromb Res* 87:559–569, 1997.

76. Ponjee GA, Janssen EM, Hermans J, van Wersch JW: Regular physical activity and changes in risk factors for coronary heart disease: A nine month prospective study, *Eur J Clin Chem Clin Biochem* 34:477–483, 1996.

77. Sasaki Y, Morimoto A, Ishii I, et al.: Preventive effect of long-term aerobic exercise on thrombus formation in rat cerebral vessels, *Haemostasis* 25:212–217, 1995.

78. Drygas WK: Changes in blood platelet function, coagulation, and fibrinolytic activity in response to moderate, exhaustive, and prolonged exercise, *Int J Sports Med* 9:67–72, 1988.

79. De JA Paz, Lasierra J, Villa JG, et al.: Changes in the fibrinolytic system associated with physical conditioning, *Eur J Appl Physiol* 65:388–393, 1992.

80. Tanaka K, Nakanishi T: Obesity as a risk factor for various diseases: Necessity of lifestyle changes for healthy aging, *Appl Human Sci* 15:139–148, 1996.

81. Jako P: The role of physical activity in the prevention of certain internal diseases, *Orv Hetil* 136:2379–2383, 1995.

82. Nolte LJ, Nowson CA, Dyke AC: Effect of dietary fat reduction and increased aerobic exercise on cardiovascular risk factors, *Clin Exp Pharmacol Physiol* 24:901–903, 1997.

83. Haskell WL, Wolffe JB: Memorial lecture. Health consequences of physical activity: Understanding and challenges regarding dose-response, *Med Sci Sports Exerc* 26:649–660, 1994.

84. Larson EB, Bruce RA: Health benefits of exercise in an aging society, *Arch Intern Med* 147:353–356, 1987.

85. Bao W, Srinivasan SR, Valdez R, et al.: Longitudinal changes in cardiovascular risks from childhood to young adulthood in offspring of parent with coronary artery disease: The Bogalusa Heart Study, *JAMA* 278:1749–1754, 1997.

86. Colombel A, Charbonnel B: Weight gain and cardiovascular risk factors in the post-menopausal woman, *Hum Reprod* 12(Suppl 1):134–145, 1997.

87. Gensini GF, Comeglio M, Colella A: Classical risk factors and emerging elements in the risk profile for coronary artery disease, *Eur Heart J* 19(Suppl A):A53–A61, 1998.

88. Anderssen SA, Holme I, Urdal P, Hjermann I: Associations between central obesity and indexes of hemostatic, carbohydrate and lipid metabolism. Results of a 1-year intervention from the Oslo Diet and Exercise Study, *Scand J Med Sci Sports* 8:109–115, 1998.

89. Shaper AG: Obesity and cardiovascular disease, *Ciba Found Symp* 201:90–103, 1996.

90. Doyle AE: Does hypertension predispose to coronary disease? Conflicting epidemiological and experimental evidence, *Am J Hypertens* 1:319–324, 1988.

91. Waters D, Craven TE, Lesperance J: Prognostic significance of progression of coronary atherosclerosis, *Circulation* 87:1067–1075, 1993.

92. Assmann G, Schulte H: The Prospective Cardiovascular Münster Study: Prevalence and prognostic significance of hyperlipidemia in men with systemic hypertension, *Am J Cardiol* 59:9G–17G, 1987.

93. Olson RE: Discovery of the lipoproteins, their role in fat transport and their significance as risk factors, *J Nutr* 128:439S–443S, 1998.

94. Pekkanen J, Linn S, Heiss G, et al.: Ten-year mortality from cardiovascular disease in relation to cholesterol level among men with and without preexisting cardiovascular disease, *N Engl J Med* 322:1700–1707, 1990.

95. Shoji T, Nishizawa Y, Kawagishi T, et al.: Atherogenic lipoprotein changes in the absence of hyperlipidemia in patients with chronic renal failure treated by hemodialysis, *Atherosclerosis* 131:229–236, 1997.

96. Chapman MJ, Guerin M, Bruckert E: Atherogenic, dense low-density lipoproteins. Pathophysiology, and new therapeutic approaches, *Eur Heart J* 19(Suppl A):A24–A30, 1998.

97. Frost PH, Havel RJ: Rationale for use of non-high-density lipoprotein cholesterol rather than low-density lipoprotein cholesterol as a tool for lipoprotein cholesterol screening and assessment of risk and therapy, *Am J Cardiol* 81:26B–31B, 1998.

98. Grundy SM, Balady GJ, Criqui MH, et al.: When to start cholesterol-lowering therapy in patients with coronary heart disease. A statement for healthcare professionals from the American Heart Association Task Force on Risk Reduction, *Circulation* 95:1683–1685, 1997.

99. Kris-Etherton PM, Krummel D, Russell ME, et al.: The effect of diet on plasma lipids, lipoproteins, and coronary heart disease, *J Am Diet Assoc* 88:1373–1400, 1988.

100. Kris-Etherton PM, Krummel D: Role of nutrition in the prevention and treatment of coronary heart disease in women, *J Am Diet Assoc* 93:987–993, 1993.

101. Smith-Schneider LM, Sigman-Grant MJ, Kris-Etherton PM: Dietary fat reduction strategies, *J Am Diet Assoc* 92:34–38, 1992.

102. Srinath U, Jonnalagadda SS, Naglak MC, et al.: Diet in the prevention and treatment of atherosclerosis. A perspective for the elderly, *Clin Geriatr Med* 11:591–611, 1995.

103. Connor SL, Gustafson JR, Artaud-Wild SM, et al.: The cholesterol/saturated-fat index: An indication of the hyper-cholesterolaemic and atherogenic potential of food, *Lancet* 1:1229–1232, 1986.

104. Connor SL, Gustafson JR, Artaud-Wild SM, et al.: The cholesterol-saturated fat index for coronary prevention: Background, use, and a comprehensive table of foods, *J Am Diet Assoc* 89:807–816, 1989.

105. Artaud-Wild SM, Connor SL, Sexton G, Connor WE: Differences in coronary mortality can be explained by differences in cholesterol and saturated fat intakes in 40 countries but not in France and Finland. A paradox, *Circulation* 88:2771–2779, 1993.

106. Gordon DJ, Probstfield JL, Garrison RJ, et al.: High-density lipoprotein cholesterol and cardiovascular disease. Four prospective American studies, *Circulation* 79:8–15, 1989.

107. Miller M, Mead LA, Kwiterovich Jr PO, Pearson TA: Dyslipidemias with desirable plasma total cholesterol levels and angiographically demonstrated coronary artery disease, *Am J Cardiol* 65:1–5, 1990.

108. Drexel H, Amann FW, Beran J, et al.: Plasma triglycerides and three lipoprotein cholesterol fractions are independent predictors of the extent of coronary atherosclerosis, *Circulation* 90:2230–2235, 1994.

109. Verdery RB: Reverse cholesterol transport from fibroblasts to high density lipoproteins: Computer solutions of a kinetic model, *Can J Biochem* 59:586–592, 1981.

110. Berger GM: High-density lipoproteins, reverse cholesterol transport and atherosclerosis—Recent developments, *S Afr Med J* 65:503–506, 1984.

111. Miller NE, La Ville A, Crook D: Direct evidence that reverse cholesterol transport is mediated by high-density lipoprotein in rabbit, *Nature* 314:109–111, 1985.

112. Gwynne JT: High-density lipoprotein cholesterol levels as a marker of reverse cholesterol transport, *Am J Cardiol* 64:10G–17G, 1989.

113. Schmitz G, Bruning T, Williamson E, Nowicka G: The role of HDL in reverse cholesterol transport and its disturbances in Tangier disease and HDL deficiency with xanthomas, *Eur Heart J* 11(Suppl E):197–211, 1990.

114. Pieters MN, Schouten D, Van Berkel TJ: In vitro and in vivo evidence for the role of HDL in reverse cholesterol transport, *Biochim Biophys Acta* 1225:125–134, 1994.

115. Assmann G, Schulte H, von Eckardstein A, Huang Y: High density lipoprotein cholesterol as a predictor of coronary heart disease risk. The PROCAM experience and pathophysiological implications for reverse cholesterol transport, *Atherosclerosis* 124(Suppl):S11–S20, 1996.

116. Hill SA, McQueen MJ: Reverse cholesterol transport—A review of the process and its clinical implications, *Clin Biochem* 30:517–525, 1997.

117. Kannel WB: Hazards, risks, and threats of heart disease from the early stages to symptomatic coronary heart disease and cardiac failure, *Cardiovasc Drugs Ther* 11(Suppl 1):199–212, 1997.

118. Chennell A, Sullivan DR, Penberthy LA, Hensley WJ: Comparability of lipoprotein measurements, total HDL cholesterol ratio and other coronary risk functions within and between laboratories in Australia, *Pathology* 26:471–476, 1994.

119. Castelli WP, Anderson K: A population at risk. Prevalence of high cholesterol levels in hypertensive patients in the Framingham Study, *Am J Med* 80:23–32, 1986.

120. Krauss RM: Atherogenicity of triglyceride-rich lipoproteins, *Am J Cardiol* 81:13B–17B, 1998.

121. Hodis HN, Mack WJ: Triglyceride-rich lipoproteins and progression of atherosclerosis, *Eur Heart J* 19(Suppl A):A40–A44, 1998.

122. Castelli WP: The triglyceride issue: A view from Framingham, *Am Heart J* 112:432–437, 1986.

123. Grundy SMN, Cleeman JI, Merez NB, et al.: ATP guidelines: Implications of recent clinical trials for the National Cholesterol Education Program Adult Treatment Panel III Guidelines, *J Am Coll Cardiol* 44:720–732, 2004.

124. Stone N, Robinson J, Lichtenstein A. 2013 ACC/AHA guideline on the treatment of blood cholesterol to reduce atherosclerotic cardiovascular risk in adults: A report of the American College of Cardiology/American Heart Association Task Force on Practice Guidelines Circulation. Published online November 12, 2013.

125. Brownlee M: The pathological implications of protein glycation, *Clin Invest Med* 18:275–281, 1995.

126. Giugliano D, Ceriello A, Paolisso G: Diabetes mellitus, hypertension, and cardiovascular disease: Which role for oxidative stress? *Metabolism* 44:363–368, 1995.

127. Duncan BB, Heiss G: Nonenzymatic glycosylation of proteins—A new tool for assessment of cumulative hyperglycemia in epidemiologic studies, past and future, *Am J Epidemiol* 120:169–189, 1984.

128. Heart Protection Study Collaborative Group: MRC/BHF Heart Protection Study of cholesterol lowering with simvastatin in 20,536 high-risk individuals: A randomised placebo-controlled trial, *Lancet* 360:7–22, 2002.

129. Akimova EV, Bogmat LF: Premature coronary heart disease: The influence of positive family history on platelet activity in vivo in children and adolescents (family study), *J Cardiovasc Risk* 4:13–18, 1997.

130. Saito T, Nanri S, Saito I, et al.: A novel approach to assessing family history in the prevention of coronary heart disease, *J Epidemiol* 7:85–92, 1997.

131. Allen JK, Blumenthal RS: Risk factors in the offspring of women with premature coronary heart disease, *Am Heart J* 135:428–434, 1998.

132. Pohjola-Sintonen S, Rissanen A, Liskola P, Luomanmaki K: Family history as a risk factor of coronary heart disease in patients under 60 years of age, *Eur Heart J* 19:235–239, 1998.

133. Khaw KT, Barrett-Connor E: Family history of heart attack: A modifiable risk factor? *Circulation* 74:239–244, 1986.

134. Barrett-Connor E, Khaw K: Family history of heart attack as an independent predictor of death due to cardiovascular disease, *Circulation* 69:1065–1069, 1984.

135. De Backer G, Ambrosioni E, Borch-Johnsen K, et al.: European guidelines on cardiovascular disease prevention in clinical practice. Third Joint Task Force of European and Other Societies on Cardiovascular Disease Prevention in Clinical Practice, *Eur Heart J* 24:1601–1610, 2003.

136. McPherson R, Frohlich J, Fodor G, et al.: Canadian Cardiovascular Society position statement—Recommendations for the diagnosis and treatment of dyslipidemia and prevention of cardiovascular disease, *Can J Cardiol* 22:913–927, 2006.

137. Taraboanta C, Wu E, Lear S, et al.: Subclinical atherosclerosis in subjects with family history of premature coronary artery disease, *Am Heart J* 155(6):1020–1026, 2008.

138. Centers for Disease Control and Prevention (CDC): Awareness of family health history as a risk factor for disease: United States, 2004, *MMWR Morb Mortal Wkly Rep* 53:1044–1047, 2004.

139. Neaton JD, Wentworth D: Serum cholesterol, blood pressure, cigarette smoking, and death from coronary heart disease. Overall findings and differences by age for 316,099 white men. Multiple Risk Factor Intervention Trial Research Group, *Arch Intern Med* 152:56–64, 1992.

140. Go A, Mozaffarian D, Roger V, et al.: on behalf of the American Heart Association Statistics Committee and Stroke Statistics Subcommittee Heart disease and stroke statistics—2013 update: A report from the American Heart Association, *Circulation* 127: e6–e245, 2013.

141. Smith Jr SC: Risk reduction therapies for patients with coronary artery disease: A call for increased implementation, *Am J Med* 104:23S–26S, 1998.

142. Grundy SM, Balady GJ, Criqui MH, et al.: Primary prevention of coronary heart disease: Guidance from Framingham: A statement for healthcare professionals from the AHA task force on risk reduction, *Circulation* 97:1876–1887, 1998.

143. Haskell WL, Alderman EL, Fair JM, et al.: Effects of intensive multiple risk factor reduction on coronary atherosclerosis and clinical cardiac events in men and women with coronary artery disease. The Stanford Coronary Risk Intervention Project (SCRIP), *Circulation* 89:975–990, 1994.

144. Williams MA: Cardiovascular risk-factor reduction in elderly patients with cardiac disease, *Phys Ther* 76:469–480, 1996.

145. McCann TJ, Criqui MH, Kashani IA, et al.: A randomized trial of cardiovascular risk factor reduction: Patterns of attrition after randomization and during follow-up, *J Cardiovasc Risk* 4:41–46, 1997.

146. Morley JE, Reese SS: Clinical implications of the aging heart, *Am J Med* 86:77–86, 1989.

147. Rodeheffer RJ, Gerstenblith G, Beard E, et al.: Postural changes in cardiac volumes in men in relation to adult age, *Exp Gerontol* 21:367–378, 1986.

148. Dahlberg ST: Gender difference in the risk factors for sudden cardiac death, *Cardiology* 77:31–40, 1990.

149. Orchard TJ: The impact of gender and general risk factors on the occurrence of atherosclerotic vascular disease in non-insulin-dependent diabetes mellitus, *Ann Med* 28:323–333, 1996.

150. Motro M, Shemesh J: Prevalence of coronary calcification in relation to age, gender and risk factor profile in the insight population, *Br J Clin Pract Suppl* 88:1–5, 1997.

151. Kitler ME: Coronary disease: Are there gender differences? *Eur Heart J* 15:409–417, 1994.

152. Murphy S, Xu J, Kochanek K: Deaths: Final data for 2010. In *National Vital Statistics Reports*, Hyattsville, MD, National Center for Health Statistics, 61: p 4, 2013, p 61:4.

153. Brochier ML, Arwidson P: Coronary heart disease risk factors in women, *Eur Heart J* 19(Suppl A):A45–A52, 1998.

154. Lunetta M, Barbagallo A, Attardo T, et al.: Coronary heart disease in type 2 diabetic patients: Common and different risk factors in men and women, *Diabetes Metab* 23:230–231, 1997.

155. Frost PH, Davis BR, Burlando AJ, et al.: Coronary heart disease risk factors in men and women aged 60 years and older: Findings from the systolic hypertension in the elderly program, *Circulation* 94:26–34, 1996.

156. Bellamy L, Casas J-P, Hingorani AD, Williams DJ: Pre-eclampsia and risk of cardiovascular disease and cancer in later life: Systematic review and meta-analysis, *BMJ* 335:974, 2007.

157. Shumaker SA, Brooks MM, Schron EB, et al.: Gender differences in health-related quality of life among postmyocardial infarction patients: Brief report. CAST Investigators. Cardiac Arrhythmia Suppression Trials, *Womens Health* 3:53–60, 1997.

158. Kambara H, Kinoshita M, Nakagawa M, Kawai C: Gender difference in long-term prognosis after myocardial infarction—Clinical characteristics in 1000 patients. The Kyoto and Shiga Myocardial Infarction (KYSMI) Study Group, *Jpn Circ J* 59:1–10, 1995.

159. Behar S, Zion M, Reicher-Reiss H, et al.: Short- and long-term prognosis of patients with a first acute myocardial infarction with concomitant peripheral vascular disease. SPRINT Study Group, *Am J Med* 96:15–19, 1994.

160. Salpeter SR, Walsh JME, Greyber E, Salpeter EE: Coronary heart disease events associated with therapy in younger and older women; a meta-analysis, *J Gen Intern Med* 21(4):363–366, 2006.

161. Grodstein F, Stampfer MJ, Manson JE, et al.: Postmenopausal estrogen and progestin use and the risk of cardiovascular disease, *N Engl J Med* 335:453–461, 1996.

162. Rossouw JE, Anderson GL, Prentice RL, et al.: Risks and benefits of estrogen plus progestin in healthy postmenopausal women: Principal results from the Women's Health Initiative randomized controlled trial, *JAMA* 288:321–333, 2002.

163. Anderson GL, Limacher M, Assaf AR, et al.: Effects of conjugated equine estrogen in postmenopausal women with hysterectomy: The Women's Health Initiative randomized controlled trial, *JAMA* 291:1701–1712, 2004.

164. Salpeter SR, Walsh JM, Greyber E, Ormiston TM, Salpeter EE: Mortality associated with hormone replacement therapy in younger and older women: A meta-analysis, *J Gen Intern Med* 19:791–804, 2004.

165. Mosca L, Banka CL, Benjamin EJ, et al.: Evidence-based guidelines for cardiovascular disease prevention in women: 2007 update, *Circulation* 115(15):e407, 2007.

166. Friedman M, Rosenman RH: Association of specific overt behavior pattern with blood and cardiovascular findings, *JAMA* 169:1286–1296, 1959.

167. Lachar BL: Coronary-prone behavior. Type A behavior revisited, *Tex Heart Inst J* 20:143–151, 1993.

168. Keltikangas-Jarvinen L, Raikkonen K, Hautanen A, Adlercreutz H: Vital exhaustion, anger expression, and pituitary and adrenocortical hormones. Implications for the insulin resistance syndrome, *Arterioscler Thromb Vasc Biol* 16:275–280, 1996.

169. King KB: Psychologic and social aspects of cardiovascular disease, *Ann Behav Med* 19:264–270, 1997.

170. Grignani G, Pacchiarini L, Zucchella M, et al.: Effect of mental stress on platelet function in normal subjects and in patients with coronary artery disease, *Haemostasis* 22:138–146, 1992.

171. Markovitz JH, Matthews KA: Platelets and coronary heart disease: Potential psychophysiologic mechanisms, *Psychosom Med* 53:643–668, 1991.

172. Superko HR, Fogelman A: *Lipoproteins and atherosclerosis—The role of HDL cholesterol, Lp(a), and LDL particle size*, New Orleans, LA, March 7–10, 1999, Presented at the American College of Cardiology, 48th Scientific Session.

173. Cohen J, Wilson WF: *Homocysteine, fibrinogen, Lp(a), small dense LDL, oxidative stress, and C. pneumoniae infection: How important are they?* New Orleans, LA, March 7–10, 1999, Presented at the American College of Cardiology, 48th Scientific Session.

174. Robinson K, Arheart K, Refsum H, et al.: Concentrations: Risk factors for stroke, peripheral vascular disease and coronary artery disease. European Comac Group, *Circulation* 97(5):437–443, 1998.

175. Glueck CJ, Shaw P, Lang JE, et al.: Evidence that homocysteine is an independent risk factor for atherosclerosis in hyperlipidemic patients, *Am J Cardiol* 75(2):132–136, 1995.

176. Rosenson RS, Kang DS: Overview of homocysteine. UpToDate In Freeman MW, Waltham MA, editors: *UpToDate*, 2015. http://www.uptodate.com/contents/overview-of-homocysteine?source=machineLearning&search=Overview+of+homocysteine&selectedTitle=1~150&sectionRank=1&anchor=H24#H24. (Accessed July 14, 2015).

177. Albert CM, Ma J, Rifai N, Stampfer MJ, Ridker PM: Prospective Study of C-reactive protein, homocysteine, and plasma lipid levels as predictors of sudden cardiac death, *Circulation* 105:2595–2599, 2002.

178. Zhao X: Pathogenesis of atherosclerosis. UpToDate In Kaski JC, Libby P, Waltham MA, editors: *UpToDate*, 2015. http://www.uptodate.com/contents/pathogenesis-of-atherosclerosis?source=search_result&search=pathogenesis+of+atherosclerosis&selectedTitle=1~150. (Accessed July 14, 2015).

179. Kannel WB, Shatzkin A: Sudden death: Lessons from subsets in population studies, *J Am Coll Cardiol* 5(Suppl 6):141B, 1985.

180. Meyerburg R, Castellanos A: Cardiac arrest and sudden cardiac death. In Braunwald E, editor: *Heart Disease: A Textbook of Cardiovascular Medicine*, ed 9, Philadelphia, 2012, Saunders.

181. White RD: Optimal access to and response by public and voluntary services, including the role of bystanders and family members, in cardiopulmonary resuscitation, *New Horiz* 5:153–157, 1997.

182. Lloyd-Jones D, Adams R, Carnethon M, et al.: Heart disease and stroke statistics 2009 update: A report from the American Heart Association Statistics Committee and Stroke Statistics Subcommittee, *Circulation* 119:e21–181, 2009.

183. Reeder GS, Kennedy HL: Criteria for the diagnosis of acute myocardial infarction. UpToDate. In Cannon CP, Hoeksra J, Jaffe AS, Waltham MA, editors: *UpToDate*, 2015. http://www.uptodate.com/contents/criteria-for-the-diagnosis-of-acute-myocardial-infarction?source=search_result&search=criteria+for+diagnosis+of+acute+myocardial&selectedTitle=1~150. (Accessed July 14, 2015).

184. Thygesen K, Alpert J, White H: Joint ESC/ACCF/AHA/WHF task force for the redefinition of myocardial infarction. Universal definition of myocardial infarction, *Eur Heart J* 28(20):2525, 2007.

185. Cannon C, Braunwald E: Unstable angina and non-ST elevation myocardial infarction. In Braunwald E, editor: *Heart Disease: A Textbook of Cardiovascular Medicine*, ed 9, Philadelphia, 2012, Saunders.

186. Hilton TC, Chaitman BR: The prognosis in stable and unstable angina, *Cardiol Clin* 9:27–38, 1991.

187. Brann WM, Tresch DD: Management of stable and unstable angina in elderly patients, *Compr Ther* 23:49–56, 1997.

188. Chierchia S, Brunelli C, Simonetti I, et al.: Sequence of events in angina at rest: primary reduction in coronary flow, *Circulation* 61:759–768, 1980.

189. Haft JI, Mariano DL, Goldstein J: Comparison of the histopathology of culprit lesions in chronic stable angina, unstable angina, and myocardial infarction, *Clin Cardiol* 20:651–655, 1997.

190. Thieme T, Wernecke KD, Meyer R, et al.: Angioscopic evaluation of atherosclerotic plaques: Validation by histomorphologic analysis and association with stable and unstable coronary syndromes, *J Am Coll Cardiol* 28:1–6, 1996.

191. Moon JC, De Arenaza DP, Elkington AG, et al.: The pathologic basis of Q-wave and non-Q-wave myocardial infarction: A cardiovascular magnetic resonance study, *J Am Coll Cardiol* 44:554, 2004.

192. Antman E, Morrow D: ST-segment elevation myocardial infarction: management. In Braunwald E, editor: *Heart Disease: A Textbook of Cardiovascular Medicine*, ed 9, Philadelphia, 2012, Saunders.

193. Swan HJ, Forrester JS, Diamond G, et al.: Hemodynamic spectrum of myocardial infarction and cardiogenic shock. A conceptual model, *Circulation* 45:1097, 1972.

194. Forrester JS, Wyatt HL, Da Luz PL, et al.: Functional significance of regional ischemic contraction abnormalities, *Circulation* 54:64, 1976.

195. McNeer JF, Wallace AG, Wagner GS, et al.: The course of acute myocardial infarction, *Circulation* 51:410, 1975.

196. Libby P, Bonow RO, Mann DL, et al.: *Braunwald's Heart Disease: A Textbook of Cardiovascular Medicine*, ed 8, Philadelphia, 2007, Saunders.

197. Rosengren A, Wilhelmsen L, Hagman M, Wedel H: Natural history of myocardial infarction and angina pectoris in a general population sample of middle-aged men: A 16-year follow-up of the Primary Prevention Study, Goteborg, Sweden, *J Intern Med* 244:495–505, 1998.

198. Lewis CE, Raczynski JM, Oberman A, Cutter GR: Risk factors and the natural history of coronary heart disease in blacks, *Cardiovasc Clin* 21:29–45, 1991.

199. Kramsch DM, Blankenhorn DH: Regression of atherosclerosis: Which components regress and what influences their reversal, *Wien Klin Wochenschr* 104:2–9, 1992.

200. Hodis HN: Reversibility of atherosclerosis—Evolving perspectives from two arterial imaging clinical trials: The cholesterol lowering atherosclerosis regression study and the monitored atherosclerosis regression study, *J Cardiovasc Pharmacol* 25:S25–S31, 1995.

201. Ornish D, Scherwitz LW, Billings JH, et al.: Intensive lifestyle changes for reversal of coronary heart disease, *JAMA* 280:2001–2007, 1998.

202. Patrono C: Prevention of myocardial infarction and stroke by aspirin: Different mechanisms? Different dosage? *Thromb Res* 92:S25–S32, 1998.

203. Mosa L, Banka CL, Benjamin EJ, et al.: Evidence-based guide for cardiovascular disease prevention in women: 2007 Update, *Circulation* 115:1481–1501, 2007.

204. Azen SP, Mack WJ, Cashin-Hemphill L, et al.: Progression of coronary artery disease predicts clinical coronary events. Long-term follow-up from the Cholesterol Lowering Atherosclerosis Study, *Circulation* 93:34–41, 1996.

205. Blankenhorn DH, Johnson RL, Nessim SA, et al.: The Cholesterol Lowering Atherosclerosis Study (CLAS): Design methods, and baseline results, *Control Clin Trials* 8:356–387, 1987.

206. Campbell NC, Thain J, Deans HG, et al.: Secondary prevention clinics for coronary heart disease: Randomised trial of effect on health, *BMJ* 316:1434–1437, 1998.

207. Chobanian AV, Bakris GL, Black HR, et al.: The seventh report of the Joint National Committee on prevention, detection, evaluation, and treatment of high blood pressure: The JNC 7 report, *JAMA* 289(19):2560–2572, 2003.

208. Pickering TG, Hall JE, Appel LJ, et al.: Recommendations for blood pressure measurement in humans and experimental animals: Part 1: Blood pressure measurement in humans: A statement for professionals from the Subcommittee of Professional and Public Education of the American Heart Association Council on High Blood Pressure Research, *Hypertension* 45(1):142–161, 2005.

209. Cushman WC: The clinical significance of systolic hypertension, *Am J Hypertens* 11:182S–185S, 1998.

210. Kannel WB: Blood pressure as a cardiovascular risk factor: Prevention and treatment, *JAMA* 275:1571–1576, 1996.

211. Cohn JN, Limas CJ, Guiha NH: Hypertension and the heart, *Arch Intern Med* 133:969–979, 1974.

212. Frohlich ED: The heart in hypertension. In Genest J, Kuchel O, Hamet P, et al.: *Hypertension: Physiopathology and Treatment*, New York, 1983, McGraw-Hill.

213. *Society of Actuaries & Association of Life Insurance Medical Directors of America. Blood Pressure Study 1979*, Chicago, 1980, Society of Actuaries & Association of Life Insurance Medical Directors of America.

214. Kannel WB: Framingham study insights into hypertensive risk of cardiovascular disease, *Hypertens Res* 18:181–196, 1995.

215. Kannel WB, Wolf PA, Verter J, McNamara PM: Epidemiologic assessment of the role of blood pressure in stroke: The Framingham Study, 1970, *JAMA* 276:1269–1278, 1996.

estimated that 5.7 million or more Americans suffer from CHF and that 670,000 new cases occur yearly, requiring 1.1 million hospitalizations each year.[4] In addition, the lifetime risk of developing heart failure for both men and women at age 40 years is 1 in 5, with the annual rate of developing heart failure over the age of 85 years is 65%.[4] Individuals with a wide variety of heart and lung diseases very likely will develop CHF at some time during their lives,[3] frequently manifested as pulmonary congestion or pulmonary edema.[1] This chapter describes the etiology, pathophysiology, clinical manifestations, medical management, prognosis of CMD and CHF, and indications for physical therapy, including patient management.

Causes and Types of Cardiac Muscle Dysfunction

Most often, CMD may not present with symptoms, but many of the signs and symptoms of CHF are the result of a "sequence of events with a resultant increase in fluid in the interstitial spaces of the lungs, liver, subcutaneous tissues, and serous cavities."[5] The etiology of CHF is varied, but it is most commonly the result of CMD.

The varied causes of CMD and subsequently CHF can be best classified according to 11 specific processes or causes, which are described in Table 4-1.[5–7]

Hypertension

The increased arterial pressure seen in systemic hypertension eventually produces left ventricular hypertrophy. An extremely elevated ventricular and occasionally elevated atrial pressure commonly seen in patients with CMD tend to produce a less effective pump as the myocardial contractile fibers become overstretched, thus increasing the work of each myocardial fiber in an attempt to maintain an adequate cardiac output.[8,9] Myocardial work continued in this manner eventually produces left ventricular hypertrophy as the contractile fibers adapt to the increased workload.[10,11] The two problems with left ventricular hypertrophy are the increase in afterload and the increased energy expenditure (metabolic cost) required for myocardial contraction because of increased myocardial cell mass.[8,10,12] The increased cell mass without an additional increase in vasculature also affects blood supply to the muscle, resulting in a decreased blood supply to some of the new muscle mass. Medical management of hypertension should begin upon diagnosis after echocardiogram is performed for baseline documentation of ventricular involvement. Medical management usually consists of angiotensin-converting enzyme (ACE) inhibitors, calcium-channel blockers, diuretics, or possibly β blockers. Chapter 14 provides detailed information on medications. Exercise training performed regularly has demonstrated changes in systolic pressure of 10 mm Hg and diastolic pressure of 8 mm Hg, but must be maintained throughout an individual's lifetime to maintain benefits.

Coronary Artery Disease (Myocardial Infarction/Ischemia)

Coronary artery disease is the second most common cause of CMD,[3] which occurs because of dysfunction of the left or right

Table 4-1 Etiology of congestive heart failure	
Causes	**Description**
Hypertension	↑ Arterial pressure leads to left ventricular hypertrophy (↑ myocardial cell mass) and ↑ energy expenditure.
Coronary artery disease (myocardial ischemia)	Dysfunction of the left or right ventricle or both as a result of injury. Scar formation and ↓ contractility may occur, as well as reduced relaxation.
Cardiac dysrhythmias	Extremely rapid or slow cardiac arrhythmias impair the functioning ventricles. Dysfunction may be reversible if arrhythmia is controlled.
Renal insufficiency	Causes fluid overload, which frequently progresses to CMD and CHF that may be reversed.
Cardiomyopathy	Contraction and relaxation of myocardial muscle fibers are impaired. Primary causes: pathologic processes in the heart muscle itself, which impair the heart's ability to contract. Secondary causes: systemic disease processes.
Heart valve abnormality	Valvular stenosis or incompetent valves (valvular insufficiency because of abnormal or poorly functioning valve leaflets) cause myocardial hypertrophy and a decrease in ventricular distensibility with mild diastolic dysfunction.
Pericardial effusion	Injury to the pericardium can cause acute pericarditis (inflammation of the pericardial sac surrounding the heart) and progress to pericardial effusion and cardiac compression as fluid fills the pericardial sac. May also develop cardiac tamponade.
Pulmonary embolism	Severe hypoxemia may result from embolus blocking a moderate to large amount of lung, resulting in elevated pulmonary artery pressures, a right ventricular work and right heart.
Pulmonary hypertension	Elevated pressures in pulmonary artery lead to increased afterload for the right ventricle and subsequently, over time, to right ventricular failure.
Spinal cord injury	Transection of the cervical spinal cord prevents the sympathetic-driven changes necessary to maintain cardiac performance.
Age-related changes	Aging appears to decrease cardiac output by altered contraction and relaxation of cardiac muscle. The two most common congenital heart defects are nonstenotic bicuspid aortic valve and the leaflet abnormality associated with mitral valve prolapse.

ventricle or both as a result of injury.[13–15] Besides the ischemic injury from disease restricting blood flow to the cardiac muscle, there could be actual injury from infarction resulting in scar formation and decreased contractility, as well as reduced relaxation. In addition, other factors can cause injury, including myocardial damage, or "stunning," following coronary angioplasty[16,17] and postperfusion (postpump) syndrome following cardiopulmonary bypass surgery.[18,19] Essentially postpump syndrome results in organ and subsystem dysfunction following abnormal bleeding, inflammation, concomitant renal dysfunction, and peripheral and central vasoconstriction.

Cardiac Arrhythmias

Cardiac arrhythmias can also cause CMD for reasons similar to those given for myocardial infarction.[5] Extremely rapid or slow cardiac arrhythmias can impair the functioning of the left or right ventricle, or both, and an overall CMD ensues. Prolonged very slow or very fast heart rates are frequently caused by a sick sinus node syndrome or heart block (producing very slow heart rates), prolonged supraventricular tachycardia (i.e., rapid atrial fibrillation or flutter), or ventricular tachycardia (both tachycardias produce very fast heart rates).[20,21] (See Chapter 9 for explanation and pictures.) Very slow heart rates or heart blocks are often an adverse reaction or side effect of a specific medication, but when medications are withheld and slow heart rates or a heart block persists, the implantation of a permanent pacemaker is generally performed.[20] This type of CMD is readily amenable to treatment and quite reversible.

Cardiac muscle dysfunction caused by very rapid heart rates is also reversible. Rapid atrial fibrillation or flutter can produce CMD and is often easily treated by the administration of verapamil or digoxin[20] (see Chapter 14). If these drugs fail, electrical cardioversion is usually performed, after which rapid heart rates frequently become much more normal as the cyclic "circus movement" propagating the rapid rhythm is disrupted and the sinoatrial node is allowed to resume control of the heart's rhythm.[20] Ventricular tachycardia and fibrillation are life-threatening cardiac arrhythmias, which, if prolonged, rapid, or both, can also produce CMD and death. The treatment of ventricular tachycardia and fibrillation is dependent on the clinical status of the patient and follows the guidelines set forth by the American Heart Association.[20] The use of implantable cardiac defibrillators (ICDs) has been a treatment of choice for patients with recurrent ventricular tachycardia or fibrillation that is unresponsive to antiarrhythmic medications.[21,22] Ventricular function is intimately related to cardiac rhythm. Any abnormally fast, slow, or unsynchronized rhythm can impair ventricular and atrial function quickly and progress to CHF and even death.[20] Many patients with CMD have preexisting arrhythmias that must be controlled, typically with medication, but sometimes by other methods (e.g., ablation, ICD)[21] to prevent further deterioration of a muscle that is already compromised.

Because antiarrhythmic agents act as cardiodepressants and often have proarrhythmic effects, they are not usually indicated in individuals with CHF.[23]

Renal Insufficiency

Acute or chronic renal insufficiency tends to produce a fluid overload, which frequently progresses to CMD and CHF that can often be reversed if it is the only underlying pathophysiologic process. However, other pathophysiologic processes may produce the fluid overload that caused CMD.[24] Consequently, CMD is seldom reversed by the correction of fluid volume alone. Nevertheless, the primary treatment is to decrease the reabsorption of fluid from the kidneys so that more fluid is eliminated (in essence, diuresed).[24] The diuretic most commonly used is furosemide (Lasix), which can be given intravenously or orally. In addition to and as a result of the administration of a diuretic, electrolyte levels are carefully monitored, ensuring that potassium and sodium levels are within the normal range to prevent further retention of fluid from high levels of potassium and sodium or the detrimental effects of low levels (e.g., cardiac arrhythmias and muscle weakness). Low-dose aldosterone antagonists are also recommended in individuals with moderately severe heart failure symptoms or with left ventricle (LV) dysfunction after acute coronary syndrome (as long as serum creatinine is <2.5 mg dL).[25]

Severe renal insufficiency, demonstrating advanced azotemia, is best treated by dialysis (peritoneal or hemodialysis), which may remove as much as 1 L of extracellular fluid per hour.[24]

Cardiomyopathy

Cardiomyopathy is a disease in which the contraction and relaxation of myocardial muscle fibers are impaired.[10] This impaired contractility can result from either primary or secondary causes.[26] The primary causes are the result of pathologic processes in the heart muscle itself, which impair the heart's ability to contract. The secondary causes of cardiomyopathy are the result of a systemic disease processes rather than of pathologic myocardial processes and can be classified according to the systemic disease that subsequently affects myocardial contraction (Table 4-2 and Fig. 4-1). They may also be subdivided into tertiary causes to allow for treatment of root causation using the most appropriate protocol available.

Cardiomyopathies are differentiated based on a functional standpoint, emphasizing three basic categories: dilated, hypertrophic, and restrictive (Fig. 4-2); or from a causal viewpoint, categorized as genetic, acquired, or mixed. Patients often present with a combination of these classifications.[10] The cardiomyopathies are distinguished from one another by echocardiographic and myocardial biopsy results.[10]

Dilated Cardiomyopathies

Dilated cardiomyopathies "probably represent a final common pathway that is the end result of myocardial damage produced by a variety of toxic, metabolic, or infectious agents."[10] Possible causes of dilated cardiomyopathies include the following:[10]

- Long-term alcohol abuse
- Systemic hypertension
- A variety of infections
- Cigarette smoking
- Pregnancy
- Carnitine deficiency

These conditions may not be primarily responsible for dilated cardiomyopathy, but may act to lower the threshold for its development. Little is known regarding the further development of dilated cardiomyopathies, but the dilation that occurs in this type of cardiomyopathy, and that sets it apart

Table 4-2 Secondary causes of cardiomyopathy

Primary Cardiomyopathies	Secondary Cardiomyopathies
Genetic (hypertrophic cardiomyopathy; conduction abnormalities: prolonged QT syndrome; Brugada syndrome)	Infiltrative (amyloidosis and Gaucher disease)
Mixed (dilated cardiomyopathy; restrictive cardiomyopathy)	Storage (haemochromatosis and Fabry disease)
Acquired (inflammatory myocarditis, peripartum, stress cardiomyopathy—"broken heart syndrome" or tako-tsubo)	Toxicity (drugs, alcohol, heavy metals, and chemicals/chemotherapy)
	Inflammatory (sarcoidosis) endocrine (diabetes mellitus; thyroid disorders; hyperparathyroidism), cardiofacial (Noonan syndrome, lentiginosis) neuromuscular/neurologic, nutritional deficiencies, and autoimmune and collagen disorders

From McCartan C, Mason R, Jayasinghe SR, et al: Cardiomyopathy classification: ongoing debate in the genomics era, review article, *Biochem Res Int* 2012:796926, 2012.

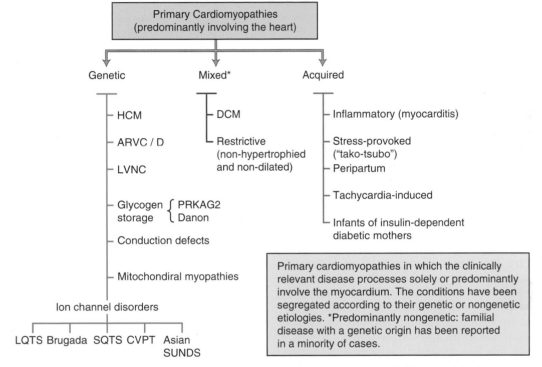

Figure 4-1 Classification of cardiomyopathy ARVC/D = arrhythmogenic right ventricular cardiomyopathy/dysplasia; CVPT = catecholaminergic polymorphic ventricular tachycardia; DCM = dilated cardiomyopathy; HCM = hypertrophic cardiomyopathy; LQTS = long-QT syndrome; LVNC = left ventricular noncompaction; PRKAG2 = gene encoding the γ2 regulatory subunit of the AMP-activated protein kinase; SQTS = short-QT syndrome; SUNDS = sudden unexplained nocturnal death syndrome. (Modified from Maron BJ, Towbin JA, Thiene G, et al: Contemporary definitions and classification of the cardiomyopathies: an American Heart Association Scientific Statement from the Council on Clinical Cardiology, Heart Failure and Transplantation Committee; quality of care and outcomes research and functional genomics and translational biology interdisciplinary working groups; and Council on Epidemiology and Prevention, *Circulation* 113:1807-1816, 2006.)

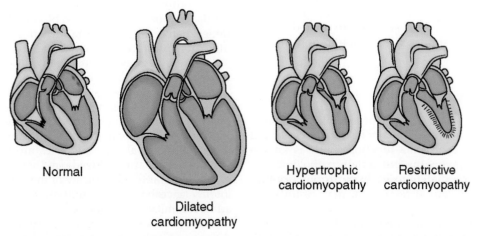

Figure 4-2 The cardiomyopathies (Courtesy Merck Manual on-line www.merck.com/mmhe/sec03/ch026/ch026a.html Accessed 12/31/05 IN Moser DK: Cardiac Nursing: A Companion to Braunwald's Heart Disease, Philadelphia, 2007, Saunders.)

from hypertrophic cardiomyopathy, appears to be a result of myocardial mitochondrial dysfunction.[10] Dysfunction of myocardial mitochondria leads to a lack of energy necessary for proper cardiac function, causing the heart to be a less effective pump.[10] Ineffective pumping increases both the left ventricular end-diastolic volume and pressure, which dilate the LV (and frequently the other heart chambers). Because of inappropriate energy sources, the LV is unable to contract properly or to relax individual muscle fibers in response to increased workload, thereby preventing myocardial hypertrophy but producing ineffective systolic (pumping) function. Cardiomyopathy as a consequence of treatment of malignancy with chemotherapy is often related to anthracycline administration. Anthracycline cardiomyopathy is dose related and, depending on the aggressiveness of treatment protocols, can be seen in 5% to 20% of patients receiving these agents.

Hypertrophic Cardiomyopathy

Hypertrophic cardiomyopathy should be thought of as the opposite of dilated cardiomyopathy, both functionally and etiologically. The hypertrophy associated with hypertrophic cardiomyopathy is inappropriate for the applied hemodynamic load and is associated with proper myocardial mitochondrial function. Furthermore, the dysfunction of hypertrophic cardiomyopathy is one of diastolic dysfunction, which impairs the filling of the ventricles during diastole.[10] This increases the left ventricular end-diastolic pressure and eventually increases left atrial, pulmonary artery, and pulmonary capillary pressures, all of which cause a hypercontractile LV. The hypercontractile myocardial muscle fibers of hypertrophic cardiomyopathy are frequently disorganized and demonstrate cellular disarray. The greater the disarray, the greater the hypertrophic cardiomyopathy.[10] In addition, hypertrophic cardiomyopathy has a high risk of sudden cardiac death.[27]

Susceptibility to hypertrophic cardiomyopathy appears to be genetically transmitted as an autosomal-dominant trait. It has been suggested that the apparent myocardial isometric contraction of hypertrophic cardiomyopathy is the result of malaligned myocardial muscle fibers[11] or an abnormal configuration of the interventricular septum in response to a genetic influence.[28] Other causes of hypertrophic cardiomyopathy have been suggested, including abnormal sympathetic stimulation, subendocardial ischemia, and abnormal calcium ion dynamics.[10]

The characteristic findings of hypertrophic cardiomyopathy are rapid ventricular emptying and high ejection fraction (EF), which are the opposite of those found in dilated cardiomyopathy but somewhat similar to those found in restrictive cardiomyopathy.[10]

Restrictive Cardiomyopathy

Restrictive cardiomyopathy, like hypertrophic cardiomyopathy, is a cardiomyopathy of diastolic dysfunction and frequently unimpaired contractile function. Little is known about restrictive cardiomyopathy, but certain pathologic processes, including myocardial fibrosis, hypertrophy, infiltration, or a defect in myocardial relaxation, may result in its development.[10]

The specific treatment of cardiomyopathy is dependent on the underlying cause, but in general includes physical,

nutritional, pharmacologic, mechanical, and surgical intervention.[10] One pharmacologic intervention worth mentioning is β-adrenergic blockade, which appears to improve symptoms and survival through five means:[10]

- Negative chronotropic effect with reduced myocardial oxygen demand
- Reduced myocardial damage because of decreased catecholamines
- Improved diastolic relaxation
- Inhibition of sympathetically mediated vasoconstriction
- Increase in myocardial β-adrenoceptor density

These factors are important because they are the basic mechanisms supporting the use of β blockers for dilated, restrictive, and hypertrophic cardiomyopathies, as well as CHF in general, because "treatment is on the same basis as that for heart failure."[10]

Heart Valve Abnormalities and Congenital/Acquired Heart Disease

Heart valve abnormalities can also cause CMD, as blocked valves (valvular stenosis), incompetent valves (valvular insufficiency caused by abnormal or poorly functioning valve leaflets), or both cause heart muscle to contract more forcefully to expel the cardiac output. This subsequently produces myocardial hypertrophy, which can decrease ventricular distensibility and produce a mild diastolic dysfunction; if untreated and prolonged, this dysfunction can lead to more profound diastolic and systolic dysfunction.[29] Incompetent valves are frequently associated with myocardial dilation in addition to hypertrophy, because regurgitant blood fills the atria or ventricles forcefully.[29] Atrial dilation often accompanies mitral and tricuspid insufficiency, whereas ventricular dilation accompanies aortic or pulmonary insufficiency. Aortic insufficiency can dilate the LV, whereas pulmonary insufficiency can dilate the right ventricle. Mitral insufficiency frequently dilates the left atrium, whereas tricuspid insufficiency dilates the right atrium. Such dilation can lengthen individual cardiac muscle fibers in the atria and ventricles to such a degree that myocardial contraction is impaired severely, but frequently the accompanying myocardial hypertrophy prevents such extreme dilation. However, the abnormal hemodynamics from hypertrophy and dilation often produce CMD.[29]

Acute heart valve dysfunction or rupture can cause rapid and life-threatening CMD because a ruptured valve impairs cardiac output and regurgitant blood fills the heart's chambers rather than exiting the aorta.[6] If left untreated, valve rupture ultimately produces pulmonary edema and eventually death.

Heart valve abnormalities that cause CMD appear to be reversible to a point. If the abnormality persists for too long, cardiac function appears to be permanently impaired.[29] Acute problems such as heart valve rupture can affect proper cardiac muscle function profoundly and, as mentioned, are fatal if not surgically repaired within a relatively short period. The most common valvular surgeries are valvular replacement, valvuloplasty (pressurized reduction of atherosclerotic plaque, similar to angioplasty of the coronary arteries), valvulotomy (incision), and commissurotomy (incision to separate adherent, thickened leaflets).[29]

Other heart valve conditions can be classified as chronic conditions and include the stenotic and regurgitant abnormalities of the aortic, pulmonary, mitral, or tricuspid valves. Prolonged valvular stenosis or regurgitation affects cardiac function and can eventually lead to CMD, but cardiac function is less likely to return to normal after valvuloplasty or surgical repair or replacement of a chronic valvular condition.[29]

Pericardial Effusion or Myocarditis

Injury to the pericardium of the heart can cause acute pericarditis (inflammation of the pericardial sac surrounding the heart), which may progress to pericardial effusion, possibly resulting in cardiac compression as fluid fills the pericardial sac.[10] Increased fluid accumulation within the pericardial space increases intrapericardial pressure and produces cardiac tamponade. Cardiac tamponade is characterized by elevated intracardiac pressures, progressively limited ventricular diastolic filling, and reduced stroke volume.[10] Thus the mechanism of CMD, which is primarily a diastolic dysfunction (limited ventricular diastolic filling because of cardiac compression), produces a secondary systolic dysfunction. The same sequence of primary diastolic CMD producing secondary systolic CMD occurs in myocarditis.

The prompt treatment of pericarditis with nonsteroidal antiinflammatory agents (aspirin or indomethacin) or corticosteroids (usually prednisone) frequently prevents pericardial effusion. Treatment of the causative inflammatory process in myocarditis (most commonly viral) should prevent the diastolic and systolic CMD of pericardial effusion and myocarditis.[10] However, patients who do not respond to this therapy must undergo more extensive treatment, including drainage of fluid from the pericardium (pericardiocentesis) for pericardial effusion; immunosuppressive, antibiotic, and possibly antiviral agents for myocarditis; and aggressive CHF management (digitalization, diuresis, and afterload or preload reduction) for both pericardial effusion and myocarditis.[10]

Pulmonary Embolism

Cardiac muscle dysfunction from a pulmonary embolism is the result of elevated pulmonary artery pressures that dramatically increase right ventricular work. Right and left ventricular failure can occur because of decreased oxygenated coronary blood flow and decreased blood flow to the LV.[30] A similar, but often less extreme, condition occurs in pulmonary hypertension.

An acute pulmonary embolism is also a potentially life-threatening condition. As previously mentioned, the primary CMD resulting from a pulmonary embolism is a result of a very high pulmonary artery pressure (because of damaged lung tissue and less area for proper pulmonary perfusion), which increases the work of the right ventricle and eventually produces right-sided heart failure. Left-sided heart failure may accompany right-sided failure because of decreased blood volume and coronary perfusion to the left ventricle, impairing the pumping ability of the heart.[30]

The treatment of a pulmonary embolism consists of the following:[30,31]

- A rapidly acting fibrinolytic agent (typically heparin) should be administered immediately. Heparin reduces the mortality rate of pulmonary embolism as it slows or prevents clot progression. Two forms of recombinant

tissue plasminogen activator (alteplase [TPA] and or reteplase [r-PA]) are commonly used.
- A sedative to decrease the patient's anxiety and pain.
- Oxygen to improve the PaO_2 (partial pressure of arterial oxygen) and decrease the pulmonary artery pressure.
- Occasionally an embolectomy.

Cardiac muscle dysfunction caused by a pulmonary embolism occasionally can be reversed (especially if treatment is initiated immediately), but quite frequently some degree of CMD ensues because of infarcted lung tissue, which increases the work of the right ventricle.[30] When such a condition exists, the pulmonary artery pressure rises and may produce pulmonary hypertension. Pulmonary hypertension can often produce CMD by increasing right ventricular work, resulting in right ventricular hypertrophy (and inefficient right ventricular performance). This may reduce the right ventricular stroke volume, thereby decreasing the left ventricular stroke volume and cardiac output.

Pulmonary Hypertension

Pulmonary hypertension is defined by mean pulmonary arterial pressure (mPAP) and is considered abnormal in individuals with primary pulmonary hypertension if higher than 25 mm Hg, and abnormal in individuals with chronic obstructive pulmonary disease (COPD) if higher than 20 mm Hg. An elevated mPAP is a predictor of poor prognosis in patients with COPD. The usual suspect accused of the development of pulmonary hypertension in COPD is hypoxia, which is undoubtedly, both acutely and chronically, associated with an increase in pulmonary vascular resistance (PVR). An increase in PVR can increase the work of the right ventricle and lead to right heart dysfunction and eventually failure. Fig. 4-3 shows the three categories of diseases that lead to elevated pressure in pulmonary circulation, right ventricular hypertrophy, and right ventricular failure. In addition, Fig. 4-4 shows survival curves for individuals with normal and low right ventricular EFs. Fig. 4-5 demonstrates how pulmonary hypertension can lead to heart failure.

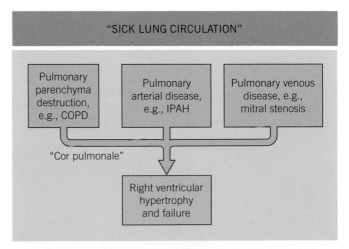

Figure 4-3 Three categories of diseases leading to an elevated pressure in the pulmonary circulation, right ventricular hypertrophy, and right ventricular failure. The common denominator is a "sick lung circulation." *COPD,* Chronic obstructive pulmonary disease; *IPAH,* idiopathic pulmonary arterial hypertension. (From Crawford MH, DiMarco JP, Paulus WJ: *Cardiology,* ed 3. Philadelphia, 2010, Saunders.)

Spinal Cord Injury

Spinal cord injury also can produce CMD when the cervical spinal cord becomes transected, which "causes an imbalance between parasympathetic and sympathetic control of the cardiovascular system."[32] Several studies have identified neurogenic pulmonary edema as a frequently fatal complication of cervical spinal cord transection.[33–35] Transection of the cervical spinal cord prevents sympathetic nervous system information from reaching the cardiovascular system (heart, lung, arterial and venous systems), thus preventing the sympathetic-driven changes necessary to maintain

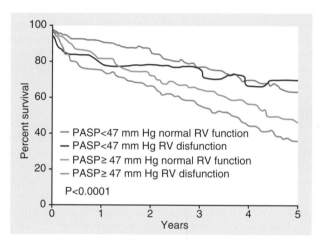

Figure 4-4 Five-year Kaplan-Meier survival curves in heart failure preserved ejection fraction according to pulmonary arterial systolic pressure (PASP) median value distribution (47 mm Hg) and right ventricular (RV) function (normal or systolic dysfunction). (Redrawn from Guazzi M. Pulmonary hypertension in heart failure preserved ejection fraction: prevalence, pathophysiology, and clinical perspectives, *Circulation Heart Failure* 7:367-377, 2014.)

cardiac performance (i.e., increased heart rate and force of myocardial contraction, constriction of venous capacitance vessels, or arterial constriction). Lacking these cardiovascular adaptations, patients with spinal cord injuries (who frequently are volume depleted because of fluid loss from multiple injuries) may develop a specific type of CMD that produces neurogenic pulmonary edema.[32] Because of the possibility of volume depletion, it has been recommended that cardiac filling pressures be monitored, that "cardiac preload be increased by giving fluids,"[32] and that construction of a ventricular function curve may be useful in guiding therapy and treatment for patients with spinal cord injuries that are at risk for neurogenic pulmonary edema.[32] It appears, then, that a slightly elevated pulmonary capillary wedge pressure (not exceeding 18 mm Hg) many facilitate optimal cardiac performance in these patients.

Age-Related Changes

Although distinctly different processes, congenital or acquired heart diseases and the aging process can produce a similar type of CMD, which is often initially well tolerated but, as the dysfunction persists, may become more symptomatic and troublesome. The adaptability of infants and children to extreme conditions is evident in congenital heart disease, which frequently can be managed for many years with specific medications before surgical intervention becomes necessary.[36,37] The CMD associated with the aging process is initially well tolerated, not because of the aged individual's ability to adapt, but because the degree of CMD is usually mild. Aging appears to decrease cardiac output by altered contraction and relaxation of cardiac muscle.[38,39] However, heart disease, hypertension, and other pathologic processes can increase CMD substantially and subsequently can impair functional

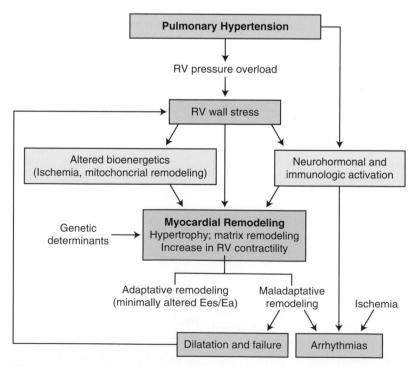

Figure 4-5 The development of heart failure as a result of pulmonary hypertension. RV, right ventricule; Ees, End-systolic elastance; Ea, arterial elastance. (Vonk-Noordegraaf, et al: Right heart adaptation to pulmonary arterial hypertension: physiology and pathobiology, *J Am Coll Cardiol* 62(25 Suppl):D22–D33, 2013.)

abilities, and these pathologic processes are more prevalent in the older population.[38,39]

Congenital and Acquired Heart Disease

Congenital heart disease is the result of "altered embryonic development of a normal structure or failure of such a structure to progress beyond an early stage of embryonic or fetal development."[36] Approximately 0.6% of live births but 1.3% live preterm births are complicated by cardiovascular malformations, such as ventricular septal defect, atrial septal defect, patent ductus arteriosus, coarctation of the aorta, and tetralogy of Fallot. The two most common cardiac anomalies are the congenital nonstenotic bicuspid aortic valve and the leaflet abnormality associated with mitral valve prolapse.[36,40]

Acquired heart disease can occur in infancy and childhood as a result of disease processes such as those outlined in Box 4-1. Although the disease processes are different in acquired and congenital heart disease, the resultant pathophysiologic processes are not unlike those seen in adults with CMD because it is dysfunctional cardiac muscle that eventually produces the clinical signs and symptoms.[36]

Age-Associated Changes in Cardiac Performance

The aging process involves several interrelated pathophysiologic processes, all of which have the potential to impair physical performance, including cardiac function. Although several earlier studies have revealed a reduced cardiac output in the elderly (at rest and with exercise),[41-43] a study that excluded subjects with ischemic heart disease demonstrated no "age effect" on cardiac performance.[44] In this study, the heart rates of the elderly were lower at most workloads, but increased stroke volume apparently compensated for the decreased heart rates and thus maintained cardiac output (cardiac output = heart rate × stroke volume).[44]

BOX 4-1   Disease processes of congenital vs. acquired heart disease

Congenital cardiac malformations
  Volume overload
    Left-to-right shunting
      Ventricular septal defect
      Patent ductus arteriosus
    Atrioventricular or semilunar valve insufficiency
      Aortic regurgitation in bicommissural aortic valve
      Pulmonary regurgitation after repair of tetralogy of Fallot
  Pressure overload
    Left-sided obstruction
      Severe aortic stenosis
      Aortic coarctation
    Right-sided obstruction
      Severe pulmonary stenosis
  Complex congenital heart disease
    Single ventricle
      Hypoplastic left heart syndrome
      Unbalanced atrioventricular septal defect
    Systemic right ventricle
      l-transposition ("corrected transposition") of the great arteries
Structurally normal heart
  Primary cardiomyopathy
    Dilated
    Hypertrophic
    Restrictive
  Secondary
    Arrhythmogenic
    Ischemic
    Toxic
    Infiltrative
Infectious

From Hsu DT, Pearson GD: Heart failure in children part I: history, etiology, and pathophysiology, *Circ Heart Fail* 2:63-70, 2009.

Clinical tip

- ↑ Systolic arterial pressure because of ↓ distensibility of arteries
- ↓ Aortic distensibility
- May develop left ventricular hypertrophy if pressure not treated; will subsequently develop diastolic dysfunction
- Other changes are caused by disease and not by the aging process

---

However, other age-associated changes, such as increased systolic arterial pressure and decreased aortic distensibility, probably contribute to the mild-to-moderate left ventricular hypertrophy commonly found in the elderly.[45] This hypertrophy preserves left ventricular systolic function but impairs left ventricular diastolic function. Diastolic dysfunction delays left ventricular filling, which is more profound in the presence of hypertension, coronary artery disease, and higher heart rates.[46] Additionally, increased norepinephrine levels (probably because of decreased catecholamine sensitivity) and decreased baroreceptor sensitivity and plasma renin concentrations have been reported in elderly subjects.[38]

These pathophysiologic processes, as well as other confounding variables such as coronary artery disease, exposure to environmental toxins (cigarette smoking, radiation), malnutrition, and other lifestyle habits, must be considered to accurately document the effects of aging on cardiac and exercise performance. Nonetheless, the consensus regarding the cardiovascular aging process is as follows:[39]

- After neonatal development, the number of myocardial cells in the heart does not increase.
- There is moderate hypertrophy of left ventricular myocardium, probably in response to increased arterial vascular stiffness and dropout of myocytes.
- When myocardial hypertrophy occurs, it is disproportionate to capillary and vascular growth. The ability of the myocardium to generate tension is well maintained as a result of prolonged duration of contraction and greater stiffness despite a modest decrease in the velocity of shortening of cardiac muscle.

- There is a selective decrease in β-adrenergic receptor-mediated inotropic, chronotropic, and vasodilating cardiovascular responses with aging.
- Increased pericardial and myocardial stiffness and delayed relaxation during aging may limit left ventricular filling during stress.

The primary cause of the changes associated with aging has been attributed to one or a combination of three theories: the genome, the physiologic, and the organ theories.[39] The genome theories are based on the programming of genes for aging, death, or both, whereas the physiologic theories (cross-linkage theory) are dependent on specific pathophysiologic processes. The organ theories (primarily immunologic and neuroendocrine) may be the most encompassing because immunologic and neurohormonal dysfunction is hypothesized to produce both general and specific aging effects.[39] Table 4-3 provides a useful overview of the effects of aging.

Cardiac Muscle

Animal studies reveal that the contraction and relaxation times of cardiac muscle are prolonged in aged rats.[47–50] This prolongation "can be attributed to alterations in mechanisms that govern excitation–contraction coupling in the heart,"[39] primarily the increase and decrease of cytosolic calcium in the myofilaments. The rate that the sarcoplasmic reticulum pumps calcium is reduced in hearts of older animals and "appears to be a major contributor to the prolonged transient and prolonged time course of cardiac muscle relaxation."[39] The diminished ability of the sarcoplasmic reticulum to pump

calcium may also be responsible for the following changes observed in elderly animals:

- Prolonged time to peak force and half relaxation time of peak stiffness[51–53]
- Lower muscular twitch force at higher stimulation rates[54]

Pathophysiology

The interdependence and interrelationship between the cardiac and pulmonary systems are demonstrated in the clinical manifestations of heart failure. One of the most common clinical manifestations is pulmonary edema, which is primarily a result of increased pulmonary capillary pressure, although other factors may contribute to its origin (Fig. 4-6). Left ventricular failure is the most common cause of such increased pulmonary capillary pressure, which produces the congestion of CHF. Consequently, the term *CMD* accurately describes the primary cause of pulmonary edema and the underlying pathophysiology of CHF because CMD essentially impairs the heart's ability to pump blood or the LV's ability to accept blood.[5]

The heart's ability to accept and pump blood depends on a number of factors of which the primary variables include total blood volume, body position, intrathoracic pressure, atrial contributions to ventricular filling, pumping action of the skeletal muscle, venous tone, and intrapericardial pressure. Many of these factors are responsible for CMD and CHF. Conversely, many of them can be used to treat the pathophysiology of CMD and CHF. Examples of this include providing supplemental oxygen to decrease myocardial ischemia and subsequently improve myocardial contraction, or using different body positions to either increase or decrease the return of blood to the heart (such as supine vs. sitting positions, respectively). Increased return of blood to the heart as a result of a supine body position could worsen CMD and CHF in a

Table 4-3 Changes and effects of aging	
Change	**Effect**
Decreased vascular elasticity	Increased blood pressure
Left ventricular hypertrophy	Decreased ventricular compliance
Decreased adrenergic responsiveness	Decreased exercise heart rate
Decreased rate of calcium pumped by the sarcoplasmic reticulum	Prolonged time for cardiac muscle relaxation
Prolonged time to peak force of cardiac muscle	Prolonged contraction time of cardiac muscle
Decreased cardiac muscle twitch force	Reduction in the velocity of the cardiac muscle shortening
Decreased rate of adenosine triphosphate (ATP) hydrolysis	Reduction in the velocity of the cardiac muscle shortening
Decreased myosin adenosine triphosphatase (ATPase) activity	Reduction in the velocity of the cardiac muscle shortening
Diastolic dysfunction	Impaired ventricular filling with potential to increase cardiac preload and congestive heart failure
Decreased lean body mass	Decreased muscle strength and peak oxygen consumption

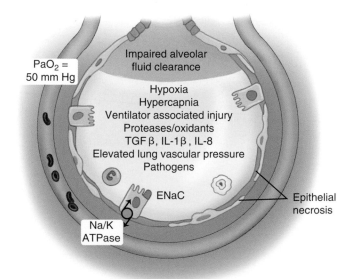

Figure 4-6 Mechanisms responsible for pulmonary edema: Shown are some of the clinically relevant mechanisms that decrease the rate of alveolar fluid clearance in patients with acute respiratory distress syndrome. Type I and type II alveolar epithelial cell necrosis is shown. The loss of epithelial barrier function and the ability to generate net alveolar epithelial sodium and fluid clearance are also depicted. (Modified from Matthay MA: Resolution of pulmonary edema: Thirty years of progress. *Am J Respir Crit Care Med* 189(11):1301-1308, 2014)

person with existing CHF and an increased volume of blood in the ventricles, but the same body position might be beneficial for a person with CHF and decreased volume of blood in the ventricles because of aggressive diuresis to remove fluid from the lungs and various parts of the body.[5]

This apparent ambiguity can be better understood by further discussing Fig. 4-7, in which the volume of blood in

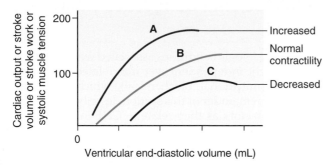

Figure 4-7 Frank–Starling law of the heart. Relationship between length and tension in the heart. End-diastolic volume determines end-diastolic length of ventricular muscle fibers and is proportional to tension generated during systole, as well as to cardiac output, stroke volume, and stroke work. A change in myocardial contractility causes the heart to perform on a different length–tension curve. **A,** Increased contractility; **B,** normal contractility; **C,** heart failure or decreased contractility. (Modified from McCance KL: *Pathophysiology: The Biologic Basis for Disease in Adults and Children,* ed 6, St. Louis, 2010, Mosby.)

the ventricle of the heart (ventricular end-diastolic volume [VEDV]) is plotted against ventricular performance. Excessive VEDV decreases ventricular performance (if extreme, shock can ensue), but lower levels of VEDV tend to improve ventricular performance. However, if the VEDV is inadequate because of decreased body fluid and blood volume or change in body position (both of which may decrease the return of blood to the heart), ventricular performance can worsen. A person with CHF typically has increased VEDV (because of a poorly contracting heart), which can increase further from the increased venous return of a supine position. Other mechanisms can also increase venous return, such as increasing venous tone and the pumping action of skeletal muscle. Even a slight increase in the VEDV of a person with CHF may worsen the CMD and CHF.[5]

Congestive heart failure is often described as a syndrome with many pathophysiologic and compensatory mechanisms that occur in an attempt to maintain an adequate ejection of blood from the ventricle each minute (cardiac output) to the organs and tissues of the body (cardiac index). The following sections help clarify the pathophysiology.

Congestive Heart Failure Descriptions

Congestive heart failure is described in numerous ways based upon the pathophysiology associated with it (Table 4-4). Right-sided or left-sided CHF simply describes which side of

Table 4-4 Co morbidities and impact on disease and prevalence in patients with heart failure diagnosis		
Comorbidity	**Bidirectional Impact on Disease Progression**	**Heart Failure Specifics**
Chronic obstructive pulmonary disease	Inflammation; hypoxia; parenchymal changes; airflow limitation, leading to pulmonary congestion; abnormal left ventricular (LV) diastolic filling; inhaled beta-agonist cardiovascular effects Elevated LV end-diastolic pressure and beta-blocker use may compromise lung function	More prevalent in preserved ejection fraction (HFpEF), compared to reduced (HFrEF) Higher mortality risk in HFpEF
Anemia	Adverse LV remodeling; adverse cardiorenal effects; increased neurohormonal and inflammatory cytokines Inflammation; hemodilution; renal dysfunction; metabolic abnormalities exacerbate	More prevalent in HFpEF Similar increased risk for mortality in both groups
Diabetes	Diabetic cardiomyopathy; mitochondrial dysfunction; abnormal calcium homeostasis; oxidative stress; renin-angiotensin-aldosterone system (RAAS) activation; atherosclerosis; coronary artery disease Incident and worsening diabetes metlitus via sympathetic and RAAS activation	More prevalent in HFpEF Similar increased risk for mortality in both groups
Renal dysfunction	Sodium and fluid retention; anemia; inflammation; RAAS and sympathetic activation Cardiorenal syndrome through low cardiac output; accelerated atherosclerosis; inflammation; increased venous pressure	Similar prevalence in both groups Similar increased risk for mortality in both groups
Sleep disordered breathing	Hypoxia; systemic inflammation; sympathetic activation; arrhythmias; hypertension (pulmonary and systemic); RV dysfunction; worsening congestion Rostral fluid movement may worsen pharyngeal obstruction; instability of ventilatory control system	Similar prevalence in both groups Unknown mortality differential associated with HFpEF vs. HFrEF
Obesity	Inflammation; reduced physical activity and deconditioning; hypertension; metabolic syndrome; diabetes mellitus Fatigue and dyspnea may limit activity; spectrum of metabolic disorders including nutritional deficiencies	More prevalent in HFpEF Obesity paradox; potential for a U-shaped association with mortality
Pathways linking several common comorbidities to disease progression in both heart failure with preserved ejection fraction (HFpEF) and heart failure with reduced ejection fraction (HFrEF) are presented, and factors exacerbating other comorbid conditions are highlighted. These comorbidities are interrelated by several common mechanisms, including inflammation and worsening congestion, as well as by sympathetic and renin-angiotensin-aldosterone system activation. Heart failure influences each of the comorbidities, demonstrating the bidirectional association. From Mentz RJ, et al: *J Am Coll Cardiol* 64(21):2281-2293, 2014.		

the heart is failing, as well as the side that is initially affected and behind which fluid tends to localize. For example, left-sided heart failure is frequently the result of left ventricular insult (e.g., myocardial infarction, hypertension, aortic valve disease), which causes fluid to accumulate behind the LV (left atrium, pulmonary veins, pulmonary capillaries, lungs). If the left-sided failure is severe, there is progressive accumulation beyond the lungs, manifesting itself as right-sided failure.[5] Thus right-sided CHF may occur because of left-sided CHF or because of right ventricular failure (e.g., secondary to pulmonary hypertension, pulmonary embolus, right ventricular infarction). In either case, fluid backs up behind the right ventricle and produces the accumulation of fluid in the liver, abdomen, and bilateral ankles and hands.

Heart failure with reduced ejection fraction (HFrEF) is the description most frequently associated with heart failure and is the result of a low cardiac output at rest or during exertion. Heart failure with preserved ejection fraction (HFpEF) usually results from a volume overload, as may occur in pregnancy, thyrotoxicosis (overactivity of the thyroid gland, such as in Graves disease), and renal insufficiency.[5–7,55–57] It is important to note that although the term *preserved* implies a greater cardiac output, it nonetheless is still lower than it was before CHF developed.

Systolic versus diastolic heart failure is perhaps the most informative and useful distinction in CHF because optimal cardiac performance is dependent on both proper systolic and diastolic functioning. The impaired contraction of the ventricles during systole that produces an inefficient expulsion of blood (low stroke volume) is termed *systolic heart failure*. Diastolic heart failure is associated with an inability of the ventricles to accept the blood ejected from the atria during rest or diastole. Both types are very important in the overall scheme of CHF and often occur simultaneously, as in the patient who suffers a massive anterior myocardial infarction (loss of contracting myocardium, producing systolic heart failure) with subsequent replacement of the infarcted area with nondistensible fibrous scar tissue, which does not readily or adequately accept the blood ejected into the LV from the left atria and produces diastolic heart failure. Despite the various descriptions of CHF just presented, the primary cause of CHF is CMD.

Specific Pathophysiologic Conditions Associated with Congestive Heart Failure

The pathophysiologic conditions associated with CMD appear to involve eight independent, yet interrelated, systems and one process (nutritional/biochemical), which are found in Table 4-5. The remainder of this section describes and explains each of these factors as they relate to CHF in CMD. Fig. 4-8 provides an overview of the specific pathophysiologic areas affected by CHF.

Cardiovascular Function

The pathophysiology of CHF can be understood best by describing the Frank–Starling mechanism. The Frank–Starling mechanism was one of the earliest efforts to better understand cardiac muscle relaxation and contraction or, in essence, "the relation between ventricular filling pressure (or end-diastolic volume) and ventricular mechanical activity,"[58] expressed as the volume output of the heart, or the stroke volume (cardiac output divided by heart rate because CO = HR × SV).

In the early 1900s, Frank and Starling discovered that the stroke volume is dependent on both diastolic cardiac muscle fiber length and myocardial contractility (force of contraction and heart rate).[59] This relationship can be better understood by studying Fig. 4-9, in which left ventricular stroke work is plotted against left ventricular filling pressure. The figure shows that an optimal range of left ventricular filling pressures exists that, when exceeded, decreases left ventricular

Table 4-5 Pathophysiologic conditions associated with congestive heart failure			
	Prevalence (%)	Related with Mortality	McSH-Search (*N* articles)
Anemia	37	Yes	1,010
Cerebral dysfunction	28-58	Yes	407
Cognitive dysfunction	50-60	Yes	116
COFD	10-50	Yes	449
Depression	22	Yes	577
Diabetes	6-44	Yes	2,100
Erectile dysfunction	85	-	36
Gout/hyperuricemia	-	Yes	34
Hypertension	60-70	Yes	4,734
Iron deficiency	50-60	Yes	168
Kidney dysfunction	Up to 55	Yes	1,610
Liver dysfunction	30-60	Yes	521
Sleep apnea	60	Yes	641
Stroke	5	Yes	720

From All comorbidities in heart failure: Summary of all comorbidities in heart failure, including prevalence, hazard ratio for mortality and number of articles by MeSH search. Van deursen VM et al: Comorbidities in heart failure, *Heart Fail Rev* 19:163-172, 2014.

stroke work considerably.[9,58] As the left ventricular filling pressure increases, so does the stretch on cardiac muscle fiber during diastole. Taken a step further, the left ventricular filling pressure is representative of the left VEDV, which determines the degree of stretch on the myocardium.[58,59] This is apparent in Fig. 4-7, which also demonstrates that an optimal range of VEDV (or filling pressure) exists, which, if exceeded or insignificant, decreases ventricular performance. In summary, the following major influences that determine the degree of myocardial stretch should be considered when examining patients with CHF and when developing interventions:[9]

- Atrial contribution to ventricular filling
- Total blood volume
- Body position
- Intrathoracic pressure

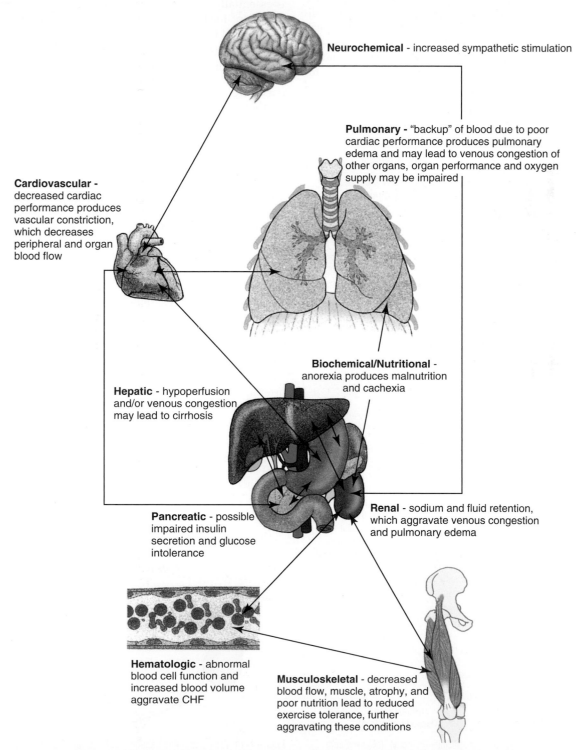

Neurochemical - increased sympathetic stimulation

Pulmonary - "backup" of blood due to poor cardiac performance produces pulmonary edema and may lead to venous congestion of other organs, organ performance and oxygen supply may be impaired

Cardiovascular - decreased cardiac performance produces vascular constriction, which decreases peripheral and organ blood flow

Biochemical/Nutritional - anorexia produces malnutrition and cachexia

Hepatic - hypoperfusion and/or venous congestion may lead to cirrhosis

Pancreatic - possible impaired insulin secretion and glucose intolerance

Renal - sodium and fluid retention, which aggravate venous congestion and pulmonary edema

Hematologic - abnormal blood cell function and increased blood volume aggravate CHF

Musculoskeletal - decreased blood flow, muscle, atrophy, and poor nutrition lead to reduced exercise tolerance, further aggravating these conditions

Figure 4-8 The compensatory and pathophysiologic interrelationships among organs and organ systems affected by congestive heart failure (CHF). (Modified from Cahalin LP: Heart failure, *Phys Ther* 76(5):516, 1996.)

- Intrapericardial pressure
- Venous tone
- Pumping action of skeletal muscle

Stroke volume is the result of the degree of myocardial stretch, as well as that of myocardial contractility. Myocardial contractility (inotropy) is influenced by many variables; Fig. 4-10 lists the major ones.

Despite these major influences, without adequate diastolic filling (and the necessary degree of myocardial stretch), stroke volume remains unchanged. The importance of diastolic filling of the ventricles is apparent in patients who have pericardial effusion (i.e., cardiac tamponade) or myocarditis, who are unable to attain adequate diastolic filling. This situation results in a decreased stroke volume that can be hemodynamically significant, producing a hypoadaptive systolic blood

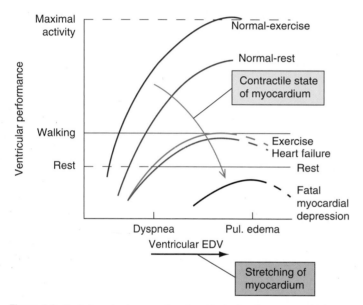

Figure 4-9 Illustration showing a number of ventricular function curves, which depict the relationship between ventricular end-diastolic volume (EDV) through stretching of the myocardium (i.e., the Frank–Starling law of the heart), and the effects of various states of contractility. Sympathetic stimulation, as normally occurs during exercise, increases stroke volume at a given level of ventricular filling, whereas heart failure results in lower stroke volume at a given level of ventricular filling, which may or may not increase during exercise. The dashed lines are the descending limbs of the ventricular performance curves, which are seen only rarely in patients. Levels of ventricular EDV associated with filling pressures that induce dyspnea and pulmonary edema are indicated, along with levels of ventricular performance required during rest, walking, and maximal activity. (Modified from Braunwald E, Ross Jr J, Sonnenblick EH. *Mechanisms of Contraction of the Normal and Failing Heart*, Boston, 1979, Little, Brown. In *Watchie Cardiovascular and Pulmonary Physical Therapy: A Clinical Manual*, ed 2, St. Louis, 2010, Saunders.)

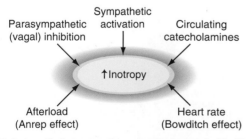

Figure 4-10 Factors affecting myocardial contractility (inotropy) (Modified from Klabunde R: *Cardiovascular Physiology Concepts*, ed 2, Philadelphia, 2012, Lippincott Williams & Wilkins/Wolters Kluwer.)

pressure response to exercise (decrease in systolic blood pressure with increased heart rate).

The left ventricular end-diastolic pressure is often referred to as the *preload*. This filling pressure (the pressure in the LV before the ejection of the stroke volume) is analogous to the pulling backward on the rubber band of a slingshot before releasing the rubber band to eject an object. The afterload is the resistance that the stroke volume encounters after it is ejected from the LV. The resistance (or afterload), therefore, is essentially the peripheral vascular resistance. Much of the treatment for CMD involves lowering both the preload and afterload of the cardiovascular system.

The left ventricular filling pressure discussed earlier can be closely approximated by the pulmonary capillary wedge pressure, which is frequently monitored in patients in coronary care or intensive care units.[60] Left ventricular systolic performance is deteriorating when the pulmonary capillary wedge pressure is greater than 15 to 20 mm Hg.

Biochemical Markers: Natriuretic Peptides Released by Cardiac Muscle

The natriuretic peptides are structurally related but genetically distinct peptides.[61] Atrial natriuretic peptide (ANP) was identified in granules in atria and discovered to also be secreted by endothelial cells. Brain natriuretic peptide (BNP) and its amino-terminal fragment N-terminal pro-B-type natriuretic peptide (NT-proBNP) is stored as proBNP and then cleaved into the inactive NT-proBNP. It was first identified in brain tissue but has now been recognized to be produced by cardiac tissue. *Dendroaspis* natriuretic peptide (DNP) is another peptide that can be measured in human blood; it is elevated with CHF and causes relaxation of isolated arteries.[62–64]

Atrial natriuretic peptide and BNP are released from arterial and cardiac myocytes, respectively, in response to increased stretch resulting from high filling pressure, high arterial pressure, or cardiac dilation (Fig. 4-11). Once released,

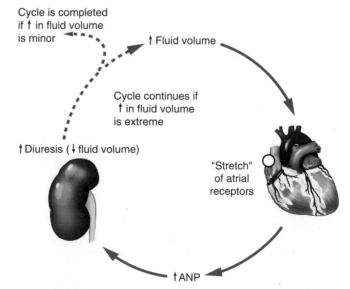

Figure 4-11 Atrial natriuretic peptide (ANP). Elevated vascular volume releases ANP, which increases the glomerular filtration rate (GFR) and facilitates natriuresis and diuresis.

both ANP and BNP bind to receptors in target tissues, such as the aorta, vascular smooth muscle, renal cortex and medulla, and adrenal zona glomerulosa.[24] Both ANP and BNP act to reduce the adverse stimulus of stretch by causing arterio- and venodilation, reduction in blood volume through natriuresis, and suppression of secretions of renin and aldosterone. Although the peptides produce these effects to reduce fluid volume, they are only minor forces, which, unfortunately, are no match for the profound fluid retention produced by the kidneys. Therefore the cause-and-effect relationship between stretch and release of ANP and BNP represents a classical physiologic negative-feedback regulatory system. In general, the natriuretic peptides cause relaxation of vascular smooth muscle but the potency varies depending on the peptide and the anatomic origin of the blood vessel.[65]

Clinicians are increasingly using biochemical markers to diagnose and manage disease states. Levels of plasma BNP are increased in patients with various forms of heart disease, especially those with heart failure.[66] Levels of plasma BNP are also increased in patients with acute coronary syndrome, where it correlates with the degree of left ventricular systolic dysfunction and survival. Although echocardiography is the most widely used method for the confirmation of the clinical diagnosis of heart failure, BNP is rapidly emerging as a very sensitive and specific adjunctive diagnostic marker.[66] Greater levels of ANP and BNP also are associated with higher morbidity and mortality rates.[67,68]

When fluid volume that typically produces increased left VEDV "backs up" into the left atrium, producing elevated atrial pressure, the elevated atrial pressure stimulates the release of a specific regulatory hormone, ANP. Atrial natriuretic peptide is released from atrial myocyte granules when atrial pressure or volume exceeds an unknown value (see Fig. 4-11).[24]

Renal Function

The subtle, yet devastating, effects of the renal system in CHF can be appreciated best in Fig. 4-12, which outlines the five major steps for the initiation and maintenance of renal sodium retention. As previously mentioned, sodium (and ultimately water) is retained in CHF because of inadequate cardiac output.[8,12] The arterial system of the body senses, via renal and extrarenal sensors, that the arterial blood flow is inadequate, often because of a poor cardiac output, and initiates a process to retain fluid (to increase arterial blood flow), which is identical to that initiated in hypovolemic states.[24] In effect, the kidneys in CHF act like those in an individual with a reduced volume of body fluid.

The subsequent retention of sodium and water is a result of several factors:[24]

- Augmented α-adrenergic neural activity;
- Circulating catecholamines (e.g., epinephrine, norepinephrine);
- Increased circulating and locally produced angiotensin II, which results in renal vasoconstriction, thus decreasing the glomerular filtration rate (GFR) and renal blood flow.

These effects increase the renal filtration fraction (the ratio of GFR to renal blood flow), which increases the protein concentration in the peritubular capillaries and results in an increased quantity of sodium reabsorbed in the proximal tubule.[69,70] Fig. 4-13 illustrates the reabsorption process and provides a thorough overview of renal function in CHF.

Laboratory findings suggestive of impaired renal function in CHF include increases in blood urea nitrogen (BUN) or other nitrogenous bodies (azotemia), as well as increased blood creatinine levels. This prerenal azotemia is the result of enhanced water reabsorption in the collecting duct, which becomes more pronounced with increased antidiuretic

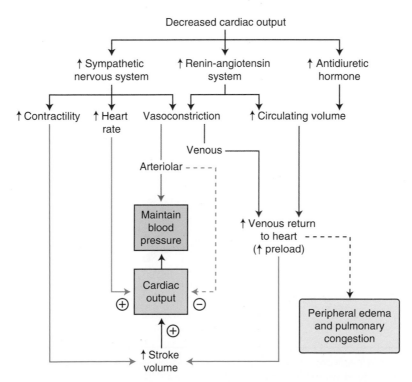

Figure 4-12 Mechanisms of congestive heart failure. Cardiac muscle dysfunction (From Lilly L: Pathophysiology of Heart Disease, ed 6, Philadelphia, 2015, Lippincott Williams & Wilkins.)

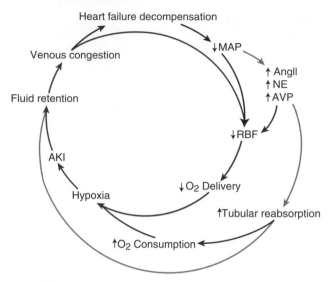

Figure 4-13 Physiologic effects of myocardial failure. The reduced cardiac output in heart failure decompensation leads to reduced mean arterial pressure (MAP), and renal blood flow (RBF), which lowers renal oxygen delivery and may lead to hypoxia and acute kidney injury (AKI). At the same time the neurohormonal signaling; e.g., angiotensin II (ANG II), sympathetic nervous activity (NE), and vasopressin (AVP), reduces RBF and increases tubular reabsorption. Reabsorption in turn increases oxygen consumption, further aggravating hypoxia, while the reabsorbed fluid and AKI exacerbates heart failure decompensation in a vicious circle. (Modified from Jonsson S, Becirovic Agic M, Melville JM, Hultstrom M: Renal neurohomronal regulation in heart failure decompensation, *Am J Physiol* 307(5):R493-R497, 2014.)

hormone levels and which augments the passive reabsorption of urea.[24] An increase in urea production, a decrease in excretion of urine, and an increased BUN may occur even before a decrease in GFR. A decreased GFR is the primary reason for the increased BUN and serum creatinine levels commonly seen in patients with CHF.[24]

> **Clinical tip**
>
> Laboratory findings of impaired renal function: increased BUN and increased blood creatinine levels.

Pulmonary Function

Pulmonary edema can be cardiogenic (hemodynamic) or noncardiogenic (caused by alterations in the pulmonary capillary membrane) in origin.[5] The differential diagnosis can be made by history, physical examination, and laboratory examination, as shown in Fig. 4-6. Despite the different origins of pulmonary edema, the sequence of liquid accumulation is similar for both and appears to consist of three distinct stages (Fig. 4-14):

- **Stage I (see Fig. 4-14, A).** Difficult to detect or quantify because it seems to represent "increased lymph flow without net gain of interstitial liquid."[71] The edema

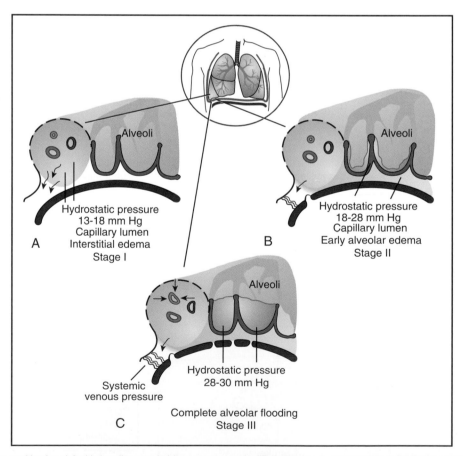

Figure 4-14 Pulmonary edema resulting from left-sided cardiac muscle failure may present in different stages. **A,** In stage I, the redistribution stage, interstitial edema results from an elevated capillary pressure (13-18 mm Hg), which forces fluid (plasma) into the interstitial area. **B,** In stage II, early alveolar edema occurs when the capillary hydrostatic pressure is significantly elevated (18-28 mm Hg), causing fluid to move from the capillary, invade the interstitium, and cross the alveolar membrane. **C,** In stage III, complete alveolar flooding occurs when the capillary hydrostatic pressure is severely elevated (>28 mm Hg), causing fluid to flood the alveoli and possibly invade the large airways.

associated with the increased lymph flow may actually improve gas exchange in the lung as more of the small pulmonary vessels are distended. However, if lymph flow continues, pulmonary edema increases, and the airways and vessels become filled with increased amounts of liquid, particularly in the gravity-dependent portions of the lung.[71]

- **Stage II (see Fig. 4-14, B).** Accumulation of liquid compromises the small airway lumina, resulting in a mismatch between ventilation and perfusion, which produces hypoxemia and wasted ventilation. Tachypnea of CHF often ensues.[71] In addition, the degree of hypoxemia appears to be correlated to the degree of elevation of the pulmonary capillary wedge pressure.[72]
- **Stage III (see Fig. 4-14, C).** As lymph flow continues, edema increases in the vascular system and interstitium, increasing the pulmonary capillary wedge pressure and eventually flooding the alveoli known as pulmonary edema, which significantly compromises gas exchange, producing severe hypoxemia and hypercapnia.[71] In addition, severe alveolar flooding can produce the following: (1) filling of the large airways with blood-tinged foam, which can be expectorated; (2) reductions in most lung volumes (e.g., vital capacity); (3) a right-to-left intrapulmonary shunt; and (4) hypercapnia with acute respiratory acidosis.[71]

Perhaps the most important principle regarding pulmonary edema is that of maintaining pulmonary capillary pressures at the lowest possible levels.[71] Pulmonary edema can be decreased by more than 50% when pulmonary capillary wedge pressures are decreased from 12 to 6 mm Hg.

The effect of repeated bouts of pulmonary edema (which is common in CHF) upon pulmonary function appears to be profound. More advanced CHF may produce a "global respiratory impairment" that is associated with varying degrees of obstructive and restrictive lung disease.[73,74]

Neurohumoral Effects

The neurohumoral system profoundly affects heart function in physiologic (fight-or-flight mechanism) and pathologic states (CMD). In general, the neural effects are much more rapid, whereas humoral effects are slower because the information sent by the autonomic nervous system via efferent nerves travels faster than the information traveling through the vascular system.[75]

Normal Cardiac Neurohumoral Function

Neurohumoral signals to the heart are perceived, interpreted, and augmented by the transmembrane signal transduction systems in myocardial cells.[75] The primary signaling system in the heart appears to be the receptor-G-protein-adenylate cyclase (RGC) complex as it regulates myocardial contractility. Fig. 4-15 illustrates the complexity of this system, which consists of (1) membrane receptors; (2) guanine nucleotide–binding regulatory proteins (the G proteins, which transmit stimulatory or inhibitory signals); and (3) adenylate cyclase, which converts adenosine triphosphate (ATP) to cyclic adenosine monophosphate (cAMP). Adenylate cyclase is an effector enzyme activated by a receptor agonist, thus enhancing cAMP synthesis. The lower portion of Fig. 4-10 shows that increased cAMP

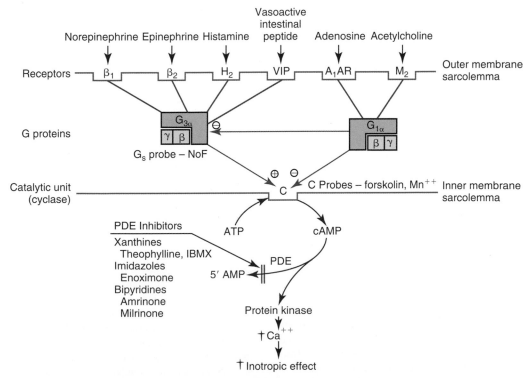

Figure 4-15 Neural control of cardiopulmonary function. The receptor-G-protein-adenylate cyclase complex and other important receptors, all of which affect the inotropic state of the heart. *ATP,* Adenosine triphosphate; *cAMP,* cyclic adenosine monophosphate; *Gs,* G-stimulatory protein; *G1,* G-inhibitory protein; *IBMX,* isobutyl methylxanthine; *PDE,* phosphodiesterase.

synthesis ultimately increases the force of myocardial contraction (the inotropic effect).[75]

The top portion of Fig. 4-15 shows the receptor agonists responsible for the initial activation of the RGC complex. These agents include norepinephrine, epinephrine, histamine, vasoactive intestinal peptide, adenosine, and acetylcholine.

Although Fig. 4-15 shows the complete system, it does not reveal the degree of influence each receptor agonist has on cardiac function. In general, the most influential receptor agonists are the sympathetic neurotransmitters norepinephrine and epinephrine, as they relay excitatory autonomic nervous system stimuli to both postsynaptic α- and β-adrenergic receptors (primarily β for norepinephrine) in the myocardium.[75] Inhibitory autonomic nervous system stimuli are transmitted by the parasympathetic nervous system via the vagus nerve and the neurotransmitter acetylcholine. The adrenergic receptors (α_1, α_2, β_1, and β_2) are discussed briefly in the next paragraphs so that Fig. 4-15 can be appreciated fully, as are the neurohumoral changes that accompany CMD.

α-Adrenergic Receptors

Stimulation of α_1-adrenergic receptors appears to activate the phosphodiesterase transmembrane signaling system,[76,77] which increases phosphodiesterase and activates protein kinase, thus marginally increasing the inotropic effect.[78] Conversely, stimulation of α_2-adrenergic receptors activates the inhibitory G protein and inhibits adenylate cyclase, which decreases the inotropic effect.[79]

β-Adrenergic Receptors

The importance of the β-adrenergic pathway cannot be overemphasized because it has been proposed that the heart is a β-adrenergic organ.[80] Two β-adrenergic receptors have been identified, β_1 and β_2, which are "distinguished by their differing affinities for the agonists epinephrine and norepinephrine." The β_2-adrenergic receptor has a 30-fold greater affinity for epinephrine than for norepinephrine.[81] In brief, β_2-adrenergic receptor stimulation promotes vasodilation of the capillary beds and muscle relaxation in the bronchial tracts, whereas β_1-adrenergic receptor stimulation increases heart rate and myocardial force of contraction.[75]

Guanine Nucleotide–Binding Regulatory Proteins

As briefly discussed, the G proteins transmit stimulatory (Gs) or inhibitory (G1) signals to the catalytic unit (inner membrane sarcolemma) of myocardial contractile tissue. The stimulatory and inhibiting signals are dependent on a very complex, and only partially understood, mechanism of receptor-mediated activation.

Catalytic Unit of Adenylate Cyclase

The activation of adenylate cyclase (and subsequent increase in myocardial force of contraction) is, unfortunately, poorly understood but has been observed to be decreased in patients with CHF. This decrease is the result of "a paradoxical diminution in the function of the RGC complex,"[75] which alters the receptor–effector coupling and "limits the ability of both endogenous and exogenous adrenergic agonists to augment cardiac contractility."[75] The inability of endogenous (produced in the body) or exogenous (medications) adrenergic agonists to increase the force of myocardial contraction is frequently seen in patients with CHF, and may be a contributing factor in CMD.[75,82]

Neurohumoral Alterations in the Failing Human Heart

Abnormalities in Sympathetic Neural Function

The sympathetic neural function of the heart is profoundly affected in CHF. The effects are primarily caused by abnormal RGC complex function, despite interstitial (in the interspaces of the myocardium), intrasynaptic, and systemwide increased concentrations of norepinephrine.[75]

The abnormal RGC complex function in CHF appears to be associated with the insensitivity of the failing heart to β-adrenergic stimulation.[75] This insensitivity to β-adrenergic stimulation is apparently the result of a decrease in β_1-adrenergic receptor density[75] and is very important because the heart contains a ratio of 3.3:1.0 β_1- to β_2-adrenergic receptors.[75] In CHF, the ratio decreases to approximately 1.5:1.0, producing a 62% decrease in the β_1-adrenergic receptors and no significant increase in β_2 density.[83,84] Although the number of β_2 receptors does not appear to change in CHF, the β_2 receptor "is partially 'uncoupled' from the effector enzyme adenylate cyclase."[82,85] This uncoupling only mildly desensitizes the β_2-adrenergic receptors, which initially are able to compensate for the decreased number of β_1 receptors by providing substantial inotropic support.[86] The duration of inotropic support appears to be short lived, and myocardial failure becomes more pronounced.[75]

> ### Clinical tip
>
> Excessive sympathetic nervous system stimulation occurs in CHF, and because of abnormalities in particular parts of the neurohumoral system, the heart becomes insensitive to β-adrenergic stimulation, which results in a decreased force of myocardial contraction and an inability to attain higher heart rates during physical exertion. This is where the role of β blockers plays a major part in treatment of CHF.

Hepatic Function

The fluid overload associated with CHF affects practically all organs and body systems, including liver function. Increased fluid volume eventually leads to hepatic venous congestion, which prevents adequate perfusion of oxygen to hepatic tissues. Subsequent hypoxemia from the hypoperfusion produces cardiac cirrhosis, which is characterized histologically by central lobular necrosis, atrophy, extensive fibrosis, and occasionally sclerosis of the hepatic veins.[10]

> ### Clinical tip
>
> Hepatomegaly, or liver enlargement, is frequently associated with CHF and can be identified readily as tenderness in the right upper quadrant of the abdomen. Patients with longstanding CHF, however, are generally not tender to palpation, although hepatomegaly is frequently present. Laboratory values showing liver involvement include abnormal aspartate aminotransferase (AST), bilirubin, and lactate dehydrogenase (LDH-5).

Hematologic Function

The normal morphology of the blood and blood-forming tissues is frequently disrupted in CHF. The most common abnormality is a secondary polycythemia (excess of red corpuscles in the blood), which is a result of either a reduction in oxygen transport or an increase in erythropoietin production.[87] Erythropoietin is an α_2-globulin responsible for red blood cell production, and its important role is demonstrated in Fig. 4-16. This figure shows that the hypoxia occasionally observed in patients with CHF may stimulate erythropoietin production, which increases not only red blood cell mass, but also blood volume, in an already compromised cardiopulmonary system (partly because of fluid volume overload). This potentially vicious circle can progress and cause cardiopulmonary function to deteriorate further.

Clinically, anemia (low hemoglobin and hematocrit), which may be present in some patients with CHF, is a paradox, for when it is severe it can cause CHF independently, but when it precedes CHF, anemia may actually allow for more efficient and effective cardiac function.[87] Improved cardiac output may occur because blood viscosity is reduced in patients with anemia, which subsequently decreases systemic vascular resistance. Consequently, anemia acts as an afterload reducer and may promote an increased cardiac output, but at the cost of lower arterial oxygen and oxygen saturation levels, as well as increased work for the heart.[87] Such a condition (and others) is termed "a shift in the oxyhemoglobin curve." The curve can be shifted to the right or left but normally follows the pattern depicted in Fig. 2-10 which represents a specific percentage of oxygen saturation for a given concentration of arterial oxygen. Oxygen saturation remains relatively stable, with arterial oxygen concentrations greater than 60 mm Hg, but below this level, the oxygen saturation drops dramatically. Table 4-6 shows the oxygen saturation levels when arterial oxygen concentrations are less than 60 mm Hg.

Various conditions move this normal curve to the right or left, and these changes subsequently affect the respective oxygen saturation. For example, anemia shifts the curve to the right, representing a lower concentration of arterial oxygen, which moves the critical point of oxygen saturation to

70 mm Hg (therefore to the right). This means that at levels of less than 70 mm Hg, the level of oxygen saturation decreases dramatically compared with the normal level of 60 mm Hg. Thus patients with anemia have less reserve before their oxygen stores desaturate.[87]

> **Clinical tip**
>
> Treatment for severe anemia often involves blood transfusion; however, a blood transfusion may increase the heart's work because of the increase in volume and subsequently increased preload on a weak heart. The patient with a poor performing heart should be monitored carefully after blood transfusions, including heart rate, dyspnea, SpO_2 (oxygen saturation measured by pulse oximetry), blood pressure, and other symptoms.

Also of concern for patients with advanced CMD is the state of hemostasis (the mechanical and biochemical aspects of platelet function and coagulation), which is frequently disrupted as a result of accompanying liver disease.[5] Inhibition of platelet function to the point at which the platelet count drops below 150,000 cells/μL is termed *thrombocytopenia* and is caused by hereditary factors or drugs, or often is acquired from systemic disease.[88] Inherited thrombocytopenia is uncommon; however, thrombocytopenia caused by drugs is much more common and frequently is an adverse reaction associated with use of aspirin, corticosteroids, antimicrobial agents (penicillins and cephalothins), phosphodiesterase inhibitors (dipyridamole), caffeine, sympathetic blocking agents (β antagonists), and heparin.[88] Acquired disorders of platelet function are a common complication of renal failure. This is usually corrected by renal dialysis, but patients with chronic CHF may demonstrate a mild-to-moderate level of platelet dysfunction.[88]

> **Clinical tip**
>
> Hematologic impairments in CHF consist of the following: possible polycythemia, possible anemia (if present, oxygen saturation should be monitored), and possible hemostasis abnormalities such as thrombocytopenia (monitoring laboratory blood values is recommended).

Skeletal Muscle Function

Skeletal muscle myopathy has been identified in patients with CHF and in those with CHF and preexisting cardiomyopathy.[89,90] Among the causes of heart failure, including coronary

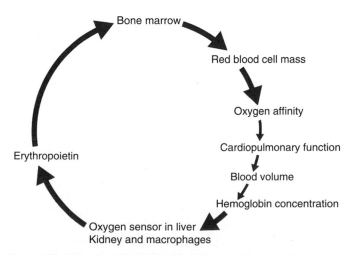

Figure 4-16 Mechanisms of hematologic function. Hematologic function is occasionally disrupted in congestive heart failure and can further impair cardiopulmonary function and patient status.

Bone marrow → Red blood cell mass → Oxygen affinity → Cardiopulmonary function → Blood volume → Hemoglobin concentration → Oxygen sensor in liver / Kidney and macrophages → Erythropoietin → Bone marrow

Table 4-6 Relationship of PaO₂ to SpO₂			
	Oxygen Saturation		
PaO₂ (mm Hg) (partial pressure of arterial oxygen)	40%	50%	60%
SpO₂ (%) (oxygen saturation measured by pulse oximetry)	70%	80%	90%

artery disease, high blood pressure, and diabetes, skeletal muscle diseases can also cause cardiomyopathy and lead to heart failure.

Skeletal muscle dysfunction in patients with CHF has been studied far less in patients without cardiomyopathy than in patients with cardiomyopathy. A review by Limongelli et al defines the link between heart and skeletal muscle dysfunction and lists the disease, noncardiac phenotype, and the corresponding cardiomyopathy. Charcot–Marie–Tooth disease; myofibrillar myopathy and degeneration; Friedreich's ataxia; glycogen storage disease; Danon disease; carnitine deficiency; Barth syndrome; myoadenylate deaminase deficiency; ocular myopathies; neuropathy, ataxia, and retinitis pigmentosa (NARP) syndrome; and Kearns–Sayre syndrome all contribute to hypertrophic, dilated cardiomyopathies and will require management of arrhythmias, including pacemaker/automatic implantable cardioverter-defibrillator (AICD) or transplantation. Muscular dystrophies of all types lead to a higher incidence of dilated cardiomyopathies and hypertrophic cardiomyopathies with a risk of sudden cardiac death. To quote Limongelli et al: "Adult and pediatric cardiologists should be aware that skeletal muscle weakness may indicate a primary neuromuscular disorder…, a mitochondrial disease…a [glycogen] storage disorder… or metabolic disorder. In such patients, skeletal muscle weakness usually precedes cardiomyopathies and dominates the clinical picture. On the other hand, skeletal involvement may be subtle, and the first symptom of a neuromuscular disorder may be the occurrence of heart failure, conduction disorders or ventricular arrhythmias due to cardiomyopathy.… Early screening with ECG and echocardiogram and eventually, a more detailed cardiovascular evaluation should be performed to diagnose early cardiac involvement in patients with skeletal muscle weakness."[91]

Skeletal muscle abnormalities caused by dilated and hypertrophic cardiomyopathies have been reported previously and have consistently revealed type I and type II muscle fiber atrophy.[92–99] Patients with CHF and cardiomyopathy have been found to have three distinct skeletal muscle abnormalities: selective atrophy of type II fibers, pronounced nonselective myopathy, and hypotrophy of type I fibers.[89] Isometric maximal muscle strength of persons with CHF appears to be reduced to nearly 50% of the value for age-, sex-, and weight-matched control subjects. Loss of muscle strength will result in each muscle fiber operating nearer to its maximal capacity for a given absolute power output. Consequently, the changes in skeletal muscle metabolism that are associated with fatigue might be expected to occur at lower absolute workloads and hence to limit maximal exercise capacity in these patients.[90]

Pancreatic Function

Severe CMD can potentially reduce blood flow to the pancreas "as a consequence of splanchnic visceral vasoconstriction, which accompanies severe left ventricular failure."[100] The reduction in blood flow to the pancreas impairs insulin secretion and glucose tolerance, which are further impaired by increased sympathetic nervous system activity and augmented circulatory catecholamines (inhibiting insulin secretion) that stimulate glycogenolysis and elevate blood sugar levels.[101]

Reduced secretion of insulin is of paramount importance because hypoxic and dysfunctional heart muscle depends a great deal on the energy from the metabolism of

glucose, which is reduced significantly if insulin secretion is impaired.[100] Ultimately, there is further deterioration of left ventricular function, creating a vicious circle.

Normally, the heart obtains 60% to 90% of its energy requirements from the oxidation of free fatty acids.[102] The oxidation of free fatty acids increases the production of acetylcoenzyme A (acetyl-CoA) limiting carbohydrate metabolism.[102] However, as previously noted, myocardial ischemia (because of the limited supply of oxygen) inhibits the oxidation of free fatty acids, thus preventing the transport of cytosolic acyl-coenzyme A (acyl-CoA) to the mitochondria for oxidation. Increased intracellular concentrations of acyl-CoA produce inhibition of adenine nucleotide translocase, which is important for myocardial energy metabolism because it transports ATP synthesized in the mitochondria to the cytosol.[102,103]

This final inhibition of adenine nucleotide translocase may be a key factor contributing to myocardial dysfunction.[102]

Finally, CMD and CHF are common in persons with diabetes and are important risk factors for the development of cardiomyopathy. Such a relationship clearly identifies the important roles nutrition and proper biochemical functions have in cardiovascular disease.

Nutritional and Biochemical Aspects

Nutritional concerns are very important when assessing and treating patients with CMD. Stomach and intestinal abnormalities are not uncommon in these patients, who frequently receive many medications with profound side effects.[104] In addition, the interrelated disease processes occurring in other organs because of CMD and CHF frequently produce anorexia, which leads ultimately to malnutrition. The primary malnutrition is a protein-calorie deficiency, but vitamin deficiencies have also been observed (folic acid, thiamine, and hypocalcemia-accompanied vitamin D deficiency).[104] These deficient states may simply be the result of decreased intake, but "abnormal intestinal absorption and increased rates of excretion may also contribute."[104]

Protein-calorie deficiency is common in chronic CHF because of cellular hypoxia and hypermetabolism that frequently produce cachexia (malnutrition and wasting).[104] A catabolic state may also develop, yielding an excess of urea or other nitrogenous compounds in the blood (azotemia). This causes a vicious circle, which, because of gastrointestinal hypoxia and decreased appetite (anorexia) and protein intake, produces cardiac atrophy and more pronounced CMD.[104]

One particular area of concern is thiamine deficiency because of improper nutrition, which can affect this population dramatically. The force of myocardial contraction and cardiac performance in general appears to be dependent on the level of thiamine, and it has been suggested that "the possibility of thiamine deficiency should be considered in many patients with heart failure of obscure origin."[55] In addition, patients undergoing prolonged treatment with furosemide (Lasix)—the first drug of choice in the treatment of CHF—have demonstrated significant thiamine deficiency, which may improve with replacement.[105]

Two other nutritional concerns include carnitine deficiency and coenzyme Q10. Skeletal muscle carnitine deficiency has been observed in a small population of patients with hypertrophic cardiomyopathy and has been linked with genetic causes.[91] When carnitine was replenished, cardiac symptoms and echocardiographic parameters apparently improved.[106] In addition, substantial literature supports the supplementation of coenzyme Q10 in persons with CHF deficient in this apparently important biochemical component, which appears to have a role in the essential function of mitochondria, antioxidation of heart muscle, and cardiostimulation.[107–111]

Individuals with CHF and renal dysfunction may also demonstrate:

- Decreased production of erythropoietin (a hormone synthesized in the kidney that is an important precursor of red blood cell production in bone marrow), causing anemia and possibly less free fatty acid oxidation[112,113]
- Potential for decreased calcium absorption from the gastrointestinal tract,[114] as well as the development of hyperparathyroidism[115]
- Impaired gluconeogenesis and lipid metabolism, as well as degradation of several peptides, proteins, and peptide hormones, including insulin, glucagon, growth hormone, and parathyroid hormone.[116]

Individuals with CHF may benefit from enteral or parenteral products to improve nutrition and the biochemical profile.

Clinical tip

There are several nutritional and biochemical aspects of CHF, including malnutrition (this may occur), thiamine and carnitine deficiency (this should be considered in patients with CHF of obscure origin), and a deficiency of coenzyme Q10 (supplementation appears to improve myocardial performance and functional status).

Clinical Manifestations of Congestive Heart Failure

Heart failure is commonly associated with several characteristic signs and symptoms (Box 4-2).

BOX 4-2 Characteristic signs and symptoms of heart failure

1. Dyspnea
2. Tachypnea
3. Paroxysmal nocturnal dyspnea (PND)
4. Orthopnea
5. Peripheral edema
6. Cold, pale, and possibly cyanotic extremities
7. Weight gain
8. Hepatomegaly
9. Jugular venous distension
10. Rales (crackles)
11. Tubular breath sounds and consolidation
12. Presence of an S_3 heart sound
13. Sinus tachycardia
14. Decreased exercise tolerance or physical work capacity

Symptoms of Congestive Heart Failure

Dyspnea

Dyspnea (breathlessness, or air hunger) is probably the most common finding associated with CHF and is frequently the result of poor gas transport between the lungs and the cells of the body. The cause of poor transport at the lungs is often excessive blood and extracellular fluid in the alveoli and interstitium, interfering with diffusion and causing a reduction in vital capacity.[5] However, the cause of poor transport at the cellular level may be less apparent. Inadequate oxygen supply either at rest or during muscular activity increases the frequency of breathing (respiratory rate) or the amount of air exchanged (tidal volume) or both.[117] For this reason, subjects with CHF characteristically complain of easily provoked dyspnea or, in severe cases of CHF, dyspnea at rest.

Paroxysmal Nocturnal Dyspnea

Another common complaint of individuals suffering from CHF is paroxysmal nocturnal dyspnea (PND), in which sudden, unexplained episodes of shortness of breath occur as patients with CHF assume a more supine position to sleep.[5] After a period of time in a supine position, excessive fluid fills the lungs. Earlier in the day, this fluid is shunted to the lower extremities and the lower portions of the lungs because upright positions and activities permit more effective minute ventilation (V) and perfusion (Q) of the lungs (correcting the V/Q mismatch) and the effects of gravity keep the lungs relatively fluid free. Individuals who suffer from PND frequently place the head of the bed on blocks or sleep with more than two pillows. Patients with marked CHF often assume a sitting position to sleep and are sometimes found sleeping in a recliner instead of a bed.[5]

Orthopnea

The term *orthopnea* describes the development of dyspnea in the recumbent position.[5] Sleeping with two or more pillows elevates the upper body to a more upright position and enables gravity to draw excess fluid from the lungs to the more distal parts of the body. The severity of CHF can sometimes be inferred from the number of pillows used to prevent orthopnea. Thus the terms *two-, three-, four-, or more pillow orthopnea* indirectly allude to the severity of CHF (e.g., four-pillow orthopnea suggests more severe CHF than two-pillow orthopnea).

Signs Associated with Congestive Heart Failure

Breathing Patterns

A rapid respiratory rate at rest, characterized by quick and shallow breaths, is common in patients with CHF. Such tachypnea is apparently not caused by hypoxemia, but rather by stimulation of stretch receptors in the interstitium stimulated by increased pressure or fluid. The quick, shallow breathing of tachypnea may assist the pumping action of the lymphatic vessels, thus minimizing or delaying the increase in interstitial liquid.[71]

A clinical finding observed in many patients with CMD is extreme dyspnea after a change in position, most frequently from sitting to standing. This response appears to be occasionally but inconsistently associated with orthostatic hypotension and increased heart rate activity. The orthostatic hypotension and dyspnea (tachypnea) may be the result of (1) lower extremity muscle deconditioning, producing a pooling of blood in the lower extremities when standing, with a subsequent decrease in blood flow to the heart and lungs, which may result in marked dyspnea and increased heart rates; and/or (2) attenuation of the natriuretic peptide factor (ANP/BNP), which may suggest advanced atrial distension and poor left ventricular function.[118] It appears that the more pronounced the dyspnea, the more severe the CMD, and vice versa. This pattern of breathing, therefore, is another clinical finding that can be timed (time for the dyspnea to subside) and occasionally measured (blood pressure and heart rate) to document progress or deterioration in patient status.

In addition, frequently associated with CHF is a breathing pattern characterized by waxing and waning depths of respiration with recurring periods of apnea. Although the Scottish physician John Cheyne and the Irish physician William Stokes first observed this breathing pattern in asthmatics and thus coined the term *Cheyne–Stokes respiration*, it has been observed in individuals who are suffering central nervous system damage (particularly those in comas) and in individuals with CMD.[5]

Clinical tip

Patients with CHF often demonstrate breathing impairments, including tachypnea, resting dyspnea, dyspnea with exertion, occasional dyspnea with positional change (with or without orthostatic hypotension), and/or waxing and waning depth of breathing (Cheyne–Stokes respiration).

Rales (Crackles)

Pulmonary rales, sometimes referred to as *crackles*, are abnormal breath sounds that, if associated with CHF, occur during inspiration and represent the movement of fluid in the alveoli and subsequent opening of alveoli that previously were closed because of excessive fluid.[5] This sound is produced in the body with the opening of alveoli and airways that previously had no air; after the sound associated with such an opening is transmitted through the tissues overlying the lungs, the characteristic sound of rales is identical to that of hair near the ears being rubbed between two fingers. Rales are frequently heard at both lung bases in individuals with CHF, but may extend upward, depending on the patient's position, the severity of CHF, or both. Therefore auscultation of all lobes should be performed in a systematic manner, allowing for bilateral comparison.

The importance of the presence and magnitude of rales was addressed in 1967 and provided data for the Killip and Kimball classification of patients with acute myocardial infarction.[119] Table 4-7 defines classes I through IV, each of which is associated with an approximate mortality rate.[120] Individuals with rales extending over more than 50% of the lung fields were observed to have a very poor prognosis.

Heart Sounds

Heart sounds can provide a great deal of information regarding cardiopulmonary status but unfortunately are ignored in most physical therapy examinations. The normal heart sounds include a first heart sound (S_1), which represents closure of the mitral and tricuspid valves, and a second sound (S_2), which represents closure of the aortic and pulmonary valves. The most common abnormal heart sounds are the third (S_3) and fourth (S_4), which occur at specific times in the cardiac cycle as a result of abnormal cardiac mechanics. An S_3 heart sound may be normal in children and young adults and is termed a *physiologic normal* S_3.[121] An S_4 is presystolic (heard before S_1), and S_3 occurs during early diastole, after S_2. The presence of an S_3 indicates a noncompliant LV and occurs as blood passively fills a poorly relaxing LV that appears to make contact with the chest wall during early diastole.[121] The presence of an S_3 is considered the hallmark of CHF.[122] There are several reasons why the left ventricle may be noncompliant, of which fluid overload and myocardial scarring (via myocardial infarction or cardiomyopathy) appear to be the most common.

The presence of an S_4 represents "vibrations of the ventricular wall during the rapid influx of blood during atrial contraction" from an exaggerated atrial contraction (atrial "kick").[121] It is commonly heard in patients with hypertension, left ventricular hypertrophy, increased left ventricular end-diastolic pressure, pulmonary hypertension, and pulmonary stenosis.[121]

Auscultation of the heart (Fig. 4-17) may also reveal adventitious (additional) sounds, most frequently murmurs. Murmurs not only are common in patients with CMD, but also appear to be of great clinical significance. Stevenson and coworkers demonstrated that the systolic murmur of secondary mitral regurgitation was an important marker in the treatment of a subgroup of patients with congestive cardiomyopathy.[123] The

---

Table 4-7 The Killip and Kimball classification of patients with acute myocardial infarction

	Definition	NSTEMI Mortality Rate at 30 Days	STEMI Mortality Rate at 30 Days	NSTEMI Mortality Rate at 5 Years	STEMI Mortality Rate at 5 Years
Class I	No clinical signs of heart failure	5	4	19	18
Class II	Rales in the lungs, third heart sound, JVD	10	10	25	28
Class III	Acute pulmonary edema	27	12	32	29
Class IV	Cardiogenic shock or arterial hypotension and evidence of peripheral vasoconstriction	35	24	58	45

Mortality rates of 1906 documented AMI patients admitted to CCU. Killip classification as a significant, sustained, consistent predictor and independent of relevant covariables
Data from Gallindo de Mello BH, et al. Validation of the Killip–Kimball Classification and Late Mortality after Acute Myocardial Infarction. *Arq Bras Cardiol* 103(2):107-117, 2014.

patients who benefited from afterload (the resistance to ventricular ejection or peripheral vascular resistance) reduction were those with a very large LV (left ventricular end-diastolic dimension >60 cm) and a resultant systolic murmur.[123] This study demonstrated the importance of auscultation of the heart at rest and immediately after exercise in persons with CHF to gain insight into the dynamics of myocardial activity.

Peripheral Edema

Peripheral edema frequently accompanies CHF, but in some clinical situations it may be absent when, in fact, a patient has significant CHF.[5] In CHF, fluid is retained and not excreted because the pressoreceptors of the body sense a decreased volume of blood as a result of the heart's inability to pump an adequate amount of blood. The pressoreceptors subsequently relay a message to the kidneys to retain fluid so that a greater volume of blood can be ejected from the heart to the peripheral tissue.[69] Unfortunately, this compounds the problem and makes the heart work even harder, which further decreases its pumping ability. The retained fluid commonly accumulates bilaterally in the dependent extracellular spaces of the periphery.[5] Dependent spaces, such as the ankles and pretibial areas, tend to accumulate the majority of fluid and can be measured by applying firm pressure to the pretibial area for 10 to 20 seconds, then measuring the resultant indentation in the skin (pitting edema). This is frequently graded as mild, moderate, or severe, or it is given a numerical value, depending on the measured scale (Table 4-8). Peripheral edema can also accumulate in the sacral area (the shape of which resembles the popular fanny packs) or in the abdominal area (ascites). By using the pitting edema scale to determine the severity and location of peripheral edema (pretibial or sacral, distal or proximal) and obtaining girth measurements of the lower extremities and the abdomen, important information regarding patient status can be obtained. However, it should be noted that peripheral edema is a sign that is associated with many other pathologies and does not by itself imply CHF.

Jugular Venous Distention

Jugular venous distension also results from fluid overload. As fluid is retained and the heart's ability to pump is further compromised, the retained fluid "backs up," not only into the lungs, but also into the venous system, of which the jugular veins are the simplest to identify and evaluate. The external jugular vein lies medial to the external jugular artery, and with an individual in a 45-degree semirecumbent position, it can be readily measured for signs of distension. Although individuals with marked CHF may demonstrate jugular venous distension in all positions (supine, semisupine, and erect), typically, jugular venous distension is measured when the head of the bed is elevated to 45 degrees.[60,121] The degree of elevation should be noted, as well as the magnitude of distension (mild, moderate, severe). Normally, the level is less than 3 to 5 cm above the sternal angle of Louis. Measurements of the internal jugular vein may be more reliable than those of the external jugular vein. Nonetheless, the highest point of visible pulsation is determined as the trunk and head are elevated, and the vertical distance between this level and the level of the sternal angle of Louis is recorded (Fig. 4-18).[71,121]

Evaluation of the jugular waveforms can also be performed in this position, but catheterization of the pulmonary artery for assessment of pulmonary arterial pressures provides the greatest amount of information. A tremendous amount of information can be projected to a hemodynamic monitor, where the pulmonary artery pressure can be assessed and specific waveforms may be observed. The A

Table 4-8 Pitting edema scale	
Edema Characteristics	**Score**
Barely perceptible depression (pit)	1+
Easily identified depression (EID) (skin rebounds to its original contour within 15 sec)	2+
EID (skin rebounds to its original contour within 15 to 30 sec)	3+
EID (rebound >30 sec)	4+

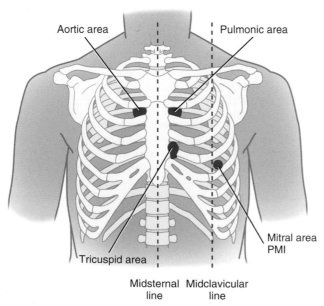

Figure 4-17 Primary auscultatory areas. Auscultation of the heart is performed in a systematic fashion using both the bell and diaphragm of the stethoscope at the indicated sites.

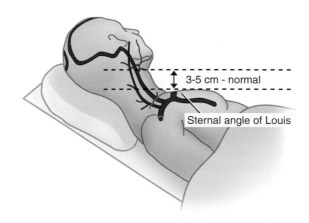

Figure 4-18 Evaluation of venous pressure. Elevated venous pressure frequently represents right-sided and left-sided heart failure, which is characterized by pulmonary congestion and distension of the external jugular vein that is greater than 3 to 5 cm above the sternal angle of Louis.

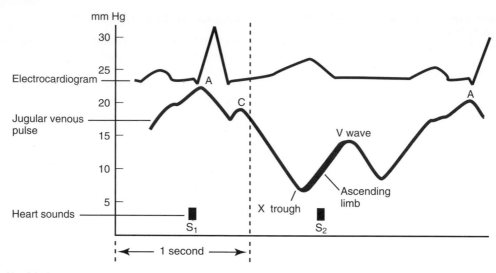

Figure 4-19 The relationship of the jugular venous pulse to the electrocardiogram and heart sounds. The jugular venous pulse (and its various component wave patterns, C, V, and A waves) can be observed in the external jugular vein or via intensive care monitoring (which is often accompanied by an electrocardiogram). The physiologic and mechanical events producing these wave patterns can be better analyzed by assessing the heart sounds and their respective location in the cardiac and venous pulse cycles.

wave of venous distension from right atrial systole, occurring just before S_1, and the V wave, frequently indicating a regurgitant tricuspid valve, are two such examples and are displayed in Fig. 4-19.[71,121] Although the assessment of hemodynamic function via pulmonary artery pressure monitoring is considered an advanced skill, it is relatively simple to interpret the typical intensive care unit monitor and thus obtain important hemodynamic information. Perhaps the most important aspect of such monitoring is identifying the pulmonary artery pressure, which is schematized in Fig. 4-19. A mean pulmonary artery pressure greater than 25 mm Hg is the definition of pulmonary hypertension and appears to be associated with a variety of pathophysiologic phenomena (hypoxia, cardiac arrhythmias, and pulmonary abnormalities).[60,121]

Pulsus Alternans

Pulsus alternans (mechanical alteration of the femoral or radial pulse characterized by a regular rhythm and alternating strong and weak pulses) can frequently identify severely depressed myocardial function and CHF in general. This is performed using light pressure at the radial pulse with the patient's breath held in midexpiration (to avoid the superimposition of respiratory variation on the amplitude of the pulse).[121] Sphygmomanometry can more readily recognize this phenomenon, which commonly demonstrates 20 mm Hg or greater alternating systolic blood pressure. Characteristically, if pulsus alternans exists, a 20 mm Hg or greater decrease in systolic blood pressure occurs during breath holding because of increased resistance to left ventricular ejection. It should be noted that a difference exists between pulsus alternans and pulsus paradoxus, which is characterized by a marked reduction of both systolic blood pressure (−20 mm Hg) and strength of the arterial pulse during inspiration. Pulsus paradoxus can also be detected by sphygmomanometry[121] and is occasionally seen in CHF. However, it is associated more frequently with cardiac tamponade and constrictive pericarditis primarily because of increased venous return and volume to the right side of the heart, which bulges the interventricular

septum into the LV, thus decreasing the amount of blood present in the LV and the amount of blood ejected from it (because of decreased left ventricular volume and opposition to stroke volume from the bulging septum).[121]

Changes in the Extremities

Occasionally, the extremities of persons with CHF will be cold and appear pale and cyanotic. This abnormal sensation and appearance are a result of the increased sympathetic nervous system activation of CHF, which increases peripheral vascular vasoconstriction and decreases peripheral blood flow.[124,125]

Weight Gain

As fluid is retained, total body fluid volume increases, as does total body weight. Fluctuations of a few pounds from day to day are usually considered normal, but increases of several pounds per day (more than 3 lb) are suggestive of CHF in a patient with CMD.[5] Body weight should always be measured from the same scale at approximately the same time of day with similar clothing and before exercise is started.

Sinus Tachycardia

Sinus tachycardia or other tachyarrhythmias may occur in CHF as the pressoreceptors and chemoreceptors of the body detect decreased fluid volume and decreased oxygen levels, respectively.[5] The body attempts (via increased heart rate) to increase the delivery of fluid and oxygen to the peripheral tissues where it is needed. Unfortunately, this only compounds the problem and makes the heart work even harder, which further impairs its ability to pump.

Decreased Exercise Tolerance

Decreased exercise tolerance is ultimately the culmination of all of the preceding pathophysiologies that produce the characteristic signs and symptoms just discussed. It is apparent that as individuals at rest become short of breath, gain weight, and develop a faster resting heart rate, their ability

Table 4-9 Weber classification of functional impairment in aerobic capacity and anaerobic threshold as measured during incremental exercise testing

Class	Degree of Impairment	VO$_2$max (mL/min/kg)	Anaerobic threshold (mL/min/kg)
A	None to mild	>20	>14
B	Mild to moderate	16 to 20	11 to 14
C	Moderate to severe	10 to 16	8 to 11
D	Severe	6 to 10	5 to 8
E	Very severe	<6	≤4

VO$_2$max, peak exercise oxygen consumption.
From Mann DL: *Heart failure: a companion to Braunwald's heart disease*, Philadelphia, 2004, Saunders.

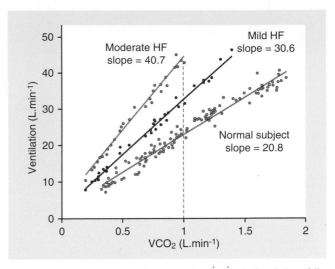

Figure 4-20 Ventilation/carbon dioxide production ($\dot{V}e/\dot{V}co_2$) slope in heart failure (HF). Note that the relation between $\dot{V}e$ and $\dot{V}co_2$ remains linear but that the slope increases with worsening heart failure. Thus, for a $\dot{V}co_2$ of 1 l/min, a normal subject has to ventilate at 22 l/min and the patient with moderate heart failure ventilates at 42 l/min. (Data from Clark AL: Origin of symptoms in chronic heart failure, *Heart* 92(1):12-16, 2006.)

to exercise is dramatically decreased. This effect has been observed repeatedly in patients with CHF and is the result of the interrelationships among the pathophysiologies briefly discussed.[5]

Individuals with heart failure demonstrate early onset anaerobic metabolism as a result of abnormalities in the skeletal muscle. The other changes in the skeletal muscle include fiber atrophy, loss of oxidative type I fibers, and an increase in glycolytic type IIB fibers.[126,127]

The methods of measuring exercise tolerance in patients with CHF have improved significantly in the past few years, but many investigators still use the criteria set forth by the New York Heart Association (NYHA) in 1964.[128] These criteria categorize patients into one of four classes, depending on the development of symptoms and the amount of effort required to provoke them. In short, patients in class I have no limitations in ordinary physical activity, whereas patients in class IV are unable to carry on any physical activity without discomfort. Patients in classes II and III are characterized by slight limitation and marked limitation in physical activities, respectively (see Table 4-7).

A great deal of investigation has been done on measuring exercise tolerance, functional capacity, and survival in persons with CHF.[128–140] Peak oxygen consumption measurements have traditionally been used to categorize persons with CHF, and numerous studies have shown that persons with lower levels of peak oxygen consumption have poorer exercise tolerance, functional capacity, and survival than persons with greater levels of peak oxygen consumption (Table 4-9).[128–135] A peak oxygen consumption threshold range of 10 to 14 mL/kg/min appears to exist, below which patients have been observed to have poorer survival.[130–135] In fact, a peak oxygen consumption below this range is frequently used to list patients for cardiac transplantation.[135]

Measurement of the anaerobic threshold (or ventilatory threshold) and the "slope of the rate of CO$_2$ output from aerobic metabolism plus the rate of CO$_2$, generated from buffering of lactic acid, as a function of the VO$_2$," as well as the change in oxygen consumption to change in work rate above the anaerobic threshold, appear to be useful and relatively reliable in determining exercise tolerance in patients with CHF (Fig. 4-20).[136–140]

Unfortunately, most physical therapists do not have access to equipment (or training in its use) to measure respiratory gases. However, simple but thorough exercise assessments that evaluate symptoms, heart rate, blood pressure, heart rhythm via electrocardiogram, oxygen saturation via oximetry, and respiratory rate at specific workloads can provide important and useful information to compare patient response from day to day. Examples of such an assessment include treadmill ambulation, bicycle ergometry, hallway ambulation, and gentle callisthenic or strength training. Through this type of assessment, progress or deterioration can be documented and appropriate therapy implemented.

The 6-minute walk test (6MWT) is a valuable tool when assessing patients with CHF.[141] It provides an insight into the functional status, exercise tolerance, oxygen consumption, and survival of persons with CHF. Although the exercise performed during the 6MWT is considered submaximal, it nonetheless closely approximates the maximal exercise of persons with CHF and is correlated to peak oxygen consumption.[141,142] Information obtained from the 6MWT has been used to predict peak oxygen consumption (unfortunately, with a modest degree of error) and survival in persons with advanced CHF awaiting cardiac transplantation (Table 4-10). Fig. 4-21 demonstrates that patients unable to ambulate greater than 468 m during the 6MWT had poorer short-term survival, but did not find a relationship with long-term survival. However, Bittner and colleagues[143] found patients unable to ambulate greater than 300 m had poorer long-term survival. Therefore not only can the cardiopulmonary response and exercise tolerance of a person with CHF be evaluated with the 6MWT, but a distance of 300 m appears to be important in determining short- and long-term survival. Several important responses observed during submaximal and maximal exercise testing in patients with CMD are also important factors of prognosis and are found in Box 4-3.[144]

Table 4-10 Multivariate equations for the prediction of peak oxygen uptake (VO_2)

	Variants	Equation Outline	Equation Sample	
1	Distance	Distance + 3.98	$[0.03 \times \text{distance (m)}]$	r = 0.64 r^2 = 0.42 P < 0.0001 SEE = 3.32
2	Distance, Age, Weight, Height, RPP	Distance - Age - Weight + Height + RPP + 2.45	$[0.02 \times \text{distance (m)}] - [0.191 \times \text{age (yr)}] - [0.07 \times \text{wt (kg)}] + [0.09 \times \text{height (cm)}] + [0.26 \times \text{RPP } (\times 10^{-3})] + 2.45$	r = 0.81 r^2 = 0.65 P < 0.0001 SEE = 2.68
3	Distance, Age, Weight, Height, RPP, FEV_1, FVC	Distance - Age - Weight + Height + RPP + FEV_1 + FVC + 7.77	$[0.02 \times \text{distance (m)}] - [0.14 \times \text{age (yr)}] - [0.07 \times \text{wt (kg)}] + [0.03 \times \text{height (cm)}] + [0.23 \times \text{RPP } (\times 10^{-3})] + [0.10 \times FEV_1 \text{(L)}] + [1.19 \times \text{FVC (L)}] + 7.77$	r = 0.83 r^2 = 0.69 P < 0.0001 SEE = 2.59
4	Distance, Age, Weight, Height, RPP, LVEF, PAP, CI	Distance - Age - Weight + Height + RPP + LVEF - PAP + CI + 8.43	$[0.02 \times \text{distance (m)}] - [0.15 \times \text{age (yr)}] - [0.05 \times \text{wt (kg)}] + [0.04 \times \text{height (cm)}] + [0.17 \times \text{RPP } (\times 10^{-3})] + [0.03 \times \text{LVEF (\%)}] - [0.04 \times \text{PAP (mm Hg)}] + [0.31 \times \text{CI (mL/min/m}^2)] + 8.43$	r = 0.85 r^2 = 0.72 P = 0.001 SEE = 2.06

CI, Cardiac index; *LVEF*, left ventricular ejection fraction; *PAP*, pulmonary artery pressure; *r* = correlation coefficient; *r*² = coefficient of determination; *RPP*, rate-pressure product; *SEE*, standard error of the estimate.

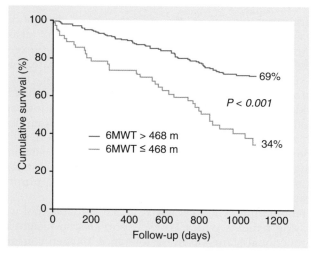

Figure 4-21 Relationship of 6MWD to long term cardiovascular survival in men with systolic heart failure. (Data from Wegrzynowska-Teodorczyk K, et al: Distance covered during a 6-minute walk test predicts long-term cardiovascular mortality and hospitalization rates in men with systolic heart failure: an observational study, *J Physiother* 59:177-187, 2013.)

Quality of Life in Congestive Heart Failure

Comprehensive instruments have been designed and consist primarily of questionnaires that measure specific attributes of life such as socioeconomic factors, psychological status, and function.

One such questionnaire was designed by Rector and associates and is titled the Minnesota Living with Heart Failure Questionnaire.[145] This questionnaire (Table 4-11) consists of 21 questions that the patient answers to the best of the patient's ability. This self-administered questionnaire appears to be more accurate and reliable with a modest degree of supervision. The Minnesota Living with Heart Failure Questionnaire has been used in several recent studies investigating the effects of various pharmacologic agents in persons with CHF, as well

---

BOX 4-3　Responses observed during submaximal and maximal exercise testing in patients with CMD

1. A more rapid heart rate rise during submaximal workloads
2. A lower peak oxygen consumption and oxygen pulse (an indirect measure of stroke volume obtained by dividing the heart rate into oxygen consumption) during submaximal and maximal work
3. A flat, blunted, and occasionally hypoadaptive (decrease) systolic blood pressure response to exercise
4. A possible increase in diastolic blood pressure
5. Electrocardiographic signs of myocardial ischemia (ST depression and/or T-wave inversion)
6. More easily provoked dyspnea and fatigue, often accompanied by angina
7. Lower maximal workloads compared with those of subjects without heart disease
8. A chronotropic (increased heart rate response) and possibly an inotropic (force of myocardial contraction) incompetence (resulting in an inability to increase the heart rate or force of myocardial contraction) during exercise in patients with severe coronary artery disease and multisystem disease that may be partially caused by an autonomic nervous system dysfunction

Data from Deboeck G, Van Muylem A, Vachiéry JL, Naeije R: Physiological response to the 6-minute walk test in chronic heart failure patients versus healthy control subjects, *Eur J Prev Cardiol* 21(8):997-1003, 2014.

---

as exercise training in CHF, and appears useful for measuring quality of life and changes in the quality of life.[146–149] These areas are two very important issues for clinical practice and research, and the information provided by this questionnaire is therefore highly desirable. Other similar questionnaires have been developed, but none have been used as extensively as the Minnesota Living with Heart Failure Questionnaire.

Significant depression is associated with an increased risk of functional decline, as well as increased morbidity and mortality independent of severity of disease.[150–153] Significant depression also is associated with more than a double increase

Table 4-11 The minnesota living with heart failure questionnaire

These questions concern how your heart failure (heart condition) has prevented you from living as you wanted during the past month. The items listed here describe different ways some people are affected. If you are sure an item does not apply to you or is not related to your heart failure, then circle 0 (No) and go on to the next item. If an item does apply to you, then circle the number rating of how much it prevented you from living as you wanted. Remember to think about ONLY THE PAST MONTH. Did your heart failure prevent you from living as you wanted during the last month by

	No	Very little			Very much	
1. Causing swelling in your ankles, legs, etc.?	0	1	2	3	4	5
2. Making your working around the house or yard difficult?	0	1	2	3	4	5
3. Making your relating to or doing things with your friends or family difficult?	0	1	2	3	4	5
4. Making you sit or lie down to rest during the day?	0	1	2	3	4	5
5. Making you tired, fatigued, or low on energy?	0	1	2	3	4	5
6. Making your working to earn a living difficult?	0	1	2	3	4	5
7. Making your walking about or climbing stairs difficult?	0	1	2	3	4	5
8. Making you short of breath?	0	1	2	3	4	5
9. Making your sleeping well at night difficult?	0	1	2	3	4	5
10. Making you eat less of the foods you like?	0	1	2	3	4	5
11. Making your going places away from home difficult?	0	1	2	3	4	5
12. Making your sexual activities difficult?	0	1	2	3	4	5
13. Making your recreational pastimes, sports, or hobbies difficult?	0	1	2	3	4	5
14. Making it difficult for you to concentrate or remember things?	0	1	2	3	4	5
15. Giving you side effects from medications?	0	1	2	3	4	5
16. Making you worry?	0	1	2	3	4	5
17. Making you feel depressed?	0	1	2	3	4	5
18. Costing you money for medical care?	0	1	2	3	4	5
19. Making you feel a loss of self-control in your life?	0	1	2	3	4	5
20. Making you stay in a hospital?	0	1	2	3	4	5
21. Making you feel you are a burden to your family or friends?	0	1	2	3	4	5

Copyright University of Minnesota, 1986. IN Rector TS, Cohn JN: Assessment of patient outcome with the Minnesota Living with Heart Failure Questionnaire: Reliability and validity during a randomized, double-blind, placebo-controlled trial of pimobendan. Pimobendan Multicenter Research Group. *Am Heart J* 124(4):1017–25, 1992..

in mortality at 3 months and with triple the rate of rehospitalization in 1 year.[150]

Cognition

Cognitive impairment is increasingly becoming recognized as an important predictor of poor clinical outcomes, repeat hospitalizations, and higher mortality rates.[154] Exercise has been established as preventing and reducing the effects of inactivity in peripheral vasculature; the effects of exercise on cerebral vasculature are starting to be studied.

Cognitive impairment is thought to be the cumulative effect of decreased cerebral perfusion and oxygenation, structural changes in the brain (particularly hippocampal damage), atrophy, loss of gray matter, and microemboli. The hippocampus is especially vulnerable to oxygen deprivation. When hippocampal tissue is damaged, the ability to perform essential self-care activities of daily living (ADLs) and routine daily tasks is diminished. Cerebral hypoperfusion has been shown to be predictive of cognitive decline from mild cognitive impairment to severe dementia.[155] In patients with heart failure, a 12-week, 3-day-per-week cardiac rehabilitation intervention demonstrated and maintained memory improvements at 12 months.[156]

Aerobic activity has been demonstrated to improve cognitive function in a number of domains, including spatial and executive functioning. The most noted improvement was in executive function; aerobic exercise was shown to reverse cognitive impairments in individuals with dementia with an overall moderate effect size of 0.57 between the exercise and control groups. Low-to-moderate-intensity aerobic exercise three or more times per week can reduce the risk of dementia by 34%. In longitudinal studies, patients who participated in exercise at age 36 and 43 had the lowest rate of memory decline at age 53.[157]

Most evidence supports that aerobic exercise benefits cognitive function. The benefits of exercise training seem to be greater for executive functioning than other cognitive processes. Exercise may also have a protective effect against cognitive decline with aging. Further research is needed to better understand the molecular mechanisms of the influence of exercise on cognitive function.

Radiologic Findings in Congestive Heart Failure

Identification of several of the signs and symptoms frequently suggests the presence of CHF, but radiologic and occasionally laboratory findings usually confirm the diagnosis and provide a baseline from which to evaluate therapy.[5] Radiologic evidence of CHF is dependent on the size and shape of the cardiac silhouette (evaluating left VEDV), as well as the presence of interstitial, perivascular, and alveolar edema (evaluating fluid in the lungs).[5] Interstitial, perivascular, and alveolar edema form the radiologic hallmark of CHF and generally occur when pulmonary capillary pressures (which reflect the left ventricular end-diastolic pressure) exceed 20 to 25 mm Hg.[5] Pleural effusions (parenchymal fluid accumulations) and atelectasis (collapsed lung segments) may also be present.

Laboratory Findings in Congestive Heart Failure

Proteinuria; elevated urine specific gravity, BUN, and creatinine levels; and decreased erythrocyte sedimentation rates (because of decreased fibrinogen concentrations resulting from impaired fibrinogen synthesis) are associated with CHF.[5] Frequently, but not consistently, PaO_2 and oxygen saturation levels are reduced and $Paco_2$ levels elevated.[158] Liver enzymes, such as AST and alkaline phosphatase, are often elevated, and hyperbilirubinemia commonly occurs, resulting in subsequent jaundice.[5] Serum electrolytes are generally normal, but individuals with chronic CHF may demonstrate hyponatremia (decreased Na+) during rigid sodium restriction and diuretic therapy or hypokalemia (decreased K+), which also may be the result of diuretic therapy.[1] Hyperkalemia can occur for several reasons, but most commonly is caused by a marked reduction in the GFR (especially if individuals are receiving a potassium-retaining diuretic) or overzealous potassium supplementation (when a non–potassium-retaining diuretic is used) (Box 4-4).[5]

Brain natriuretic peptide and its amino-terminal fragment NT-proBNP have an established role in the diagnosis of patients presenting with dyspnea of uncertain etiology and possibly in determining decompensation in CHF.[66]

Echocardiography

Echocardiography (including Doppler flow studies) is the most useful diagnostic test for evaluation of anatomy, possible etiology, and severity of heart failure. The following three major concerns regarding heart failure can be answered with echocardiography:

- Is the left ventricular LEVF preserved or reduced?
- What is the structure of the LV (hypertrophy, dilated, normal)?
- Are other structural abnormalities present (pericardial, valvular functioning, right ventricle) that would affect LV functioning?[23]

The echocardiography report should include EF, ventricular dimensions, ventricular volume, wall thickness measurement, chamber geometry, and regional wall motion.[23]

Medical Management

The treatment of CHF, in general, is directed at the underlying cause or causes. The fundamental treatment for CHF involves controlling the pathophysiologic mechanisms responsible for its existence. By improving the heart's ability to pump and reducing the workload and controlling sodium intake and water retention, CHF can be relatively well controlled.[159] Table 4-12 outlines these measures. In addition, Box 4-5 defines common predisposing factors causing decompensated heart failure.

The specific treatments for CHF include the restriction of sodium intake, use of medications (diuretics, digitalis, and other positive inotropic agents, dopamine, dobutamine, amrinone, vasodilator therapy, venodilators, ACE inhibitors, and β-adrenergic blockers), other special measures, and properly prescribed physical activity. Fig. 4-22 outlines these treatments, and a brief discussion of each reveals how the pathophysiology of CHF is affected with each of the following measures.

Dietary Changes and Nutritional Supplementation

Because of the associated dietary and nutritional deficiencies, supplementation of vitamins, minerals, and amino acids is often provided to persons with CHF. Vitamins C and E, as well as various minerals, have shown some promise as important supplements to the diet of persons with CHF.[160–163]

Dietary changes are also important for persons with CHF and include decreasing sodium intake, fluid restrictions, and eating heart-healthy foods that are low in cholesterol and fat. Such changes have been observed to decrease hospital readmissions in persons with CHF. Also, dietary counseling alone has been found to produce similar reductions in hospital readmissions and to improve patient outcomes.[164,165]

Pharmacologic Treatment

See Chapter 14 for detailed description of the following medications.

Table 4-12 Outline of treatment of chronic congestive heart failure

Treatment/Prescription		Common Factors in Decompensated Heart Failure
Proper prescription of physical activity	Decrease or discontinue exhaustive activities Decrease or discontinue full-time work or equivalent activity, introducing rest periods during the day Gradual progressive exercise training that fluctuates frequently from day to day Exercise intensity determined by level of dyspnea or adverse physiologic effort (i.e., angina or decrease in systolic blood pressure)	Not participating in rehabilitation
Restriction of sodium intake	Institute a low-sodium diet	Not changing diet
Digitalis glycoside and other inotropic agents	Dopamine Dobutamine Amrinone	Toxicity can cause arrhythmia
Diuretics	Moderate diuretic (thiazide) Loop diuretic (furosemide) Loop diuretic plus distal tubular (potassium-sparing) diuretic Loop diuretic plus thiazide and distal tubular diuretic	Not watching water intake, weighing daily
Aldosterone antagonists	Spironolactone	Noncompliance with medications can cause uncontrolled hypertension
Vasodilators or venodilators	Captopril, enalapril, or combination of hydralazine plus isosorbide dinitrate Intensification of oral vasodilator regimen Intravenous nitroprusside	Noncompliance with medications can cause uncontrolled hypertension
Angiotensin-converting enzyme	Captopril—may prevent cardiac dilation Enalapril maleate Lisinopril	Noncompliance with medications can cause uncontrolled hypertension
β Blockers	Metoprolol Bucindolol Xamoterol	Noncompliance with medications can cause uncontrolled arrhythmias
Special measures	Dialysis and ultrafiltration Assisted circulation (intraaortic balloon, left ventricular assist device, artificial heart) Cardiac transplantation	

BOX 4-5 Common precipitating factors in decompensated heart failure

- Medicine and dietary noncompliance
- Cardiac causes
- Ischemia
- Arrhythmia
- Uncontrolled hypertension
- Noncardiac causes
- Infection (pneumonia with or without hypoxia)
- Exacerbation of comorbidity (chronic obstructive pulmonary disease)
- Pulmonary embolus
- Toxins (nonsteroidal antiinflammatory drugs)
- Volume overload

The specific medications discussed here are used for the pharmacologic treatment of CHF, including diuretics, digitalis and other positive inotropic agents, dopamine, dobutamine, amrinone, vasodilator therapy, venodilators, ACE inhibitors, and β-adrenergic blockers. Three classes of drugs can exacerbate the syndrome of heart failure and should be avoided in most patients, including:

- Antiarrhythmic agents, which act as cardiodepressants and often have proarrhythmic effects. Only amiodarone and dofetilide have been shown to not adversely affect survival.
- Calcium-channel blockers can lead to worsening heart failure and are associated with increased risk of cardiovascular events.
- Nonsteroidal antiinflammatory drugs often increase sodium retention, cause peripheral vasoconstriction,[23] and impair the action of diuretics and ACE inhibitors.

Diuretics

Diuretics remain the cornerstone of treatment for CHF.[159] As outlined in Table 4-12, moderate diuretics and loop diuretics are commonly used to reduce the fluid overload of CHF by increasing urine flow. Most of these diuretics act directly on kidney function by inhibiting solute (substances dissolved in a solution) and water reabsorption. As previously discussed, furosemide (Lasix) is the most commonly used diuretic, inhibiting the cotransport of sodium, potassium, and chloride.[159] As a result, individuals on Lasix need to be on K+ supplements.

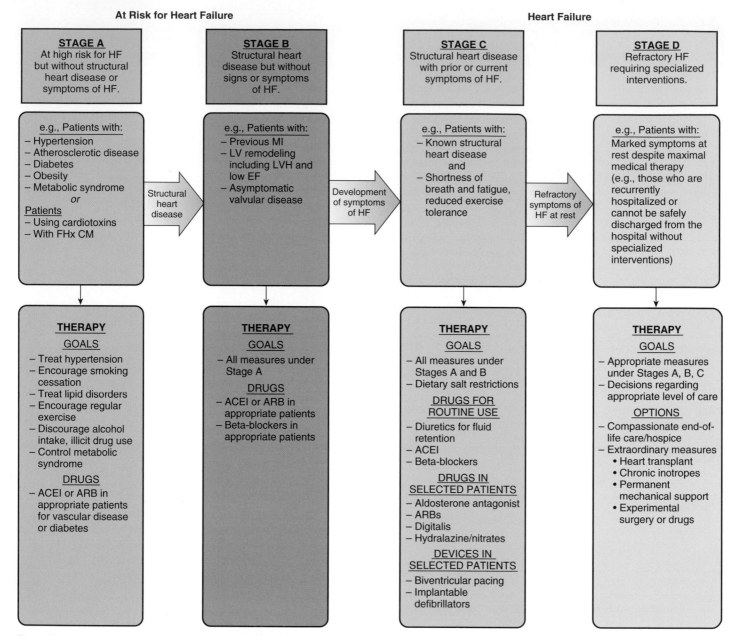

Figure 4-22 Stages in the development of heart failure (HF) and recommended therapy by stage. ACEI, angiotensin-converting enzyme inhibitor; ARB, angiotensin receptor blocker; EF, ejection fraction; FHx CM, family history of cardiomyopathy; LV, left ventricular; LVH, left ventricular hypertrophy; MI, myocardial infarction. (From Jessup M, Abraham WT, Casey DE, et al. 2009 Focused update: ACCF/AHA Guidelines for the Diagnosis and Management of Heart Failure in Adults: A report of the American College of Cardiology Foundation/American Heart Association Task Force on Practice Guidelines: developed in collaboration with the International Society for Heart and Lung Transplantation. *Circulation* 119(14):1977–2016, 2009.)

The major principles of diuretic use are as follows:

- Higher doses are required to restore than to maintain optimal volume status.
- Doses should generally be doubled when an increased effect is desired.
- The addition of metolazone or intravenous thiazides frequently resolves apparent "diuretic resistance" but should be reserved for intermittent rather than chronic use.
- Adequacy of oral diuretic dosing should be demonstrated before discharge.

With these considerations, furosemide (in bolus or continuous infusion) is generally effective to achieve diuresis, sometimes with the addition of intravenous thiazides.[129]

Aldosterone Antagonists

Aldosterone antagonists (e.g., spironolactone) are often added to the medical regimen of individuals with mild-to-moderate symptoms of heart failure in addition to other diuretics.[23]

Digoxin (Lanoxin) and Other Positive Inotropic Agents

Digoxin (digitalis) is one of medicine's oldest drugs, and most of the digitalis drugs in use today are steroid glycosides derived from the leaves of the flowering plant foxglove, or *Digitalis purpurea*. Despite its long history, there is still controversy over its use in patients with CHF and normal sinus rhythm.[166–168] However, several studies demonstrate favorable hemodynamic and clinical responses in selected patients.[169–173] The most significant clinical observations tend to be related to the positive inotropic (increased force of contraction) effect evidenced by an increased LVEF.[174] In addition, the electrophysiologic effects of digoxin on the heart help control rapid supraventricular arrhythmias (primarily atrial fibrillation or flutter) by increasing the parasympathetic tone in the sinus and atrioventricular nodes, thereby slowing conduction.[174] Current standard treatment recommendations involve the four-drug approach (digoxin, diuretics, ACE inhibitors, and β blockers) for all patients with left ventricular dysfunction and symptomatic heart failure, regardless of cause.[129]

Results from the Prospective Randomized Study of Ventricular Function and Efficacy of Digoxin (PROVED) and the Randomized Assessment of Digoxin and Inhibitors of Angiotensin-Converting Enzyme (RADIANCE) trials indicate that digoxin increases LVEF more in patients with dilated cardiomyopathy than in patients with ischemic heart disease and that withdrawal of digoxin leads to a significantly greater likelihood of clinical deterioration in patients with dilated cardiomyopathy.[175]

Dopamine

Dopamine hydrochloride is a chemical precursor of norepinephrine, which stimulates dopaminergic, β_2-adrenergic, and α-adrenergic receptors, as well as the release of norepinephrine. This results in increased cardiac output and, at doses greater than 10 µg/kg/min, markedly increased systemic vascular resistance and preload.[20] For this reason, the primary indication for dopamine is hemodynamically significant hypotension in the absence of hypovolemia.[20] Dopamine is also useful for patients with refractory CHF, in which case it is carefully titrated until urine flow or hemodynamic parameters improve. In such patients, the hemodynamic and renal effects of dopamine can be profound. Frequently, dopamine is infused together with nitroprusside or nitroglycerin to counteract the vasoconstricting action. In addition, dopamine is frequently administered (as are dobutamine and amrinone) during and after cardiac surgery to improve low cardiac output states.[20]

Dobutamine

Dobutamine is a sympathomimetic amine that stimulates β_1 receptors in the myocardium, with very little effect on α-adrenergic receptors. It provides potent inotropic effects, but is only given via intravenous infusion.[176] Like dopamine, dobutamine increases cardiac output and decreases the peripheral resistance; with the use of dopamine, there is a potentially significant increase in peripheral resistance. For this reason, dobutamine in addition to a moderate increase in volume is the treatment of choice in patients with hemodynamically significant right ventricular infarction.[20]

Amrinone/Milrinone

Amrinone and milrinone are phosphodiesterase inhibitors that lead to increased cAMP by preventing its breakdown, thereby producing rapid inotropic and vasodilatory effects. Some of the side effects can include exacerbation of myocardial ischemia if coronary occlusion exists,[177] hypotension as a result of intense vasodilation, elevation in heart rate, and increase in atrial and ventricular tachyarrhythmias. Amrinone can also cause thrombocytopenia in 2% to 3% of patients, as well as a variety of other side effects (e.g., gastrointestinal dysfunction, myalgia, fever, hepatic dysfunction, cardiac arrhythmias). Milrinone has a prolonged half-life, and its physiologic half-life may be excessive in individuals with renal dysfunction. More has been learned about the long-term effects of milrinone than about the other intravenous inotropic drugs in current use. Mortality from both heart failure and sudden death was increased with chronically administered milrinone compared with placebo without any significant improvement in symptoms.[178] Despite these adverse effects, amrinone is recommended and has proved to be therapeutic for patients with severe CHF that is refractory to diuretics, vasodilators, and other inotropic agents.[179] In addition, an increase in exercise tolerance has been observed with the use of milrinone.[180]

Vasodilators and Venodilators

Vasodilators (nesiritide, nitroglycerin, nitroprusside) are given to patients with CHF or CMD to relax smooth muscle in peripheral arterioles and to produce peripheral vasodilation that reduces filling pressures, decreases the afterload, lessens the work of the heart, decreases symptoms, and potentially decreases the degree of CMD. These medications include calcium-channel blockers and α-blockers. The clinical management of patients with CHF and CMD frequently combines vasodilators, venodilators, and ACE inhibitors.

Angiotensin-Converting Enzyme Inhibitors and α-Receptor Blockers

The combined use of ACE inhibitors, vasodilators, and venodilators has been demonstrated to be very effective in reducing symptoms and improving exercise tolerance.[181] The primary mechanism of action of these inhibitors is probably via the reduction of angiotensin II, a hormone that causes vasoconstriction,[174] but other less well-defined actions may be responsible for the therapeutic effects of ACE inhibitors in patients with CHF. Other poorly understood mechanisms of such inhibitors include "nonspecific vasodilation with unloading of the ventricle, inhibition of excessive sympathetic drive and perhaps modulation of tissue receptor systems."[174]

A great deal of interest has focused on the "prevention" hypothesis regarding the use of ACE inhibitors and the prevention of progressive CMD (dilation and CHF).[182–185] Notably, captopril may prevent such progressive cardiac dilation.[182,183] Recent studies have focused on the addition of β blockers to ACE inhibitors (and sometimes α-receptor blockers) and demonstrated a greater improvement in symptoms and reduction in the risk of death than when ACE inhibitors were used alone and the dosage was increased.[186]

α-Adrenergic Antagonists and Partial Agonists

Perhaps one of the most confusing groups of medications used in treating CHF and CMD is the β-adrenergic blockers group. One of the many uses of β blockers is to lower blood pressure, primarily via a reduction in cardiac output.[174] This reduction in cardiac output is the result of a decrease in heart rate and stroke volume, which causes an increase in end-diastolic volume and end-diastolic pressure (the slowing of the heart rate allows more time for the ventricles to fill before the next myocardial contraction with more time for the coronary arteries to fill) but somewhat paradoxically reduces the myocardial oxygen requirement.[187] This paradoxical reduction in oxygen requirement probably is the result of a decrease in sympathetic nervous system stimulation because of the blocking of the β receptors. Sympathetic (catecholamine-driven) increases in heart rate, force of myocardial contraction, velocity, and extent of myocardial contraction, as well as systolic blood pressure, are prevented by β blockade.[188,189]

β Blockers interfere with the sustained activation of the nervous system and therefore block the adrenergic effects on the heart.

Although there are a number of potential benefits to blocking all three receptors (β₁, β₂, and α), most of the deleterious effects of sympathetic activation are mediated by the β₁-adrenergic receptor. β Blockers are usually prescribed in conjunction with ACE inhibitors and in combination have demonstrated a reversal of the LV remodeling that occurs with injury and longstanding muscle dysfunction, improves symptoms, prevents rehospitalizations, and prolongs life. Consequently, β blockers are indicated for patients with symptomatic or asymptomatic heart failure and a depressed EF of lower than 40%. Three β blockers have been shown to be effective in reducing mortality in patients with chronic heart failure, including metoprolol succinate (Toprol), bisoprolol, and carvedilol.[190–192]

In the Metoprolol CR/XL Randomized Intervention Trial in Congestive Heart Failure (MERIT-HF), a 34% reduction in mortality was reported in individuals with mild-to-moderate heart failure and moderate-to-severe systolic dysfunction who were taking metoprolol CR/XL compared with placebo.[193] In addition, metoprolol CR/XL reduced mortality from both sudden death and progressive pump failure.[193]

In patients with dilated cardiomyopathy who were supported with a left ventricular assist device (LVAD) and given a specific pharmacologic regimen consisting of an ACE inhibitor, an angiotensin receptor blocker, an aldosterone antagonist, and a β blocker, followed by treatment with a β₂-adrenergic receptor agonist (clenbuterol), improvement in the myocardium resulted in explantation of the LVAD, as well as an improvement in quality of life and absence of recurrent heart failure for 1 to 4 years.[194] Thus β blockers, in addition to other pharmacologic agents like ACE inhibitors, play a significant role in LV remodeling. Recent studies indicate that β blockers can be started as early as during the hospitalization after an acute injury and should be continued for a minimum of 1 year postinjury date to optimize the ventricular remodeling.[190–192]

Anticoagulation

The patient hospitalized with heart failure is at increased risk for thromboembolic complications and deep venous thrombosis and should receive prophylactic anticoagulation with either intravenous unfractionated heparin or subcutaneous preparations of unfractionated or low-molecular-weight heparin, unless contraindicated.[195]

Mechanical Management

Implantable Cardiac Defibrillator Implantation

Implantable cardiac defibrillator implantation is recommended in the 2013 American Heart Association guidelines for the treatment of CHF for patients with an EF less than or equal to 35% and mild-to-moderate symptoms of heart failure and in whom survival with good functional capacity is otherwise anticipated to extend beyond 1 year.[196] Implantable cardiac defibrillator implantation should not be considered until medical therapy has been maximized and the patient's EF is measured under the current medical therapy.[196] Implantable cardiac defibrillators are not indicated in patients with refractory symptoms of heart failure (stage D) or in patients with concomitant diseases that would shorten their life expectancy independent of CHF.[196]

Cardiac Resynchronization Therapy

In individuals with heart failure with abnormalities in the chamber size, ventricular dyssynchrony often exists. The consequences of dyssynchrony include suboptimal ventricular filling, a reduction in the rate of rise of ventricular contractile force or pressure, prolonged duration of mitral regurgitation, and paradoxical septal wall motion.[176,177,179] These same individuals may demonstrate a prolonged QRS on the electrocardiogram (>0.12 seconds). Ventricular dyssynchrony has also been associated with increased mortality in heart failure patients.[197] As a result, electrical stimulation (activation) of the right and left ventricles in a synchronized manner can be provided by a biventricular pacemaker device. This approach, called *cardiac resynchronization therapy* (CRT), may improve ventricular contraction and reduce the degree of secondary mitral regurgitation.[58,59] In addition, the short-term use of CRT is associated with improvements in cardiac function and hemodynamics without an accompanying increase in oxygen use.[198] When CRT was added to patients on optimal medical therapy who continued to have symptoms, significant improvement was noted in quality of life, functional class, exercise capacity and 6MWD, and EF.[68,69,146] In a meta-analysis of several CRT trials, heart failure hospitalizations were reduced by 32% and all-cause mortality by 25%.[69,197]

Special Measures

Patients who respond unfavorably to the aforementioned methods of treatment for CHF and CMD and who demonstrate signs and symptoms of severe CHF are frequently managed using several rather extreme methods. As noted in Table 4-12, there are three "special measures" categories for treating CHF and CMD: dialysis and ultrafiltration, assisted circulation, and cardiac transplantation.

Dialysis and Ultrafiltration

The mechanical removal of fluid from the pleural and abdominal cavities of patients with CHF is usually unnecessary, but patients unresponsive to diuretic therapy because of severe CHF or insensitivity to diuretics may be in need of peritoneal dialysis or extracorporeal ultrafiltration.[23,159] The mechanical removal of fluid in patients with acute respiratory distress because of large pleural effusions or diaphragms elevated by ascites (both of which compress the lungs) frequently brings rapid relief of dyspnea. However, mechanical removal of fluid (primarily peritoneal dialysis) may be associated with risk of pneumothorax, infection, peritonitis, hypernatremia, hyperglycemia, hyperosmolality, and cardiac arrhythmias.[159,199] Cardiovascular collapse may also occur if too

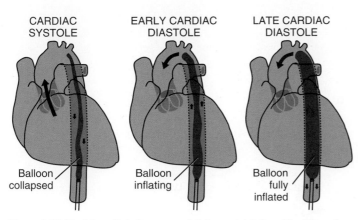

CARDIAC SYSTOLE	EARLY CARDIAC DIASTOLE	LATE CARDIAC DIASTOLE
Balloon collapsed	Balloon inflating	Balloon fully inflated

Figure 4-23 The intraaortic balloon pump. Inflation and deflation of the intraaortic balloon pump improve diastolic and systolic heart function, respectively.

much fluid is removed or if removal takes place too rapidly. It is recommended that no more than 200 mL of fluid per hour be removed and no more than 1500 mL of pleural fluid be removed during dialysis.[159,199]

For these reasons, as well as for simplicity, cost effectiveness, and long-lasting effects, ultrafiltration has become the treatment of choice for patients in need of mechanical fluid removal.[199] Extracorporeal ultrafiltration removes plasma water and sodium via an ultrafiltrate (a blend of water, electrolytes, and other small molecules with concentrations identical to those in plasma) from the blood by convective transport through a highly permeable membrane. Ultrafiltration can be performed vein to vein using an extracorporeal pump or with an arteriovenous approach.[199]

Although hemodynamic side effects (hypotension, organ malperfusion, and hemolysis) are also possible with ultrafiltration, proper monitoring of the rate of blood flow through the filter (rates above 150 mL/min or below 500 mL/hr are tolerated without side effects), as well as right atrial pressure (ultrafiltration should be discontinued when the right atrial pressure falls to 2 or 3 mm Hg)[200] and hematocrit levels (should not exceed 50%), should, for the most part, prevent them.[199]

Assisted Circulation

Several methods of treatment assist the circulation of blood throughout the body. Perhaps the most widely used is intraaortic balloon counterpulsation via the intraaortic balloon pump (IABP). The IABP catheter is positioned in the thoracic aorta just distal to the left subclavian artery via the right or left femoral artery (Fig. 4-23). Inflation of the balloon occurs at the beginning of ventricular diastole, immediately after closure of the aortic valve. This increases intraaortic pressure and diastolic pressure in general and forces blood in the aortic arch to flow in a retrograde direction into the coronary arteries. This mechanism of action is referred to as *diastolic augmentation* and profoundly improves oxygen delivery to the myocardium.[201] In addition to this physiologic assist (greater availability of oxygen for myocardial energy production) to improve cardiac performance, hemodynamic assistance is also obtained as the balloon deflates just before systole, which decreases left ventricular afterload by forcing blood to move from an area of higher pressure to one of lower pressure to fill the space previously occupied

by the balloon.[201] Consequently, the intraaortic balloon pump causes "a 10% to 20% increase in cardiac output as well as a reduction in systolic and an increase in diastolic arterial pressure with little change in mean pressure. There is also a diminution of heart rate and an increase in urine output."[201] In addition, intraaortic balloon counterpulsation produces a reduction in myocardial oxygen consumption "and decreased myocardial ischemia and anaerobic metabolism,"[201] all of which are very important in the management of CHF and CMD.

The IABP is occasionally used in conjunction with a slightly different but similar treatment called *pulmonary artery balloon counterpulsation* (PABC) in the pulmonary artery versus the thoracic aorta, which is helpful in treating right ventricular and biventricular failure unresponsive to inotropic drugs and the IABP alone.[201]

Ventricular Assist Devices

A ventricular assist device (VAD) is a mechanical pump that provides support to a failing ventricle, either the LV, right ventricle, or both (Fig. 4-24). The VAD can act as a bridge to transplant or bridge to recovery for those patients in whom ventricular function is expected to return, as a bridge to decision for patients whose status is declining and a decision on transplant eligibility is pending, or as a destination therapy for patients ineligible for heart transplant. First-generation VADs consisted of a flexible polyurethane blood sac and diaphragm placed within a rigid case outside the body that provided a pulsatile flow of blood. Second-generation VADs, which provide a continuous flow of blood, utilize a rotary pump implanted in the thoracic cavity to divert blood from the LV and propel it directly to the ascending aorta and the rest of the body. A drive line exits the patient's abdomen and attaches to a system controller that controls pump operations. Third-generation VADs are now employing a bearingless rotary pump implanted directly into the apex of the heart. Therapists working with patients who have a VAD must be aware of special precautions and safety mechanisms related to the VAD, including low-flow alarms, low-pressure alarms, and loss of standard vital signs. See Chapter 12 for more information on VADs.

Surgical Management

Reparative, reconstructive, excisional, and ablative surgeries are sometimes performed in the treatment of CHF and CMD. Reparative procedures correct cardiac malfunctions such as ventricular septal defect, atrial septal defect, and mitral stenosis, and frequently improve cardiac hemodynamics, resulting in improved cardiac performance. Coronary artery bypass graft surgery is probably the most common reconstructive surgery because myocardial ischemia and infarction are the primary causes of CMD and CHF.[202] Its effects are often profound, improving cardiac muscle function and eliminating CHF. Reconstruction of incompetent heart valves is also common.[18] Excisional procedures in patients with atrial myxomas (tumors) and large LVs are employed less often. The excision of a tumor or aneurysm is occasionally performed, and the excised area is replaced with Dacron patches.[18] Ablative procedures are also used less frequently, but for patients with persistent and symptomatic

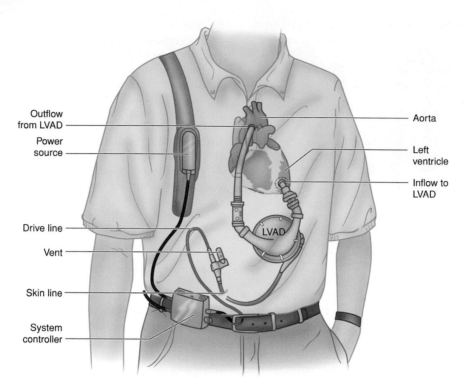

Figure 4-24 Left ventricular assist device (LVAD). The left ventricular assist device provides myocardial assistance until heart transplantation or corrective measures are taken. (From Monahan FD, Sands JK, Neighbors M: Phipps' Medical-Surgical Nursing, Health and Illness Perspectives, ed 8, St. Louis, 2007, Mosby.)

Wolff–Parkinson–White syndrome or intractable ventricular tachycardia, ablation (e.g., via laser or cryotherapy) of the reentry pathways appears to be very therapeutic.[18] The surgical implantation of automatic implantable defibrillators is increasingly common and appears to be of great therapeutic value for those with ventricular tachycardia that is unresponsive to medications and ablative procedures.[18]

Abandoned Procedures

Although somewhat unusual, the use of muscle flaps (cardiomyoplasty), usually dissected from the latissimus dorsi or trapezius muscle, had been an alternative treatment for a limited number of patients with severe CMD and CHF.[203] The muscle flap is wrapped around the LV and attached to a pacemaker, which stimulates the flap to contract, thus contracting the LV. Also, initial investigations appeared to indicate that the removal of dilated, noncontracting myocardium (partial left ventriculectomy or Batista procedure) of persons with CHF and subsequent suturing of remaining viable myocardial tissue decreased the left ventricular chamber size and improved myocardial performance. These procedures have been largely abandoned due to lack of evidence for clinical benefit.[204–207]

Cardiac Transplantation

Cardiac transplantation is the last treatment effort for a patient with CHF and CMD because "potential recipients of cardiac transplants must have end-stage heart disease with severe heart failure and a life expectancy of less than 1 year."[159] Heart transplantation can be heterologous (or xenograft, from a nonhuman primate) or, more commonly, homologous (or allograft, from another human).[159]

Orthotopic homologous cardiac transplantation is performed by removing the recipient's heart and leaving the posterior walls of the atria with their venous connections on which the donor's atria are sutured. In heterotopic homologous cardiac transplantation, the recipient's heart is left intact and the donor heart is placed in parallel, with anastomoses between the two right atria, pulmonary arteries, left atria, and aorta. Orthotopic heart transplantation is most commonly performed.

Chapter 12 provides a more complete description of cardiac transplantation.

Prognosis

As a result of multivariate analysis of clinical variables, the most significant predictors of survival in individuals with CHF have been identified and include decreasing LVEF, worsening NYHA functional status, degree of hyponatremia, decreasing peak exercise oxygen uptake, decreasing hematocrit, widened QRS on 12-lead electrocardiogram, chronic hypotension, resting tachycardia, renal insufficiency, intolerance to conventional therapy, and refractory volume overload.[208,209] In addition, elevated circulating levels of neurohormonal factors are associated with high mortality rates, but routine laboratory assessment of norepinephrine or endothelin is neither practical nor helpful in managing the patient's clinical status. Likewise, elevated BNP (or NT-proBNP) levels predict higher risk of heart failure and other events after myocardial infarction, whereas marked elevation in BNP levels during hospitalization for heart failure may predict rehospitalization and death. However, controversy still exists regarding BNP measurement and its prognostic value.[208,209]

Currently, a few mathematical models exist to help predict outcome in heart failure patients for clinicians managing treatment. Aaronson and colleagues developed a noninvasive risk stratification model based upon clinical findings and peak VO$_2$ that includes seven variables: presence of ischemia, resting heart rate, LVEF, presence of a QRS duration greater than 200 msec, mean resting blood pressure, peak VO$_2$, and serum sodium.[210] A heart failure score was then developed and related to subsequent morbidity and mortality. The model defined low-, medium-, and high-risk groups based upon 1-year event-free survival rates of 93%, 72%, and 43%, respectively. Interestingly, adding invasive data did not improve the prediction. Campana and coworkers developed a model using cause of heart failure, NYHA functional class, presence of an S$_3$ gallop, cardiac output, mean arterial pressure, and either pulmonary artery diastolic pressure or pulmonary capillary wedge pressure.[211] Patients were risk stratified into low-, intermediate-, and high-risk groups for 1-year event-free survival rates of 95%, 75%, and 40%, respectively.[211]

For three other clinical scoring systems for evaluation of heart failure (Framingham, Boston, and National Health and Nutritional Examination Surveys [NHANES]), see Box 4-6 and Table 4-13.

Physical Therapy Assessment

Because of the increase in number of patients with CHF, physical therapists in all practice settings are seeing these individuals and are responsible for assessing functional status and providing optimal treatment to improve the quality of their lives and possibly decrease morbidity and mortality. Although Chapter 16 provides cardiopulmonary assessment in detail and Chapter 18 provides detailed interventions, a brief overview of assessment and interventions for individuals with CHF is provided here.

A thorough assessment includes an interview that should include a series of questions:

- When did your symptoms start?
- Are your symptoms stable or are they getting worse?
- Are symptoms provoked or do they occur at rest?
- Are there accompanying symptoms such as chest pain or calf claudication?
- Is orthopnea or PND present?
- How far can you walk?
- Do you retain fluid?
- Do you restrict sodium in your diet?
- What sorts of activities can you no longer do?
- Are you losing or gaining weight?
- How do you sleep?

After the interview, a physical examination should involve an assessment of the patient's cardiopulmonary status, including:

- Notation of symptoms of CHF (dyspnea, PND, and orthopnea)
- Evaluation of pulse and electrocardiogram to determine heart rate and rhythm
- Evaluation of respiratory rate and breathing pattern
- Auscultation of the heart and lungs with a stethoscope

BOX 4-6 Comparison of NHANES, Boston and Framingham Criteria

Criteria	NHANES	Boston	Framingham
Dyspnea		X	
Orthopnea		X	X
Paroxysmal nocturnal dyspnea	X		X
Heart rate	X	X	X
JVD (combined with hepatomegaly or edema)	X	X	X
Rales	X	X	X
Crackles	X	X	
Wheezing		X	
S$_3$ gallop		X	X
Alveolar pulmonary edema		X	X
Alveolar fluid plus pleural fluid	X		
Interstitial pulmonary edema	X	X	X
Interstitial edema plus pleural fluid	X		
Cardiothoracic ratio >0.5 (PA projection)		X	
Upper zone flow redistribution	X	X	
Weight loss			X
Vital capacity decreased 50% from maximal capacity			X

- Evaluation of radiographic findings to determine the existence and magnitude of pulmonary edema
- Performance of laboratory blood studies to determine the PaO$_2$ and PaCO$_2$ levels
- Evaluation of the oxygen saturation levels via oximetry
- Palpation for fremitus and percussion of the lungs to determine the relative amount of air or solid material in the underlying lung
- Performance of sit-to-stand test to evaluate heart rate and blood pressure (orthostatic hypotension) and dyspnea
- Objective measurement of other characteristic signs produced by fluid overload, such as peripheral edema, weight gain, and jugular venous distension
- Assessment of cardiopulmonary response to exercise (e.g., heart rate, blood pressure, electrocardiogram)
- Administration of a questionnaire to measure quality of life

Upon the collection of data and the determination of a treatment diagnosis and prognosis, a plan of care is developed for the patient with CHF that details the interventions that are used to achieve the optimal outcome.

Table 4-13 Boston and NHANES-1 clinical scoring systems for heart failure

Categories	Criteria		NHANES	Boston
History	Dyspnea	At rest		4
		On level ground	1	2
		On climbing	1	1
		Stop when walking at own pace or on level ground after 100 yards	2	3
	Orthopnea			4
	Paroxysmal nocturnal dyspnea		3	
Physical examination	Heart rate	91–110 bpm	1	1
		>110 bpm	2	2
	Jugular venous pressure (>6 cm H_2O)			
		Alone	1	2
		Plus hepatomegaly or edema	2	3
	Rales	Basilar crackles	1	1
	Crackles	More than basilar crackles	2	2
	Wheezing			3
	S_3 gallop			3
Chest radiography	Alveolar pulmonary edema			4
	Alveolar fluid plus pleural fluid		3	
	Interstitial pulmonary edema		2	3
	Interstitial edema plus pleural fluid		3	
	Bilateral pleural effusion			3
	Cardiothoracic ratio >0.5 (PA projection)			3
	Upper zone flow redistribution		1	2

Diagnosis of heart failure Boston criteria: Definite (8–12 points); Possible (5–7 points); Unlikely (≤4 points).
Diagnosis of heart failure NHANES-1 criteria: ≥3 points.
NHANES, National Health and Nutrition Examination Surveys.
Data from Mosterd A, Deckers JW, Hoes AW, et al: Classification of heart failure in population based research: An assessment of six heart failure scores. *Eur J Epidemiol* 13(5):491–502, 1997.

Physical Therapy Interventions

Exercise Training

Exercise training is a therapeutic modality that should be considered for all patients with ventricular dysfunction (Table 4-14). Patients who are prescribed exercise training and other interventions need to be without any overt signs of decompensated heart failure, and should be monitored during treatment to observe for abnormal responses and symptoms. Increased levels of physical activity do not appear to have adverse effects on subsequent cardiac mortality or on ventricular function in patients with ventricular dysfunction. In addition, these patients derive psychological benefits from participation in exercise training, and the close medical surveillance available in the content of a supervised exercise program may facilitate better clinical decisions concerning pharmacologic therapy, interpretation of symptoms, or the necessity for and timing of operative procedures.[202]

Specific benefits of exercise training for individuals with heart failure include improvement in symptoms, clinical status, and exercise duration.[212,213] Other studies have reported improved functional capacity and quality of life and reduced hospitalizations for heart failure.[214] There also is indication that exercise training may have beneficial effects on ventricular structure and remodeling.[215] The most recent Heart Failure Action Study reported that exercise training was associated with modest significant reductions for both all-cause mortality or hospitalization and cardiovascular mortality or heart failure hospitalization.[216,217]

Guidelines for Exercise Training

Studies that have demonstrated improvements in exercise tolerance and patient symptoms were all performed using different methodologies—varying modes, intensities, durations, and frequencies of exercise (see Table 4-15). Specific guidelines for exercise training of patients with CHF are difficult to implement because patient status frequently changes. Despite a lack of specific guidelines for exercising persons with

Table 4-14 Summary of interventions for CHF

Intervention	Guidelines
Exercise training (in general)	Low level, low-impact exercise (e.g., walking) for 5 to 10 min/day gradually increasing duration to 30 min. Intensity should be monitored via level of dyspnea or perceived exertion. Frequency: 1 to 2×/day for 5 to 7 days/wk.
Exercise training with intravenous inotropic agents	Progressive increase in low-impact exercise with monitoring of blood pressure response. If patient has an ICD, monitor for ICD firing, especially with exercise.
Exercise with LVADs	Progressive increase in exercise; should demonstrate normal responses. May have flow limitations (10 to 12 L/min), or cardiovascular function from the mechanically driven cardiac output, and the effects of a 6-lb mass resting below the diaphragm that may alter ventilatory performance.
Exercise with continuous positive airway pressure (CPAP)	CPAP may function to reduce preload and afterload on heart, and decrease the workload on inspiratory muscles, which may also increase lung compliance.
Breathing exercises	Exercise program set at a specific percentage of the maximal inspiratory pressure or maximal expiratory pressure (similar to aerobic exercise training) with a device that resists either inspiration or expiration.
Expiratory muscle training	Performed in a variety of ways; most commonly with weights upon the abdomen and hyperpneic breathing. Results in improved symptoms, functional status, and pulmonary function and reduced pulmonary complications. May also use positive end-expiratory pressure devices.
Inspiratory muscle training	One protocol: Threshold inspiratory muscle trainer at 20% of maximal inspiratory pressure, 3 times a day, for 5 to 15 min.
Instruction in energy-conservation techniques	Balancing activity and rest, and performing activities in an energy-efficient manner; scheduling activities and rest.
Self-management techniques	Incorporate individuals into the management of the disease by making them responsible for their own health.

Table 4-15 Rehabilitation and exercise in HF

Exercise training in patients with HF	Supervised, tailored program with experienced clinician evaluating appropriateness, stability for exercise
Cardiac rehabilitation programs for patients with recently decompensated or advanced HF	Gradual mobilization and/or small muscle group strength/flexibility should be considered as soon as possible with experienced HF team
Exercise prescription and exercise modalities in HF	Moderate-intensity continuous aerobic exercise training (walking, jogging, cycling) at modified Borg rating of perceived exertion 3 to 5/10 65% to 85% max heart rate or 50% to 75% of peak VO_2 (need experienced evaluator for peak or max testing), keep heart rate 20 bpm below ICD firing range

Data from Moe GW, et al: The 2013 Canadian Cardiovascular Society heart failure management guidelines update: focus on rehabilitation and exercise and surgical coronary revascularization, *Can J Cardiol* 30: 249-263, 2014.

CHF, the U.S. Department of Health and Human Services Agency for Health Care Policy and Research outlined the importance of exercise training in treatment of CHF.[216–218] Exercise training was recommended "as an integral component of the symptomatic management" of persons with CHF "to attain functional and symptomatic improvement but with a potentially higher likelihood of adverse events." This recommendation was based upon significant scientific evidence from previously published investigations that were reviewed by experts in the field of cardiac rehabilitation.[218]

Patients with decompensated (uncontrolled) CHF are typically very dyspneic and therefore should not begin aerobic exercise training until the CHF is compensated. Table 4-16 lists specific exercise training guidelines, which include the attainment of a cardiac index of 2.0 L/min/m² or greater (for invasively monitored patients in the hospital) before aerobic exercise training is implemented and the maintenance of an adequate pulse pressure (not less than a 10 mm Hg difference between the systolic and diastolic blood pressure) during exercise. The development of marked dyspnea and fatigue, S_3 heart sound, or crackles during exercise requires the modification or termination of exercise.[219]

For most patients, ambulation may be the most effective and functional mode of exercise to administer and prescribe, beginning with frequent short walks and progressing to less frequent, longer bouts of exercise. Occasionally, patients may be so deconditioned that gentle strengthening exercises, restorator cycling, or ventilatory muscle training is the preferred mode of exercise conditioning. As strength and endurance improve, patients can be progressed to upright cycle ergometry or ambulating with a rolling walker.

Because dyspnea is the most common complaint of patients with CHF, the level of dyspnea or Borg rating of perceived exertion appears to be an acceptable method to prescribe and evaluate an exercise program.[202] This is supported by the observation that these subjective indices correlate well with training heart rate ranges in this patient population.[220] Therefore a basic guideline of increasing the exercise intensity to a level that produces a moderate degree of dyspnea (conversing with modest difficulty, ability to count to 5 without taking a breath, or a Borg rating of 3 on a scale of 10) may be the simplest and most effective method to prescribe exercise for patients with CHF. It also appears to be the most effective method to progress a patient's exercise prescription. The exercise prescription of patients with CHF can be progressed when (1) the cardiopulmonary response to exercise is adaptive (see Table 4-15) and (2) workloads that previously produced moderate dyspnea (e.g., Borg rating of 3/10) produce mild dyspnea (e.g., Borg rating of 2/10 or less). Because an increasing number of patients with CMD and CHF are being prescribed β blockers, which often cause little or no change in resting and exercise heart rates, the Borg rating scale again is a good clinical tool.

Table 4-16 Exercise training guidelines for patients with CHF

I. Relative criteria necessary for the initiation of an aerobic exercise training program: compensated CHF	Ability to speak without signs or symptoms of dyspnea (able to speak comfortably with a respiratory rate <30 breaths/min) <Moderate fatigue Crackles present in <one-half of the lungs Resting heart rate <120 bpm Cardiac index ≥2.0 L/min/m² (for invasively monitored patients) Central venous pressure <12 mm Hg (for invasively monitored patients)
II. Relative criteria indicating a need to modify or terminate exercise training	Marked dyspnea or fatigue (e.g., Borg rating > 3/10) Respiratory rate >40 breaths/min during exercise Development of an S_3 heart sound or pulmonary crackles Increase in pulmonary crackles Significant increase in the sound of the second component of the second heart sound (P_2) Poor pulse pressure (<10 mm Hg difference between the systolic and diastolic blood pressure) Decrease in heart rate or blood pressure of >10 bpm or mm Hg, respectively, during continuous (steady state) or progressive (increasing workloads) exercise Increased supraventricular or ventricular ectopy Increase of >10 mm Hg in the mean pulmonary artery pressure (for invasively monitored patients) Increase or decrease of >6 mm Hg in the central venous pressure (for invasively monitored patients) Diaphoresis, pallor, or confusion

From Cahalin LP: Heart failure, *Phys Ther* 76(5):516, 1996.

In addition, instructing patients to increase the respiratory rate to a level that allows one to converse comfortably may be another method for prescribing exercise training in patients with CHF ("talk test").[202]

The end result of such exercise assessments and exercise training is an improved quality of life for patients with CHF.

Exercise Training and Quality of Life

The quality of life of persons with CHF appears to be related to the ability to exercise.[145,147,148,214,221-227] Two recent studies have investigated the effects of exercise training upon the quality of life of persons with CHF. Kavanagh and associates[147] and Keteyian and associates[224] found significant improvements in exercise capacity, symptoms, and quality of life after 24 and 52 weeks of exercise training, respectively. A recent meta-analysis found that exercise training improved functional capacity and quality of life in patients with HFpEF.[228] An overview of Cochrane systematic reviews also found that quality of life does appear to be improved after exercise training in persons with CHF.[229]

Exercise Training During Continuous Intravenous Dobutamine Infusion

Many patients with severe CHF are hospitalized for prolonged periods, receiving continuous IV dobutamine infusion for inotropic support (to improve cardiac muscle contraction) while awaiting cardiac transplantation.[230] Also, it is becoming common practice for patients with severe CHF to be occasionally hospitalized for IV dobutamine infusion ("dobutamine holiday") to transiently improve myocardial performance.[231] Many patients are also being sent home on portable IV dobutamine pumps; their physical activity is less restricted when the large IV pumps are not used.[232] However, exercise training during continuous IV dobutamine infusion has received little attention.[233]

Individuals receiving inotropic support have only recently been prescribed exercise training programs.[234] Kataoka and associates[233] presented the results of a single case study in which a 53-year-old man with CHF was prescribed an exercise training program while receiving 10 μg/kg/min IV dobutamine (which he had been prescribed for 10 months before exercise training). Positive training adaptations were observed without complication and resulted in the patient being weaned from dobutamine.[234] In the ESSENTIAL trial, no adverse effects occurred when exercising patients with heart failure on enoximone, yet clinically significant differences were not reported between the treatment and the placebo groups.[235] The 6MWD was increased in the group with the inotrope support, but was not statistically significant, and no improvement in other clinical outcomes were reported.[235]

Exercise Training with Ventricular Assist Devices

Particular adjuncts to exercise conditioning in CHF include mechanical support of severe CMD via IABP and left or right VADs. Although individuals with IABPs are limited to breathing exercises and gentle exercise with upper extremities and the noncatheterized leg, individuals with VADs have enjoyed the freedom to exercise with minimal limitation. Improved technology has enabled patients who otherwise were immobilized because of IABP placement or nonmobile VAD placement to become mobile and ambulate with a cart or electric belt system that provides left ventricular assistance via portable pumping of the heart.[236-238] Patients using LVADs underwent 1173.6 hours of exercise conditioning without major complication and with only four minor complications (3.4 incidents per 1000 patient hours). The four minor complications were quickly corrected and resulted from an acute decrease in pump flow from venous pooling, decreased driveline air volume, and hypovolemia. Improvements in exercise tolerance and functional capacity continued until week 6 of conditioning, after which further improvements were minimal. It has been suggested that delay in cardiac transplantation until 6 weeks of exercise conditioning have been performed may improve postoperative recovery and surgical success.[239]

The reason for a lack of further improvement in exercise tolerance and functional capacity after week 6 was most likely because of the mechanical constraints of the LVAD. Cardiopulmonary exercise testing has demonstrated that LVAD patients demonstrate a modest training effect from chronic exercise training and appear to be limited at maximal exercise by the mechanics of the LVAD.[240] The mechanical constraints of the LVAD appear to prevent maximal levels of exercise from being attained and result in no substantial change in peak oxygen consumption after a mean of 16 weeks of aerobic exercise training. Possible mechanical constraints of the LVAD include flow limitations (10 to 12 L/min), altered cardiovascular function from the mechanically driven cardiac output, and the effects of a 6-lb mass resting below the diaphragm that may alter ventilatory performance. Limited training adaptations may also be a result of the same mechanism, but the reductions in submaximal heart rate and blood pressure, as well as increases in exercise duration, ventilation, and oxygen consumption at the ventilatory threshold, support the benefits that can be attained by exercising patients on LVAD.[237,238,240]

Exercise Training During Continuous Positive Airway Pressure Ventilation

Continuous positive airway pressure (CPAP) and bilevel positive airway pressure (BiPAP) have been observed to improve the exercise performance of patients with obstructive lung disease.[241–243] Despite the lack of research on the effect of CPAP or BiPAP upon the exercise performance of patients with CHF, resting myocardial performance has repeatedly been observed to improve with CPAP in patients with CHF[244–246] and patients with CHF and coexistent obstructive or central sleep apnea.[247–249] The beneficial effect of CPAP upon cardiac performance is postulated to be caused by increased intrathoracic pressure, which reduces cardiac preload (by impeding cardiac filling) and afterload (by reducing left ventricular transmural pressure),[244,245,249–251] as well as unloading the inspiratory muscles by providing positive pressure ventilation that may increase lung compliance.[246] The effects of CPAP or BiPAP upon exercise performance in patients with CHF are unknown, but several studies cited here have noted an improvement in dyspnea and functional status and exercise tolerance.[252]

Ventilation

Ventilatory Muscle Training

Breathing Exercises

Persons with CHF appear to benefit from breathing exercises.[253,254] Breathing exercises can be simple or complex and should be provided after a measurement of breathing strength is obtained. Such measurements include the maximal inspiratory pressure (MIP) and the maximal expiratory pressure (MEP), which are frequently measured with a manometer in centimeters of water. After strength measurements are obtained, patients are provided a breathing exercise program at a specific percentage of the MIP or MEP (similar to aerobic exercise training) with a device that resists either inspiration or expiration. The methods of measuring MIP and MEP and implementing a ventilatory muscle training program are provided.[253,254]

Facilitation of diaphragmatic breathing and inhibition of excessive accessory muscle use may decrease the work of breathing for a person with CHF and in conjunction with pursed-lip breathing may improve respiratory performance and, possibly, cardiac performance. Pursed-lip breathing is beneficial for persons with COPD by maintaining airway patency via increased positive end-expiratory pressure (PEEP).[255,256] In view of recent research, the same maintenance of airways from increased PEEP may be helpful for persons with CHF.[257,258] Furthermore, the increased PEEP and associated increase in intrathoracic pressure from varying degrees of pursed-lip breathing may decrease venous return, which could possibly decrease the left VEDV and pressure and improve myocardial performance for persons with severe CHF.[259]

Expiratory Muscle Training

The majority of studies investigating the effects of expiratory muscle training have involved persons with spinal cord injury or other neurologic disorders. In the majority of these studies, expiratory muscle training (performed in a variety of ways, but most commonly with weights on the abdomen and hyperpneic breathing) improved symptoms, functional status, and pulmonary function and reduced pulmonary complications. There is recent interest in expiratory muscle training of persons with various forms of COPD using PEEP devices, but very little literature exists. Likewise, there is little literature regarding expiratory muscle training alone in CHF. A study by Mancini and associates evaluated the effects of inspiratory and expiratory muscle training in CHF and found significant improvements in ventilatory muscle force and endurance, submaximal and maximal exercise performance, and dyspnea after 3 months of aggressive ventilatory muscle training in eight patients with chronic CHF.[254]

Despite a lack of research in expiratory muscle training alone in CHF, the observations of Mancini and associates[254] and others suggest that expiratory muscle training may be beneficial for persons with CHF by (1) increasing expiratory muscle strength to improve pulmonary function; (2) increasing PEEP to improve airway compliance; and (3) possibly decreasing venous return and the left VEDV to improve myocardial performance.[259] These changes may improve the exercise tolerance and functional status of persons with CHF. However, further investigation is needed in this area.

Inspiratory Muscle Training

Inspiratory muscle training has previously been shown to be helpful for patients with pulmonary disease by increasing ventilatory muscle strength and endurance and by decreasing dyspnea, need for medications, emergency room visits, and number of hospitalizations.[260,261] Individuals with chronic CHF have been found to have poor ventilatory muscle strength,[262–264] yet after inspiratory muscle training demonstrated significant improvements in ventilatory muscle strength and endurance, as well as dyspnea.[254,265]

Significant improvements in maximal inspiratory and expiratory pressures and degree of dyspnea were recently observed as soon as 2 weeks after ventilatory muscle training was initiated with the threshold inspiratory muscle trainer at 20% of MIP, three times a day, for 5 to 15 minutes (Fig. 4-25).[253] The improvement in ventilatory muscle strength was associated with significantly less dyspnea at rest and with exercise.

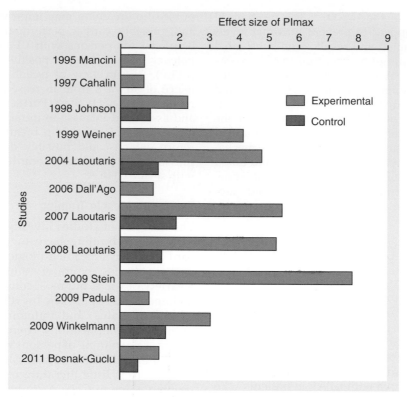

Figure 4-25 Demonstrates the effect size of inspiratory muscle training compared with control groups. These studies worked at a percentage of maximum inspiratory pressure at gradually increasing resistances. It is recommended to start working at 20% to 30% of PI_{max}. (Data from Lin SJ1, McElfresh J, Hall B, et al: Inspiratory muscle training in patients with heart failure: a systematic review. *Cardiopulm Phys Ther J* 23(3):29-36, 2012.)

However, the effects of ventilatory muscle training upon ventilatory muscle endurance, which may be the most important effect of ventilatory muscle training in this patient population, were not evaluated. Nonetheless, improvement in ventilatory muscle strength may decrease the dependency, impairment, and possibly even cost associated with chronic CHF. Increased ventilatory muscle strength may also enhance early postoperative recovery in patients undergoing cardiac transplantation or other cardiac surgery.

Instruction in Energy Conservation

Energy conservation techniques should be included in the interventions for individuals with heart failure to decrease the workload on the heart without loss of function. An analysis of all the activities an individual performs helps to develop an inventory to set priorities and organize the individual's day. Particular attention should be paid to activities that create fatigue or increased dyspnea. Box 4-7 provides suggestions for conserving energy for patients with heart failure.

Self-Management Techniques

Chronic disease management programs should identify the patients who are at high risk for morbidity and mortality and incorporate the individual into the management of the disease by making him or her responsible for his or her own health. Disease management programs for heart failure should include components that not only improve the management of the disease, but also demonstrate improved outcomes and reduction of costs. These components include:[266]

BOX 4-7　Energy conservation techniques for individuals with heart failure

- Sit while working whenever possible.
- Before you get tired, stop and rest.
- Spread tedious tasks out throughout the week.
- Do the tasks that require the most energy at times that you have the most energy.
- Alternate easy tasks with difficult tasks, and plan a rest period.
- Devote a portion of your day to an activity you enjoy and find relaxing.
- Keep items within easy reach.
- Plan ahead so you don't have to rush or push yourself hard.
- Decide activities that are not necessary for you to do, and delegate to other family members or caregivers; share the work.

- Individualized, comprehensive patient and family or caregiver education and outpatient counseling
- Optimization of medical therapy
- Vigilant follow-up
- Increased access to health care professionals
- Early attention to fluid overload
- Coordination with other agencies as appropriate
- Physician-directed care (and/or use of nurse coordinators or nurse-managed care)
- Specific content for patient and family education and counseling should include:
  - Discussion of limitation of dietary sodium to 1500 mg/day
  - Adherence to medication regimen

- Regular flu and pneumococcal immunizations
- Importance of daily weighing and monitoring of symptoms (shortness of breath, dizziness, or swelling)
- Instruction in signs/symptoms of decompensation (excessive shortness of breath, fatigue, peripheral swelling, waking at night with dyspnea or cough, etc.)
- Instruction in importance of seeking assistance when necessary
- Adherence to regular exercise program
- Limitation of alcohol intake
- Control of comorbid conditions (diabetes, elevated blood pressure, elevated lipids)

This educational content is much better received and remembered if given when the patient is in an outpatient versus an inpatient setting. Inpatient education is usually inadequate as well, as individuals do not retain what they are taught in the hospital. Individuals who are in the hospital are usually ill, anxious, distracted, or in poor condition to listen, learn, and retain any instructions. Instruction in self-management techniques after a critical event resulting in hospitalization results in improved adherence, if the patient is ready and able to learn, and in improved management of the disease.

Summary

- Causes of CMD include:
  - Myocardial infarction or ischemia
  - Cardiomyopathy
  - Cardiac arrhythmias
  - Heart valve abnormalities
  - Pericardial effusion or myocarditis
  - Pulmonary embolus
  - Pulmonary hypertension
  - Renal insufficiency
  - Spinal cord injury
  - Congenital abnormalities
  - Aging
- The term *cardiac muscle dysfunction* accurately describes the primary cause of pulmonary edema, as well as the underlying pathophysiology, which essentially impairs the heart's ability to pump blood or the LV's ability to accept blood.
- Cardiomyopathy, congenital abnormalities, renal insufficiency, and aging are associated more commonly with chronic heart failure, whereas the other factors tend to cause acute CHF.
- Right-sided or left-sided CHF simply describes which side of the heart is failing, as well as the side initially affected and behind which fluid tends to localize.
- Heart failure with reduced EF is the description associated with heart failure and is the result of a low cardiac output at rest or during exertion. Heart failure with preserved EF usually results from a volume overload.
- The impaired contraction of the ventricles during systole that produces an inefficient expulsion of blood is termed *systolic heart failure*. Diastolic heart failure is associated with an inability of the ventricles to accept the blood ejected from the atria.

- Hypertension and coronary artery disease are the most common causes of CMD.
- Cardiac arrhythmias and renal insufficiency can also cause CMD for reasons similar to those of myocardial infarction.
- Cardiomyopathies are classified from a functional standpoint, emphasizing three categories: dilated, hypertrophic, and restrictive.
- Heart valve abnormalities can also cause CMD as blocked or incompetent valves, or both, cause heart muscle to contract more forcefully to expel the cardiac output.
- Injury to the pericardium can cause acute pericarditis, which may progress to pericardial effusion.
- Cardiac muscle dysfunction from a pulmonary embolus is the result of elevated pulmonary artery pressures, which dramatically increase right ventricular work.
- Spinal cord injury can also produce CMD because of cervical spinal cord transection, which causes an imbalance between sympathetic and parasympathetic control of the cardiovascular system.
- Congestive heart failure is commonly associated with several characteristic signs and symptoms, including dyspnea, tachypnea, PND, orthopnea, hepatomegaly, peripheral edema, weight gain, jugular venous distension, rales, tubular breath sound and consolidation, presence of an S_3 heart sound, sinus tachycardia, and decreased exercise tolerance.
- Proteinuria; elevated urine specific gravity, BNP, BUN, and creatinine levels; and decreased erythrocyte sedimentation rates are associated with CHF.
- Dyspnea is probably the most common finding associated with CHF.
- A rapid respiratory rate at rest, characterized by quick and shallow breaths, is common in patients with CHF.
- The presence of an S_3 heart sound indicates a noncompliant left ventricle and occurs as blood passively fills a poorly relaxing LV.
- The retention of sodium and water is caused by (1) augmented α-adrenergic neural activity; (2) circulating catecholamines; and (3) increased levels of circulating and locally produced angiotensin II, resulting in renal vasoconstriction.
- Laboratory findings suggestive of impaired renal function in CHF include increases in BUN, as well as blood creatinine levels and BNP.
- Pulmonary edema can be cardiogenic or noncardiogenic in origin.
- The most common hematologic abnormality is a secondary polycythemia, which is caused by either a reduction in oxygen transport or an increase in erythropoietin production.
- Skeletal muscle abnormalities caused by dilated and hypertrophic cardiomyopathies have been reported previously and consistently reveal type I and type II fiber atrophy. Genetic causes may also contribute to muscle atrophy.
- Severe CMD has the potential to reduce blood flow to the pancreas, which impairs insulin secretion and glucose tolerance.
- The primary malnutrition in CHF is a protein-calorie deficiency, but vitamin deficiencies have also been observed.

- The specific treatments for CHF include restriction of sodium intake, use of medications, and self-management techniques.

- Many patients with CHF apparently have lower anaerobic thresholds, and the resultant anaerobic metabolism (because of acidosis) becomes the limiting factor in exercise performance.

- Although echocardiography is the most widely used method for the confirmation of the clinical diagnosis of heart failure, BNP is rapidly emerging as a very sensitive and specific adjunctive diagnostic marker.[66] It may also be an important prognostic marker and can be used as a rapid screening test in the urgent care setting.[65,66] Greater levels of ANP and BNP have also been found to be associated with higher morbidity and mortality rates.

- Plasma BNP, although consistently increased in patients with heart failure because of systolic dysfunction, is also increased in some patients with aortic stenosis, chronic mitral regurgitation, diastolic heart failure, and hypertrophic cardiomyopathy.

- The most significant predictors of survival in individuals with CHF have been identified and include decreasing LVEF, worsening NYHA functional status, degree of hyponatremia, decreasing peak exercise oxygen uptake, decreasing hematocrit, widened QRS on 12-lead electrocardiogram, chronic hypotension, resting tachycardia, renal insufficiency, intolerance to conventional therapy, and refractory volume overload.

Case study 4-1

An 85-year-old woman had a medical history of coronary artery bypass graft surgery in 1992 to the right coronary artery and left anterior diagonal artery, cholecystectomy, hiatal hernia, gastritis, and peptic ulcer disease. She was admitted August 9, 2010, with angina (a myocardial infarction was ruled out) and underwent cardiac catheterization on August 16, 2010, which revealed 99% occlusion of the right coronary artery graft, 85% occlusion of the left anterior diagonal artery graft, 95% stenosis of the circumflex artery, moderate mitral regurgitation, dilated left atrium, inferior hypokinesis, and an EF of approximately 30%. Echocardiographic study revealed severe left ventricular hypertrophy with a small left ventricular chamber size, inferior hypokinesis, calcified mitral valve with moderate mitral regurgitation, abnormal left ventricular compliance (left ventricular stiffness), and a dilated left atrium.

The referral for cardiac rehabilitation was written on August 11, 2010, at which time the patient was assessed and complained of left scapular pain that increased with deep breathing (different from previous angina and altered with breathing pattern). Physical examination revealed normal sinus rhythm and slightly decreased breath sounds in the left lower lobe. The patient ambulated approximately 250 feet with an adaptive heart rate and blood pressure response, without angina. The patient continued with twice-daily cardiac rehabilitation, increasing the distance ambulated to 800 feet, and underwent a thallium treadmill stress test on August 13, 2010. The patient completed 2 minutes 25 seconds of the modified Bruce protocol (attaining a maximal heart rate of 104 bpm, 67% of the

age-predicted maximal heart rate), which was terminated because of leg fatigue. The patient experienced no angina and demonstrated no ECG changes consistent with myocardial ischemia. The thallium scan demonstrated moderately severe stress-induced ischemic change in the inferior and septal areas.

Cardiac rehabilitation was performed August 14, 2010, through August 16, 2010, during which the patient walked 5 to 10 minutes (500 to 1000 feet) with adaptive heart rate and blood pressure responses to exercise, without angina. On August 17, 2010, while resting in bed, the patient developed severe angina and dyspnea, which required morphine sulfate, nitroglycerin, and heparin, suggesting impending graft occlusion. In view of these findings, coronary artery bypass graft surgery was repeated on August 20, 2010, after which the patient developed numerous complications, requiring intraaortic balloon pump assistance from which weaning was difficult. In addition, the patient experienced a postoperative anterolateral myocardial infarction as a result of a third-degree heart block that decreased the blood supply to the myocardium, respiratory failure that required full ventilatory support, congestive heart failure, and severe abdominal distension.

The patient's status further deteriorated as she became anemic and was unable to maintain adequate nutritional requirements. However, a radiograph on August 24, 2010, revealed no evidence of CHF, and ventilatory measurements demonstrated improved pulmonary function. In addition, hemoglobin and hematocrit levels were slightly increased (10.7 and 29.4, respectively). The patient was extubated on August 25, 2010, and began ambulation with nursing on August 26, 2010, during which she complained of severe abdominal pain and a feeling of increased abdominal swelling. Because of persistent abdominal pain and distension, an exploratory laparotomy was performed on August 28, 2010, resulting in resection of the small bowel.

The patient remained on bed rest for 3 days, after which she began ambulating with nursing. On September 4, 2010, the patient ambulated 50 feet with physical therapy, during which she complained of severe dyspnea and mild-to-moderate abdominal discomfort. For this reason, physical therapy discontinued ambulation but continued chest physical therapy and bedside exercise to the upper and lower extremities. However, nursing continued to ambulate the patient approximately four times per day despite her complaints of severe shortness of breath and abdominal discomfort. On September 6, 2010, immediately after walking, she developed severe abdominal discomfort associated with nausea and vomiting. Nonetheless, that evening, the patient was ambulated 200 feet, walking approximately 15 minutes, at which time she complained of severe abdominal pain; her respiratory rate was noted to be in the high 50s. On September 7, 2010, the patient was again walked approximately 75 feet with a walker and maximal assist of three, at which time she became unresponsive. Physician examination at this time revealed severe tachypnea and abdominal distension. On September 10, 2010, the patient's status further deteriorated with effusion and atelectasis of the left lung base, ischemic bowel, possible abdominal infection, anemia, and azotemia. She expired on September 11, 2010.

Discussion

This case study is an example of an 85-year-old patient who underwent bypass surgery after the following occurred:

1. She remained asymptomatic during prolonged cardiac rehabilitation exercise assessments with adaptive heart rate and blood pressure responses, but somewhat paradoxically developed angina at rest.

2. A thallium treadmill stress test demonstrated moderately severe ischemic change.

3. A cardiac catheterization revealed occluded grafts to the right coronary artery and left anterior diagonal artery and high-grade occlusion of the circumflex artery, inferior hypokinesis, and depressed EF (approximately 30%).

Unfortunately, after bypass surgery was performed, the patient developed numerous complications caused primarily by pump failure and improper exercise training that was not appropriately adjusted to the patient's needs. At no time should a patient be ambulated with moderate-to-severe pain (whatever the location or cause), as it most likely represents a pathologic process (in this case, ischemia of the small intestine). In addition, inappropriate responses to exercise training, such as a rapid heart rate or respiratory rate with minimal exercise, must be reassessed and treated before subsequent exercise is performed, or at least changes must be made in the type of exercise performed. Sitting lower extremity exercise would have been much more appropriate for this patient, who demonstrated many interrelated pathophysiologic processes that were exacerbated by improper exercise training and ultimately led to her death.

References

1. The European "Corwin" Study Group: Xamoterol in mild to moderate heart failure: A subgroup analysis of patients with cardiomegaly but no concomitant angina pectoris, *J Clin Pharmacol Suppl* 1:67S–69S, 1989.

2. Kannel WB: Epidemiological aspects of heart failure, *Cardiol Clin* 7(1):1–9, 1989.

3. Kannel WB, Belanger AJ: Epidemiology of heart failure, *Am Heart J* 121(3 Pt 1):951–957, 1991.

4. Lloyd-Jones D, Adams R, Carnethon M, et al.: Heart disease and stroke statistics 2009 update: A report from the American Heart Association Statistics Committee and Stroke Statistics Subcommittee, *Circulation* 108; 119:e21–e181, 2008.

5. Braunwald E: Clinical manifestations of heart failure. In Braunwald E, editor: *Heart Disease: A Textbook of Cardiovascular Medicine*, Philadelphia, 1988, Saunders.

6. Cheng TO: Cardiac failure in coronary heart disease, *Am Heart J* 120(2):396–412, 1990.

7. Hildner FJ: Pulmonary edema associated with low, left ventricular filling pressures, *Am J Cardiol* 44(7):1410–1411, 1979.

8. Auchincloss JH, Gilbert R, Morales R, et al.: Reduction of trial and error in the equilibrium rebreathing cardiac output method, *J Cardiopulm Rehabil* 9(2):85, 1989.

9. Braunwald E, Sonnenblick EH, Ross Jr J: Mechanisms of cardiac contraction and relaxation. In Braunwald E, editor: *Heart Disease: A Textbook of Cardiovascular Medicine*, Philadelphia, 1988, Saunders.

10. Wynne J, Braunwald E: The cardiomyopathies and myocarditides. In Braunwald E, editor: *Heart Disease: A Textbook of Cardiovascular Medicine*, Philadelphia, 1988, Saunders.

11. McCartan C1, Mason R, Jayasinghe SR, Griffiths LR: Cardiomyopathy classification: Ongoing debate in the genomics era, *Biochem Res Int* 2012:796926, 2012.

12. Braunwald E: Pathophysiology of heart failure. In Braunwald E, editor: *Heart Disease: A Textbook of Cardiovascular Medicine*, Philadelphia, 1988, Saunders.

13. Goldberger JJ, Peled HB, Stroh JA, et al.: Prognostic factors in acute pulmonary edema, *Arch Intern Med* 146(3):489–493, 1986.

14. Baigrie RS, Haq A, Morgan CD, et al.: The spectrum of right ventricular involvement in inferior wall myocardial infarction, *J Am Coll Cardiol* 1(6):1396–1404, 1983.

15. Cintron GB, Hernandez E, Linares E, et al.: Bedside recognition, incidence and clinical course of right ventricular infarction, *Am J Cardiol* 47(2):224–227, 1981.

16. Klein LW, Kramer BL, Howard E, et al.: Incidence and clinical significance of transient creatinine kinase elevations and the diagnosis of non-Q wave myocardial infarction associated with coronary angioplasty, *J Am Coll Cardiol* 17(3):621–626, 1991.

17. Fischell TA, Derby G, Tse TM, et al.: Coronary artery vasoconstriction routinely occurs after percutaneous transluminal coronary angioplasty. A quantitative arteriographic analysis, *Circulation* 78:1323, 1988.

18. Kirklin JW, Blackstone EH, Kirklin JK: Cardiac surgery. In Braunwald E, editor: *Heart Disease: A Textbook of Cardiovascular Medicine*, Philadelphia, 1988, Saunders.

19. Breisblatt WM, Stein KL, Wolfe CJ, et al.: Acute myocardial dysfunction and recovery: A common occurrence after coronary bypass surgery, *J Am Coll Cardiol* 15(6):1261–1269, 1990.

20. Zipes DP, Camm AJ, Borggrefe M, et al.: ACC/AHA/ESC 2006 guidelines for management of patients with ventricular arrhythmias and the prevention of sudden cardiac death-executive summary. A report of the American College of Cardiology/American Heart Association Task Force and the European Society of Cardiology Committee for Practice Guidelines, *Circulation* 114(10):1088–1132, 2006.

21. Cruz FES, Cheriex EC, Smeets JL, et al.: Reversibility of tachycardia-induced cardiomyopathy after cure of incessant supraventricular tachycardia, *J Am Coll Cardiol* 16(3):739–744, 1990.

22. Epstein AE, DiMarco JP, Ellenbogen KA, et al.: ACC/AHA/HRS 2008 guidelines for device-based therapy of cardiac rhythm abnormalities: Executive summary, *Circulation* 117(21):2820–2840, 2008.

23. Jessup M, Abraham WT, Casey DE, et al.: 2009 Focused update: ACCF/AHA guidelines for the diagnosis and management of heart failure in adults: a report of the American College of Cardiology Foundation/American Heart Association Task Force on practice management of heart failure in adults, *Circulation* 119(14):1977–2016, 2009.

24. Pastan SO, Braunwald E: Renal disorders and heart disease. In Braunwald E, editor: *Heart Disease: A Textbook of Cardiovascular Medicine*, Philadelphia, 1988, Saunders.

25. Pitt B, Williams G, Remme W, et al.: The EPHESUS trial: Eplerenone in patients with heart failure due to systolic dysfunction complicating acute myocardial infarction. Eplerenone Post-AMI Heart Failure Efficacy and Survival Study, *Cardiovasc Drugs Ther* 15(1):79–87, 2001.

26. Abelmann WH: Classification and natural history of primary myocardial disease, *Prog Cardiovasc Dis* 27(2):73–94, 1984.

27. Maron BJ, Fananapazir L: Sudden cardiac death in hypertrophic cardiomyopathy, *Circulation* 85(1 Suppl):I57–I63, 1992.

28. Silverman KJ, Hutchins GM, Weiss JL, et al.: Catenoidal shape of the interventricular septum in idiopathic hypertrophic subaortic stenosis: Two-dimensional echocardiographic confirmation, *Am J Cardiol* 49(1):27–32, 1982.

29. Braunwald E: Valvular heart disease. In Braunwald E, editor: *Heart Disease: A Textbook of Cardiovascular Medicine*, Philadelphia, 1988, Saunders.

30. Goldhaber SZ, Braunwald E: Pulmonary embolism. In Braunwald E, editor: *Heart Disease: A Textbook of Cardiovascular Medicine*, Philadelphia, 1988, Saunders.

31. Geerts WH, Bergqvist D, Pineo GF, et al.: Prevention of venous thromboembolism: American College of Chest Physicians evidence-based clinical practice guidelines (8th edition), *Chest* 133(6 Suppl):381S–453S, 2008.

32. MacKenzie CF, Shin B, Krishnaprasad D, et al.: Assessment of cardiac and respiratory function during surgery on patients with acute quadriplegia, *J Neurosurg* 62(6):843–849, 1985.

33. Woolman L: The disturbance of circulation in traumatic paraplegia in acute and late stages. A pathological study, *Paraplegia* 2:213–226, 1965.

34. Meyer GA, Berman IR, Doty DB, et al.: Hemodynamic responses to acute quadriplegia with or without chest trauma, *J Neurosurg* 34(2 Pt 1):168–177, 1971.

35. Bellamy R, Pitts FW, Stauffer ES: Respiratory complications in traumatic quadriplegia. Analysis of 20 years' experience, *J Neurosurg* 39(5):596–600, 1973.

36. Friedman WF: Congenital heart disease in infancy and childhood. In Braunwald E, editor: *Heart Disease: A Textbook of Cardiovascular Medicine*, Philadelphia, 1988, Saunders.

37. Borow KM, Braunwald E: Congenital heart disease in the adult. In Braunwald E, editor: *Heart Disease: A Textbook of Cardiovascular Medicine*, Philadelphia, 1988, Saunders.

38. Moser M: Physiological differences in the elderly. Are they clinically important? *Eur Heart J* 9(Suppl D):55–61, 1988.

39. Weisfeldt ML, Lakatta KG, Gerstenblith G: Aging and cardiac disease. In Braunwald E, editor: *Heart Disease: A Textbook of Cardiovascular Medicine*, Philadelphia, 1988, Saunders.

40. Tanner K, Sabrine N, Wren C: Cardiovascular malformations among preterm infants, *Pediatrics* 116(6):e833–e838, 2005.

41. Brandfonbrener M, Landowne M, Shock NW: Changes in cardiac output with age, *Circulation* 12(4):557–566, 1955.

42. Strandell T: Circulatory studies on healthy old men. With special reference to the limitation of the maximal physical working capacity, *Acta Med Scand* 175:1, 1964.

43. Conway I, Wheeler R, Sannerstedt R: Sympathetic nervous activity during exercise in relation to age, *Cardiovasc Res* 5(4):577–581, 1971.

44. Rodeheffer RJ, Gerstenblith G, Becker LC, et al.: Exercise cardiac output is maintained with advancing age in healthy human subjects: Cardiac dilatation and increased stroke volume compensate for a diminished heart rate, *Circulation* 69(2):203–213, 1984.

45. Sjögren AL: Left ventricular wall thickness determined by ultrasound in 100 subjects without heart disease, *Chest* 60(4):341–346, 1971.

46. Gerstenblith G, Fleg JL, Becker LC, et al.: Maximum left ventricular filling rate in healthy individuals measured by gated blood pool scans: Effect of age, *Circulation* 68:91–101, 1983.

47. Capasso JM, Malhotra A, Remily R, et al.: Effects of age on mechanical and electrical performance of rat myocardium, *Am J Physiol* 245(1):H72–H81, 1983.

48. Lakatta KG, Yin FCP: Myocardial aging: Functional alterations and related cellular mechanisms, *Am J Physiol* 242(6):H927–H941, 1982.

49. Bhatnagar GM, Walford GD, Beard ES, et al.: ATPase activity and force production in myofibrils and twitch characteristics in intact muscle from neonatal, adult, and senescent rat myocardium, *J Mol Cell Cardiol* 16(3):203–218, 1984.

50. Wei JY, Spurgeon HA, Lakatta KG: Excitation-contraction in rat myocardium: Alterations with adult aging, *Am J Physiol* 246(6 Pt 2):H784–H791, 1984.

51. Spurgeon HA, Steinbach MF, Lakatta KG: Chronic exercise prevents characteristic age-related changes in rat cardiac contraction, *Am J Physiol* 244(4):H513–H518, 1983.

52. Spurgeon HA, Thorne PR, Yin FCP, et al.: Increased dynamic stiffness of trabeculae carneae from senescent rats, *Am J Physiol* 232(4):H373–H380, 1977.

53. Yin FCP, Spurgeon HA, Weisfeldt ML, et al.: Mechanical properties of myocardium from hypertrophied rat hearts. A comparison between hypertrophy induced by senescence and by aortic banding, *Circ Res* 46(2):292–300, 1980.

54. Orchard CH, Lakatta KG: Intracellular calcium transients and developed tensions in rat heart muscle. A mechanism for the negative interval-strength relationship, *J Gen Physiol* 86(5):637–651, 1985.

55. Grossman W, Braunwald E: High-cardiac output states. In Braunwald E, editor: *Heart Disease: A Textbook of Cardiovascular Medicine*, Philadelphia, 1988, Saunders.

56. Perloff JK: Pregnancy and cardiovascular disease. In Braunwald E, editor: *Heart Disease: A Textbook of Cardiovascular Medicine*, Philadelphia, 1988, Saunders.

57. Mentz RJ, et al.: Noncardiac comorbidities in heart failure with reduced versus preserved ejection fraction, *J Am Coll Cardiol* 64(21):2281–2293, 2014.

58. Braunwald E: Assessment of cardiac function. In Braunwald E, editor: *Heart Disease: A Textbook of Cardiovascular Medicine*, Philadelphia, 1988, Saunders.

59. Parmley WW: Hemodynamic monitoring in acute ischemic disease. In Fishman AP, editor: *Heart Failure*, New York, 1978, McGraw-Hill.

60. Andreoli KG, Fowkes VH, Zipes DP, et al.: *Comprehensive Cardiac Care*, ed 4, St. Louis, 1979, Mosby.

61. D'Souza SP, Davis M, Baxter GF: Autocrine and paracrine actions of natriuretic peptides in the heart, *Pharmacol Ther* 101(2):113–129, 2004.

62. Collins E, Bracamonte MP, Burnett Jr JC, et al.: Mechanism of relaxations to dendroaspis natriuretic peptide in canine coronary arteries, *J Cardiovasc Pharmacol* 35(5):614–618, 2000.

63. Best PJ, Burnett JC, Wilson SH, et al.: Dendroaspis natriuretic peptide relaxes isolated human arteries and veins, *Cardiovasc Res* 55(2):375–384, 2002.

64. Richards AM, Lainchbury JG, Nicholls MG, et al.: Dendroaspis natriuretic peptide: Endogenous or dubious? *Lancet* 359(9300):5–6, 2002.

65. Creager MA, Dzau V, Loscalzo J: *Vascular Medicine. A Companion to Braunwald's Heart Disease*, Philadelphia, 2006, Saunders.

66. Maisel A: B-type natriuretic peptide levels: A potential novel "white count" for congestive heart failure, *J Card Fail* 7(2):183–193, 2001.

67. Wallén T, Landahl S, Hedner T, et al.: Atrial natriuretic peptides predict mortality in the elderly, *J Intern Med* 241(4):269–275, 1997.

68. Iivanainen AM, Tikkanen I, Tilvis R, et al.: Associations between atrial natriuretic peptides, echocardiographic findings and mortality in an elderly population sample, *J Intern Med* 241(4):261–268, 1997.

69. Skorecki KL, Brenner BM: Body fluid homeostasis in congestive heart failure and cirrhosis with ascites, *Am J Med* 72(2):323–338, 1982.

70. Hostetter TH, Pfeffer JM, Pfeffer MA, et al.: Cardiorenal hemodynamics and sodium excretion in rats with myocardial infarction, *Am J Physiol* 245(1):H98–H103, 1983.

71. Ingram Jr RH, Braunwald E: Pulmonary edema: Cardiogenic and noncardiogenic. In Braunwald E, editor: *Heart Disease: A Textbook of Cardiovascular Medicine*, Philadelphia, 1988, Saunders.

72. Fillmore SJ, Giumaraes AC, Scheidt AC, et al.: Blood gas changes and pulmonary hemodynamics following acute myocardial infarction, *Circulation* 45(3):583–591, 1972.

73. Light RW, George RB: Serial pulmonary function in patients with acute heart failure, *Arch Intern Med* 143(3):429–433, 1983.

74. Wright RS, Levine S, Bellamy PE, et al.: Ventilatory and diffusion abnormalities in potential heart transplant recipients, *Chest* 98(4):816–820, 1990.

75. Feldman AM, Bristow MR: The beta-adrenergic pathway in the failing human heart: Implications for inotropic therapy, *Cardiology* 77(Suppl 1):1–32, 1990.

76. Lefkowitz RJ, Caron MG: Adrenergic receptors: Models for the study of receptors coupled to guanine nucleotide regulatory proteins, *J Biol Chem* 263(11):4993–4996, 1988.

77. Exton JH: Molecular mechanisms involved in alpha-adrenergic responses, *Mol Cell Endocrinol* 23(3):233–264, 1981.

78. Scholz A, Schaefer B, Schmitz W, et al.: Alpha-1 adrenoceptor-mediated positive inotropic effect and inositol trisphosphate increase in mammalian heart, *J Pharmacol Exp Ther* 245(1):327–335, 1988.

79. Gilman AG: G proteins: Transducers of receptor-generated signals, *Annu Rev Biochem* 56:615–649, 1987.

80. Bristow MR: The beta-adrenergic receptor. Configuration, regulation, mechanism of action, *Postgrad Med* 29(Spec No):19–26, 1988.

81. Bristow MR, Minobe W, Rasmussen R, et al.: Alpha-1 adrenergic receptors in the nonfailing and failing human heart, *J Pharmacol Exp Ther* 247(3):1039–1045, 1989.

82. Feldman MA, Copelas L, Gwathney JK, et al.: Deficient production of cyclic AMP. Pharmacologic evidence of an important cause of contractile dysfunction in patients with end-stage heart failure, *Circulation* 75(2):331–339, 1987.

83. Bristow MR, Ginsburg R, Umans V, et al.: Beta1-and beta2-adrenergic-receptor subpopulations in nonfailing and failing human ventricular myocardium: Coupling of both receptor subtypes to muscle contraction and selective beta 1-receptor down-regulation in heart failure, *Circ Res* 59(3):297–309, 1986.

84. Fowler MB, Laser JA, Hopkins GL, et al.: Assessment of the beta-adrenergic receptor pathway in the intact failing human heart: Progressive receptor down-regulation and subsensitivity to agonist response, *Circulation* 74(6):1290–1302, 1986.

85. Bristow MR, Hershberger RE, Port D, et al.: Beta 1- and beta 2-adrenergic receptor-mediated adenylate cyclase stimulation in nonfailing and failing human ventricular myocardium, *Mol Pharmacol* 35(3):295–303, 1989.

86. Cardellach F, Galofre J, Cusso R, et al.: Decline in skeletal muscle mitochondrial respiration chain function with aging [letter], *Lancet* 334(8653):44–45, 1989.

87. Rosenthal DS, Braunwald E: Hematological-oncological disorders and heart disease. In Braunwald E, editor: *Heart Disease: A Textbook of Cardiovascular Medicine*, Philadelphia, 1988, Saunders.

88. Jandl JH: *Blood: Textbook of Hematology*, Boston, 1987, Little, Brown.

89. Shafig SA, Sande MA, Carruthers RR, et al.: Skeletal muscle in idiopathic cardiomyopathy, *J Neurol Sci* 15(3):303–320, 1972.

90. Poole-Wilson PA: The origin of symptoms in patients with chronic heart failure, *Eur Heart J* 9(Suppl H):49–53, 1988.

91. Limongelli G, et al.: Skeletal muscle involvement in cardiomyopathies, *J Cardiovasc Med 2013* 14(12):837–861, 2013.

92. Isaacs H, Muncke G: Idiopathic cardiomyopathy and skeletal muscle abnormality, *Am Heart J* 90(6):767–773, 1975.

93. Dunnigan A, Pierpont ME, Smith SA, et al.: Cardiac and skeletal myopathy associated with cardiac dysrhythmias, *Am J Cardiol* 53(6):731–737, 1984.

94. Dunnigan A, Staley NA, Smith SA, et al.: Cardiac and skeletal muscle abnormalities in cardiomyopathy: Comparison of patients with ventricular tachycardia or congestive heart failure, *J Am Coll Cardiol* 10:608–618, 1987.

95. Smith ER, Heffernan LP, Sangalang VE, et al.: Voluntary muscle involvement in hypertrophic cardiomyopathy: A study of 11 patients, *Ann Intern Med* 85(5):566–572, 1976.

96. Hootsmans WJM, Meerschwam IS: Electromyography in patients with hypertrophic obstructive cardiomyopathy, *Neurology* 21(8):810–816, 1971.

97. Meerschwam IS, Hootsmans WJM: An electromyographic study in hypertrophic obstructive cardiomyopathy. In Wolsterholme GEW, O'Connor M, London J, Churchill A, editors: *Hypertrophic Obstructive Cardiomyopathy. Ciba Foundation Study Group No. 37*, New York, 1971, Wiley.

98. Przybosewki JZ, Hoffman HD, Graff AS, et al.: A study of family with inherited disease of cardiac and skeletal muscle. Part 1: Clinical electrocardiographic, echocardiographic, hemodynamic, electrophysiological and electron microscopic studies, *S Afr Med J* 59(11):363–373, 1981.

99. Lochner A, Hewlett RH, O'Kennedy A, et al.: A study of a family with inherited disease of cardiac and skeletal muscle. Part 2: Skeletal muscle morphology and mitochondrial oxidative phosphorylation, *S Afr Med J* 59(13):453–461, 1981.

100. Massie B, Conway M, Yonge R, et al.: Skeletal muscle metabolism in patients with congestive heart failure: Relation to clinical severity and blood flow, *Circulation* 76(5):1009–1019, 1987.

101. Massie B, Conway M, Yonge R, et al.: 31P nuclear magnetic resonance evidence of abnormal skeletal muscle metabolism in patients with congestive heart failure, *Am J Cardiol* 60(4):309–315, 1987.

102. Braunwald E, Sobel BE: Coronary blood flow and myocardial ischemia. In Braunwald E, editor: *Heart Disease: A Textbook of Cardiovascular Medicine*, Philadelphia, 1988, Saunders.

103. Neely JR, Rovetto MJ, Whitmer JT, et al.: Effects of ischemia on ventricular function and metabolism in the isolated working rat heart, *Am J Physiol* 225(3):651–658, 1973.

104. Williams GH, Braunwald E: Endocrine and nutritional disorders and heart disease. In Braunwald E, editor: *Heart Disease: A Textbook of Cardiovascular Medicine*, Philadelphia, 1988, Saunders.

105. Yui Y, Fujiwara H, Mitsui H, et al.: Furosemide-induced thiamine deficiency, *Jpn Circ J* 14(9):537–540, 1978.

106. Bautista J, Rafel E, Marunez A, et al.: Familial hypertrophic cardiomyopathy and muscle carnitine deficiency, *Muscle Nerve* 13(3):192–194, 1990.

107. Folkers K: Heart failure is a dominant deficiency of coenzyme Q10 and challenges for future clinical research on CoQ10, *Clin Investig* 71(8 Suppl):S51–S54, 1993.

108. Lampertico M, Comis S: Italian multicenter study on the efficacy and safety of coenzyme Q10 as adjuvant therapy in heart failure, *Clin Investig* 71(8 Suppl):S129–S133, 1993.

109. Morisco C, Trimarco B, Condorelli M: Effect of coenzyme Q10 therapy in patients with congestive heart failure: A long-term multicenter randomized study, *Clin Investig* 71(8 Suppl):S134–S136, 1993.

110. Jameson S: Statistical data support prediction of death within 6 months on low levels of coenzyme Q10 and other entities, *Clin Investig* 71(8 Suppl):S137–S139, 1993.

111. Langsjoen PH, Folkers K: Isolated diastolic dysfunction of the myocardium and its response to CoQ10 treatment, *Clin Investig* 71(8 Suppl):S140–S144, 1993.

112. Eschbach JW, Adamson JW: Anemia of end-stage renal disease (ESRD), *Kidney Int* 28(1):1–5, 1985.

113. Eschbach JW, Egrie JC, Downing MR, et al.: Correction of the anemia of end-stage renal disease with recombinant human erythropoietin: Results of a combined phase I and II clinical trial, *N Engl J Med* 316(2):73–78, 1987.

114. Wilson L, Felsenfeld A, Drezner MK, et al.: Altered divalent ion metabolism in early renal failure: Role of 1,25(OH)2D, *Kidney Int* 27(3):565–573, 1985.

115. Madsen S, Olgaard K, Ladefoged J: Suppressive effect of 1,25-dihydroxyvitamin D3 on circulating parathyroid hormone in acute renal failure, *J Clin Endocrinol Metab* 53(4):823–827, 1981.

116. Klahr S: Nonexcretory functions of the kidney. In Klahr S, editor: *The Kidney and Body Fluids in Health and Disease*, New York, 1983, Plenum Medical Publishing.

117. Wasserman K, Hansen JE, Sue DY, et al.: *Principles of Exercise Testing and Interpretation*, Philadelphia, 1987, Lea & Febiger.

118. Moe GW, Canepa-Anson R, Howard RJ, et al.: Response of atrial natriuretic factor to postural change in patients with heart failure versus subjects with normal hemodynamics, *J Am Coll Cardiol* 16(3):599–606, 1990.

119. Killip T, Eimball JT: Treatment of myocardial infarction in a coronary care unit. A two-year experience with 250 patients, *Am J Cardiol* 20(4):457–464, 1967.

120. Mello BH, et al.: Validation of the Killip–Kimball Classification and late mortality after acute myocardial infarction, *Arq Bras Cardiol* 103(2):107–117, 2014.

121. Braunwald E: The physical examination. In Braunwald E, editor: *Heart Disease: A Textbook of Cardiovascular Medicine*, Philadelphia, 1988, Saunders.

122. Chezner MA: Cardiac auscultation: Heart sounds, *Cardiol Pract*, 1984. Sept/Oct:141.

123. Stevenson LW, Brunken RC, Belil D, et al.: Afterload reduction with vasodilators and diuretics decreases mitral regurgitation during upright exercise in advanced heart failure, *J Am Coll Cardiol* 15:174–180, 1990.

124. Constant J: *Bedside Cardiology*, Boston, 1985, Brown, Little.

125. Guyton AC: The relationship of cardiac output and arterial pressure control, *Circulation* 64(6):1079–1088, 1981.

126. Sullivan MJ, Green HJ, Cobb FR: Skeletal muscle biochemistry and histology in ambulatory patients with long-term heart failure, *Circulation* 81(2):518–527, 1990.

127. Drexler H, Riede U, Munzel T, et al.: Alterations of skeletal muscle in chronic heart failure, *Circulation* 85(5):1751–1759, 1992.

128. Criteria Committee, New York Heart Association: *Diseases of the Heart and Blood Vessels*, ed 6, Boston, 1964, Little, Brown.

129. Mann DL: *Heart Failure: A Companion to Braunwald's Heart Disease*, Philadelphia, 2004, Saunders.

130. Mancini D, Eisen H, Kussmaul W, et al.: Value of peak exercise oxygen consumption for optimal timing of cardiac transplantation in ambulatory patients with heart failure, *Circulation* 83(3):778–786, 1991.

131. Cohn J, Rector T: Prognosis of congestive heart failure and predictors of mortality, *Am J Cardiol* 62(2):25A–30A, 1988.

132. Slazchic J, Massie B, Kramer B, et al.: Correlates and prognostic implication of exercise capacity in chronic congestive heart failure, *Am J Cardiol* 55(8):1037–1042, 1985.

133. Likoff M, Chandler S, Kay H: Clinical determinants of mortality in chronic congestive heart failure secondary to idiopathic dilated or ischemic cardiomyopathy, *Am J Cardiol* 59(6):634–638, 1987.

134. Cohn J, Johnson G, Shabetai R, et al.: Ejection fraction, peak exercise oxygen consumption, cardiothoracic ratio, ventricular arrhythmias, and plasma norepinephrine as determinants of prognosis in heart failure. The V-HeFT VA Cooperative Studies Group, *Circulation* 87(6 Suppl):VI5–V16, 1993.

135. Aaronson KD, Mancini DM: Is percentage of predicted maximal exercise oxygen consumption a better predictor of survival than peak exercise oxygen consumption for patients with severe heart failure? *J Heart Lung Transplant* 14(5):981–989, 1995.

136. Sullivan MJ, Cobb FR: The anaerobic threshold in chronic heart failure. Relation to blood lactate, ventilatory basis, reproducibility, and response to exercise training, *Circulation* 81(1 Suppl):II47–II58, 1990.

137. Tavazzi L, Gattone M, Corra U, et al.: The anaerobic index: Uses and limitations in the assessment of heart failure, *Cardiology* 76(5):357–367, 1989.

138. Wasserman K, Beaver WL, Whipp BJ: Gas exchange theory, and the lactic acidosis (anaerobic) threshold, *Circulation* 81(1 Suppl): II14–II30, 1990.

139. Koike A, Itoh H, Taniguchi K, et al.: Relationship of anaerobic threshold (AT) to AVO2/WR in patients with heart disease [abstract], *Circulation* 78(Suppl 11):624, 1988.

140. Wenger NK: Left ventricular dysfunction, exercise capacity and activity recommendations, *Eur Heart J* 9(Suppl F):63–66, 1988.

141. Cahalin LP, Mathier MA, Semigran MJ, et al.: The six-minute walk test predicts peak oxygen uptake and survival in patients with advanced heart failure, *Chest* 110(2):325–332, 1996.

142. Faggiano P, D'Aloia A, Gualeni A, et al.: Assessment of oxygen uptake during the six-minute walk test in patients with heart failure [letter], *Chest* 111(4):1146, 1997.

143. Bittner V, Weiner DH, Yusuf S, et al.: Prediction of mortality and morbidity with a 6-minute walk test in patients with left ventricular dysfunction, *JAMA* 270(14):1702–1707, 1993.

144. Deboeck G, Van Muylem A, Vachiéry JL, Naeije R: Physiological response to the 6-minute walk test in chronic heart failure patients versus healthy control subjects, *Eur J Prev Cardiol* 21(8):997–1003, 2013.

145. Rector TS, Kubo SH, Cohn JN: Patients' self-assessment of their congestive heart failure: II. Content, reliability and validity of a new measure—The Minnesota Living with Heart Failure Questionnaire, *Heart Fail* 3:198, 1987.

146. Kavanagh T, Myers MG, Baigrie RS, et al.: Quality of life and cardiorespiratory function in chronic heart failure: Effects of 12 months' aerobic training, *Heart* 76:42–49, 1996.

147. Tyni-Lenné R, Cordon A, Sylvén C: Improved quality of life in chronic heart failure patients following local endurance training with leg muscles, *J Card Fail* 2(2):111–117, 1996.

148. Guyatt GH: Measurement of health-related quality of life in heart failure, *J Am Coll Cardiol* 22(4 Suppl A):185A–191A, 1993.

149. Ball E, Michel T, Cahalin LP. Quality of life in elderly heart failure patients is related to quadriceps muscle performance [abstract], *J Cardiopulm Rehabil* 17(5):329, 1997.

150. Jiang W, Alexander J, Christopher E, et al.: Relationship of depression to increased risk of mortality and rehospitalization in patient with congestive heart failure, *Arch Intern Med* 161(15):1849–1856, 2001.

151. Rumsfeld JS, Havranek E, Masoudi FA, et al.: Depressive symptoms are the strongest predictors of short-term declines in health status in patients with heart failure, *J Am Coll Cardiol* 42(10):1811–1817, 2003.

152. Fulop G, Strain HH, Stettin G: Congestive heart failure and depression in older adults: Clinical course and health services use 6 months after hospitalization, *Psychosomatics* 44(5):367–373, 2003.

153. Havranek EP, Ware MG, Lowes BD: Prevalence of depression in congestive heart failure, *Am J Cardiol* 84(3):348–350, A9, 1999.

154. Gary RA, Brunn K: Aerobic exercise as an adjunct therapy for improving cognitive function in heart failure. Review Article, *Cardiol Res Pract*, 2014: 157508, 2014.

155. Colcombe S, Kramer AF: Fitness effects on the cognitive function of older adults: A meta-analytic study, *Psychol Sci* 14(2):125–130, 2013.

156. Richards M, Hardy R, Wadsworth MEJ: Does active leisure protect cognition? Evidence from a national birth cohort, *Soc Sci Med* 56(4):785–792, 2003.

157. Alosco ML, et al.: Cardiac rehabilitation is associated with lasting improvements in cognitive function in older adults with heart failure, *Acta Cardiol* 69(4):407–414, 2014.

158. Wilson JR, Fink L, Maris J, et al.: Evaluation of energy metabolism in skeletal muscle of patients with heart failure with gated phosphorus-31 nuclear magnetic resonance, *Circulation* 71(1):57–62, 1985.

159. Smith TW, Braunwald E, Kelly RA: The management of heart failure. In Braunwald E, editor: *Heart Disease: A Textbook of Cardiovascular Medicine*, Philadelphia, 1988, Saunders.

160. Burton KP: Evidence of direct toxic effects of free radicals on the myocardium, *Free Radic Biol Med* 4(1):15–24, 1988.

161. Padh H: Vitamin C: Newer insights into its biochemical functions, *Nutr Rev* 49(3):65–70, 1991.

162. Belch JJ, Bridges AB: Oxygen free radicals and congestive heart failure, *Br Heart J* 65(5):245–248, 1991.

163. Gaziano JM: Antioxidant vitamins and coronary artery disease risk, *Am J Med* 97(3A):18S–21S, 1994.

164. Dracup K, Baker DW, Dunbar SB, et al.: Management of heart failure. II. Counseling, education, and lifestyle modifications, *JAMA* 272(18):1442–1446, 1994.

165. Fonarow CC, Stevenson LW, Walden JA, et al.: Impact of a comprehensive heart failure management program on hospital readmission and functional status of patients with advanced heart failure, *J Am Coll Cardiol* 30(3):725–732, 1997.

166. Parmley WW: Should digoxin be the drug of first choice after diuretics in chronic congestive heart failure? *J Am Coll Cardiol* 12(1):265–273, 1988.

167. Pitt B: Clot-specific thrombolytic agents: Is there an advantage? *J Am Coll Cardiol* 12(3):588, 1988.

168. Mulrow CD, Feussner JR, Velez R: Reevaluation of digitalis efficacy. New light on an old leaf, *Ann Intern Med* 101(1):113–117, 1984.

169. Arrold SB, Byrd RC, Meister W, et al.: Long-term digitalis therapy improves left ventricular function in heart failure, *N Engl J Med* 303(25):1443–1448, 1980.

170. Lee DC-S, Johnson RA, Gingham JB, et al.: Heart failure in outpatients. A randomized trial of digoxin versus placebo, *N Engl J Med* 306(12):699–705, 1982.

171. Gheorghiade M, St. Clair J, St. Clair C, et al.: Hemodynamic effects of intravenous digoxin in patients with severe heart failure initially treated with diuretics and vasodilators, *J Am Coll Cardiol* 9(4):849–857, 1987.

172. Guyatt GH, Sullivan MD, Fallen EL, et al.: A controlled trial of digoxin in congestive heart failure, *Am J Cardiol* 61(4):371–375, 1988.

173. The Captopril-Digoxin Multicenter Research Group: Comparative effects of therapy with captopril and digoxin in patients with mild to moderate heart failure, *JAMA* 259(4):539–544, 1988.

174. Francis GS: Which drug for what patients with heart failure, and when? *Cardiology* 76(5):374–383, 1989.

175. Adams Jr K, Gheorghiade M, Uretsky B, et al.: Patients with mild heart failure worsen during withdrawal from digoxin therapy, *J Am Coll Cardiol* 30(1):42–48, 1997.

176. Leier CV: Acute inotropic support. In Leier CV, editor: *Cardiotonic Drugs: A Clinical Survey*, New York, 1986, Marcel Dekker.

177. Rude RE, Kloner RA, Maroko PR, et al.: Effects of amrinone on experimental acute myocardial ischemic injury, *Cardiovasc Res* 14(7):419–427, 1980.

178. Packer M, Carver JR, Rodeheffer RJ, et al.: Effect of oral milrinone on mortality in severe chronic heart failure. The PROMISE Study Research Group, *N Engl J Med* 325(21):1468–1475, 1991.

179. Taylor SH, Verma SP, Hussain M, et al.: Intravenous amrinone in left ventricular failure complicated by acute myocardial infarction, *Am J Cardiol* 56(3):29B–32B, 1985.

180. DiBianco R, Shabetai R, Kostuk W, et al.: Oral milrinone and digoxin in heart failure: Results of a placebo-controlled, prospective trial of each agent and the combination [abstract], *Circulation* 76(Suppl IV):IV256, 1978.

181. Gattis WA, O'Connor CM, Gallup DS, et al.: Predischarge initiation of carvedilol in patients hospitalized for decompensated heart failure: Results of the Initiation Management Predischarge: Process for Assessment of Carvedilol Therapy in Heart Failure (IMPACT-HF) trial, *J Am Coll Cardiol* 43(9):1534–1541, 2004.

182. Sharpe N, Smith H, Murphy J, et al.: Treatment of patients with symptomless left ventricular dysfunction after myocardial infarction, *Lancet* 1(8580):255–259, 1988.

183. Pfeffer MA, Lamas GA, Vaughan DA, et al.: Effect of captopril on progressive ventricular dilatation after anterior myocardial infarction, *N Engl J Med* 319(2):80–86, 1988.

184. Pfeffer JM, Pfeffer MA, Braunwald E: Hemodynamic benefits and prolonged survival with long-term captopril therapy in rats with myocardial infarction and heart failure, *Circulation* 75(Suppl 1):1149, 1987.

185. Pfeffer MA, Pfeffer JM: Ventricular enlargement and reduced survival after myocardial infarction, *Circulation* 75(Suppl IV):93, 1987.

186. Douglas LM: Pathophysiology of heart failure. In Libby P, Bonow RO, Mann DL, et al.: *Braunwald's Heart Disease: A Textbook of Cardiovascular Medicine*, ed 8, Philadelphia, 2008, Saunders.

187. Massie BM, Packer M, Hanlon JT, et al.: Combined captopril and hydralazine for refractory heart failure: A feasible and efficacious regimen, *J Am Coll Cardiol* 2:338, 1983.

188. Rutherford JD, Braunwald E, Cohn PF: Chronic ischemic heart disease. In Braunwald E, editor: *Heart Disease: A Textbook of Cardiovascular Medicine*, Philadelphia, 1988, Saunders.

189. Cahalin LP: Cardiovascular medications. In Malone T, editor: *Physical and Occupational Therapy: Drug Implications for Practice*, Philadelphia, 1989, Lippincott.

190. Packer M, Bristow M, Cohn J, et al.: The effect of carvedilol on morbidity and mortality in patients with chronic heart failure. U.S. Carvedilol Heart Failure Study Group, *N Engl J Med* 334:1349–1355, 1996.

191. Costanzo MR, Johannes RS, Pine M, et al.: The safety of intravenous diuretics alone versus diuretics plus parenteral vasoactive therapies in hospitalized patients with acutely decompensated heart failure: A propensity score and instrumental variable analysis using the Acutely Decompensated Heart Failure National Registry (ADHERE) database, *Am Heart J* 154(2):267–277, 2007.

192. Douglas LM: Management of heart failure patients with reduced ejection fraction. In Libby P, Bonow RO, Mann DL, et al.: *Braunwald's Heart Disease: A Textbook of Cardiovascular Medicine*, ed 8, Philadelphia, 2008, Saunders.

193. Hunt SA, Abraham WT, Chin MH, et al.: ACC/AHA 2005 guideline update for the diagnosis and management of chronic heart failure in the adult: A report of the American College of Cardiology/American Heart Association Task Force on Practice Guidelines, *Circulation* 112:e154, 2005.

194. Birks EJ, Tansley PD, Hardy J, et al.: Left ventricular assist device and drug therapy for the reversal of heart failure, *N Engl J Med* 355:1873, 2006.

195. Cullen MJ, Appleyard ST, Bindoff L: Morphologic aspects of muscle breakdown and lysosomal activation, *Ann N Y Acad Sci* 317:440, 1979.

196. Yancy CW, et al.: 2013 ACCF/AHA guideline for the management of heart failure, *Circulation* 128:e240–e327, 2013.

197. McAlister FA, Ezekowitz JA, Wiebe N, et al.: Systematic review: Cardiac resynchronization in patients with symptomatic heart failure, *JAMA* 297(22):2502–2514, 2007.

198. Laragh JH: Atrial natriuretic hormone, the renin-aldosterone axis, and blood pressure-electrolyte homeostasis, *N Engl J Med* 313:1330, 1985.

199. L'Abbate A, Emdin M, Piacenh M, et al.: Ultrafiltration: A rational treatment for heart failure, *Cardiology* 76:384, 1989.

200. Rimondini A, Cipolla CM, Della Bella P, et al.: Hemofiltration as short-term treatment for refractory congestive heart failure, *Am J Med* 83:43, 1987.

201. Poole-Wilson PA, Buller NP, Lipkin DP: Regional blood flow, muscle strength and skeletal muscle histology in severe congestive heart failure, *Am J Cardiol* 62(8):49E–52E, 1988.

202. William RS: Exercise training of patients with ventricular dysfunction and heart failure. In Wenger NK, editor: *Exercise and the Heart*, ed 2, Philadelphia, 1985, FA Davis.

203. El Oakley RM, Jarvis JC: Cardiomyoplasty: A Critical review of experimental and clinical results, *Circulation* 90(4):2085–2092, 1994.

204. Franco-Cereceda A, McCarthy PM, Blackstone EH, et al.: Partial left ventriculectomy for dilated cardiomyopathy: Is this an alternative to transplantation? *J Thorac Cardiovasc Surg* 121:879, 2001.

205. Stolf NA, Moreira LF, Bocchi EA, et al.: Determinants of midterm outcome of partial left ventriculectomy in dilated cardiomyopathy, *Ann Thorac Surg* 66:1585, 1998.

206. Starling RC, McCarthy PM, Buda T, et al.: Results of partial left ventriculectomy for dilated cardiomyopathy: hemodynamic, clinical and echocardiographic observations, *J Am Coll Cardiol* 36:2098, 2000.

207. Leier CV: Cardiomyoplasty: is it time to wrap it up? *J Am Coll Cardiol* 28:1181, 1986.

208. Aaronson KD, Schwartz JS, Chen TM, et al.: Development and prospective validation of a clinical index to predict survival in ambulatory patients referred for cardiac transplant evaluation, *Circulation* 95:2660–2667, 1997.

209. Levy WC, Mozaffarian D, Linker DT, et al.: The Seattle heart failure model: Prediction of survival in heart failure, *Circulation* 113:1424–1433, 2006.

210. Bart BA, Shaw LK, McCants CV, et al.: Clinical determinants of mortality in patients with angiographically diagnosed ischemic or nonischemic cardiomyopathy, *J Am Coll Cardiol* 30:1002–1008, 1997.

211. Kellerman JJ, Shemesh J: Exercise training of patients with severe heart failure, *J Cardiovasc Pharmacol* 10:S172–S183, 1987.

212. Keteyian SJ, Levine AB, Brawner CA, et al.: Exercise training in patients with heart failure: A randomized, controlled trial, *Ann Intern Med* 124:1051–1057, 1996.

213. Coats AJ: Exercise training for heart failure: Coming of age, *Circulation* 99:1138–1140, 1999.

214. Belardinelli R, Georgiou D, Cianci G, et al.: Randomized, controlled trial of long-term moderate exercise training in chronic heart failure: Effects on functional capacity, quality of life, and clinical outcome, *Circulation* 99:1173–1182, 1999.

215. Giannuzzi P, Temporelli PL, Corra U, et al.: Antiremodeling effect of long-term exercise training in patients with stable chronic heart failure: Results of the Exercise in Left Ventricular Dysfunction and Chronic Heart Failure (ELVD-CHF) Trial, *Circulation* 108:554–559, 2003.

216. Whellan DJ, O'Connor CM, Lee KL, et al.: HF-ACTION Trial Investigators. Heart failure and a controlled trial investigating outcomes of exercise training (HF-ACTION) design and rationale, *Am Heart J* 153(2):201–211, 2007.

217. O'Connor CM, Whellan DJ, Lee KL, et al.: Efficacy and safety of exercise training in patients with chronic heart failure: HF-ACTION randomized controlled trial, *JAMA* 301(14):1439–1450, 2009.

218. *Cardiac Rehabilitation: Clinical Practice Guideline, Number 17*, Washington, DC, 1995, U.S. Department of Health and Human Services. Public Health Service. Agency for Health Care Policy and Research. National Heart, Lung, and Blood Institute.

219. Cahalin LP: Heart failure, *Phys Ther* 76(5):516, 1996.

220. Whaley MH, Brubaker PH, Kaminsky LA, et al.: Validity of rating of perceived exertion during graded exercise testing in apparently healthy adults and cardiac patients, *J Cardiopulm Rehabil* 17(4):261–267, 1997.

221. Cahalin LP, Certo C, LaFiandra M, et al.: Exercise training increases the oxygen uptake-work rate relationship in advanced heart failure, *Chest* 112:49S, 1997.

222. Keteyian SJ, Marks CRC, Brawner CA, et al.: Responses to arm exercise in patients with compensated heart failure, *J Cardiopulm Rehabil* 16:366, 1996.

223. Barlow CW, Qayyum MS, Davey PP, et al.: Effect of physical training on exercise-induced hyperkalemia in chronic heart failure: Relation with ventilation and catecholamines, *Circulation* 89:1144, 1994.

224. Keteyian SJ, Levine TB, Levine AB, et al.: Quality of life and exercise training in patients with heart failure: A randomized trial, *Circulation* 96:1–84, 1997.

225. Franciosa JA, Park M, Levine TB: Lack of correlation between exercise capacity and indexes of resting left ventricular performance in heart failure, *Am J Cardiol* 47:33, 1981.

226. Franciosa JA, Ziesche S, Wilen M: Functional capacity of patients with chronic left ventricular failure, *Am J Med* 67:460, 1979.

227. Jafri SM, Lakier JB, Rosman HS, et al.: Symptoms and tests of ventricular performance in the evaluation of chronic heart failure, *Am Heart J* 112(1):194–196, 1986.

228. Fukuta H, Goto T, Wakami K, Ohte N: Effects of drug and exercise intervention on functional capacity and quality of life in heart failure with preserved ejection fraction: A meta-analysis of randomized controlled trials, *Eur J Prev Cardiol*, 2014: 2047487314564729, 2016 Jan, 23(1):75–85.

229. Anderson L, Taylor RS: Cardiac rehabilitation for people with heart disease: an overview of Cochrane systematic reviews, *Cochrane Database Syst Rev* 12:CD011273, 2014.

230. Pickworth KK: Long-term dobutamine therapy for refractory congestive heart failure, *Clin Pharm* 11(7):618–624, 1992.

231. Coats AJS, Adamopoulos S: Physical and pharmacological conditioning in chronic heart failure: A proposal for pulsed inotrope therapy, *Postgrad Med J* 67(Suppl 1):S69–S72, 1991.

232. Miller LW: Outpatient dobutamine for refractory congestive heart failure: Advantages, techniques, and results, *J Heart Lung Transplant* 10(3):482–487, 1991.

233. Kataoka T, Keteyian SJ, Marks CRC, et al.: Exercise training in a patient with congestive heart failure on continuous dobutamine, *Med Sci Sports Exerc* 26(6):678–681, 1994.

234. Applefeld MM, Newman KA, Grove WR, et al.: Intermittent, continuous outpatient dobutamine infusion in the management of congestive heart failure, *Am J Cardiol* 51(3):455–458, 1983.

235. Metra M, Eichhorn E, Abraham WT, et al.: Effects of low-dose oral enoximone administration on mortality, morbidity, and exercise capacity in patients with advanced heart failure: The randomized, double-blind placebo-controlled, parallel group ESSENTIAL trials, *Eur Heart J* 30(24):3015–3026, 2009.

236. McCarthy PM: HeartMate implantable left ventricular assist device: Bridge to transplantation and future applications, *Ann Thorac Surg* 59(2 Suppl):S46–S51, 1995.

237. Kennedy MD, Haykowsky M, Humphrey R: Function, eligibility, outcomes and exercise capacity associated with left ventricular assist devices: Exercise rehabilitation and training for patients with ventricular assist devices, *J Cardiopulm Rehabil* 23(3):208–217, 2003.

238. Mettauer B, Geny B, Lonsdorfer-Wolf E, et al.: Exercise training with a heart device: A hemodynamic, metabolic, and hormonal study, *Med Sci Sports Exerc* 33(1):2–8, 2001.

239. Morrone T, Buck L, Catanese K, et al.: Early progressive mobilization of left ventricular assist device patients is safe and optimizes recovery prior to cardiac transplant, *J Heart Lung Transplant* 15(5):423–429, 1996.

240. Buck L, Morrone T, Goldsmith R, et al.: Exercise training of patients with left ventricular assist devices: A pilot study of physiologic adaptations [abstract], *J Cardiopulm Rehabil* 17(5):324, 1997.

241. O'Donnell DE, Sanii R, Younes M: Improvement in exercise endurance in patients with chronic airflow limitation using continuous positive airway pressure, *Am Rev Respir Dis* 138(6):1510–1514, 1988.

242. Henke KG, Regnis JA, Bye PTP: Benefits of continuous positive airway pressure during exercise in cystic fibrosis and relationship to disease severity, *Am Rev Respir Dis* 148(5):1272–1276, 1993.

243. Cahalin LP, Cannan J, Prevost S, et al.: Exercise performance during assisted ventilation with bi-level positive airway pressure (BiPAP), *J Cardiopulm Rehabil* 14(5):323, 1994.

244. Baratz DM, Westbrooke PR, Shah PK, et al.: Effect of nasal continuous positive airway pressure on cardiac output and oxygen delivery in patients with congestive heart failure, *Chest* 102(5):1397–1401, 1992.

245. Bradley TD, Holloway RM, McLaughlin PR, et al.: Cardiac output responses to continuous positive airway pressure in congestive heart failure, *Am Rev Respir Dis* 145(2 Pt 1):377–382, 1992.

246. Naughton MT, Rahman MA, Hara K, et al.: Effect of continuous positive airway pressure on intrathoracic and left ventricular transmural pressures in patients with congestive heart failure, *Circulation* 91(6):1725–1731, 1995.

247. Malone S, Liu PP, Hollway R, et al.: Obstructive sleep apnoea in patients with dilated cardiomyopathy: Effects of continuous positive airway pressure, *Lancet* 338(8781):1480–1484, 1991.

248. Takasaki Y, Orr D, Popkin J, et al.: Effect of nasal continuous positive airway pressure on sleep apnea in congestive heart failure, *Am Rev Respir Dis* 140(6):1578–1584, 1989.

249. Naughton MT, Liu PP, Benard DC, et al.: Treatment of congestive heart failure and Cheyne-Stokes respiration during sleep by continuous positive airway pressure, *Am J Respir Crit Care Med* 151(1):92–97, 1995.

250. Pinsky MR, Summer WR, Wise RA, et al.: Augmentation of cardiac function by elevation of intrathoracic pressure, *J Appl Physiol* 84(4):370–375, 1983.

251. Pinsky MR, Summer WR: Cardiac augmentation by phasic high intrathoracic pressure support in man, *Chest* 84:370, 1983.

252. Cahalin LP, Zambernardi L, Dec GW: Multiple systems assessment during inpatient cardiopulmonary rehabilitation [abstract], *J Cardiopulm Rehabil* 13(5):344, 1993.

253. Cahalin LP, Semigran MJ, Dec GW: Inspiratory muscle training in patients with chronic heart failure awaiting cardiac transplantation: Results of a pilot clinical trial, *Phys Ther* 77(8):830–838, 1997.

254. Mancini DM, Henson D, LaManca J, et al.: Benefit of selective respiratory muscle training on exercise capacity in patients with chronic congestive heart failure, *Circulation* 91(2):320–329, 1995.

255. Barach AL: Physiologic advantages of grunting, groaning, and pursed-lip breathing: Adaptive symptoms related to the development of continuous positive pressure breathing, *Bull N Y Acad Med* 49(8):666–673, 1973.

256. Tiep BL, Burns M, Kao D, et al.: Pursed lips breathing training using ear oximetry, *Chest* 90(2):218–221, 1986.

257. Mancini DM, Henson D, LaManca J, et al.: Respiratory muscle function and dyspnea in patients with chronic congestive heart failure, *Circulation* 86(3):909–918, 1992.

258. Mancini DM, LaManca J, Donchez L, et al.: The sensation of dyspnea during exercise is not determined by the work of breathing in patients with heart failure, *J Am Coll Cardiol* 28(2):391–395, 1996.

259. Collins SM, Cahalin LP, Semigran MJ, et al.: Strength or Endurance? *Phys Ther* 77(8):1764–1766, 1997.

260. Larson JL, Kim MJ, Sharp JT, et al.: Inspiratory muscle training with a pressure threshold breathing device in patients with chronic obstructive pulmonary disease, *Am Rev Respir Dis* 138(3):689–696, 1988.

261. Weiner P, Azgad Y, Ganam R, et al.: Inspiratory muscle training in patients with bronchial asthma, *Chest* 102(5):1357–1361, 1992.

262. McParland C, Krishnan B, Wang E, et al.: Inspiratory muscle weakness and dyspnea in congestive heart failure, *Am Rev Respir Dis* 146(2):467–472, 1992.

263. Aubuer M, Trippenbach T, Rousso C: Respiratory muscle fatigue during cardiogenic shock, *J Appl Physiol* 51(2):499–508, 1981.

264. Hammond MD, Bauer KA, Sharp JT, et al.: Respiratory muscle strength in congestive heart failure, *Chest* 98(5):1091–1094, 1990.

265. Winkelmann ER, Chiappa GR, Lima COC, et al.: Addition of inspiratory muscle training to aerobic training improves cardiorespiratory responses to exercise in patients with heart failure and inspiratory muscle weakness, *Am Heart J* 158(5): 768.e1–768.e7, 2009.

266. Ham RJ, Sloane PD, Washaw GA, et al.: *Primary Care Geriatrics: A Case-Based Approach*, ed 5, St. Louis, 2007, Mosby.

5

Restrictive lung dysfunction

Ellen Hillegass, Tamara Klintworth-Kirk, and Karlyn Schiltgen

Pulmonary pathology can be organized and discussed in a number of ways. Within this text, pulmonary function abnormalities have been divided into two main categories: obstructive dysfunction and restrictive dysfunction. If the flow of air is impeded, the defect is obstructive. If the volume of air or gas is reduced, the defect is restrictive (Fig. 5-1).[1]

Although this organization of pulmonary pathology may in some ways clarify the discussion, it must be remembered that a number of diseases and conditions result in both obstructive and restrictive lung impairment (mixed impairment). This chapter discusses those pathologies and interventions that result in restrictive lung dysfunction (Table 5-1).

Etiology

Restrictive lung dysfunction (RLD) is an abnormal reduction in pulmonary ventilation due to restriction of expansion by the chest wall or the lungs. Lung expansion is restricted, and therefore the volume of air or gas moving in and out of the lungs is decreased.[2]

Restrictive lung dysfunction is not a disease. In fact, this dysfunction may result from many different diseases arising from the pulmonary system or almost any other system in the body.

Restrictive lung dysfunction differs from obstructive lung dysfunction in several important aspects. These differences are summarized in Table 5-2.

Pathogenesis

Three major aspects of pulmonary ventilation must be considered to understand the pathophysiology of RLD. They are (1) compliance of both the lung and the chest wall; (2) lung volumes and capacities; and (3) the work of breathing.

In order to classify pulmonary disease into one of the two categories (obstructive vs. restrictive), pulmonary function testing (PFT) needs to be performed. With RLD, PFTs will typically show a decrease in almost all volumes and capacities with fairly normal flow rates, along with a decrease in diffusion capacity (Fig. 5-2).[3]

Compliance

Pulmonary compliance encompasses both lung and chest wall compliance. It is the physiologic link that establishes a relationship between the pressure exerted by the chest wall or the lungs and the volume of air that can be contained within the lungs.[2] With RLD, chest wall or lung compliance, or both, is decreased.

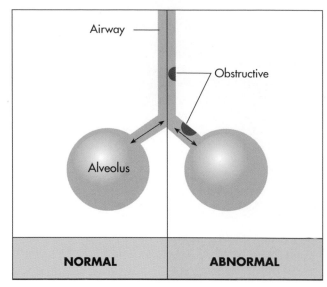

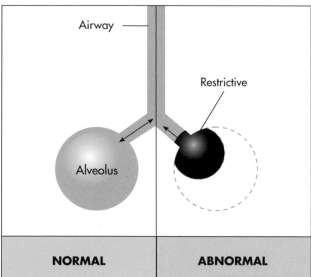

Figure 5-1 Pathophysiologic aspects of lung disease. (From Kacmarek R, Stoller J, Heuer A: *Egan's Fundamentals of Respiratory Care*, ed 10, St. Louis, 2013, Mosby.)

As discussed in Chapter 2, a decrease in compliance of the lungs indicates that they are becoming stiffer and thus more difficult to expand. It takes a greater transpulmonary pressure to expand the lung to a given volume in a person with decreased lung compliance.[3] If the amount of pressure used to move air into the lungs is constant, the volume of air would be decreased. A chest wall low in compliance limits thoracic expansion and, therefore lung inflation, even if the lung itself has normal compliance.

Because pulmonary compliance is decreased in RLD, resistance to lung expansion is increased. In other words, decreased pulmonary compliance requires an increase in pressure just to maintain adequate lung expansion and ventilation. This means the patient has to work harder just to move air into the lungs.

Lung Volumes

Restrictive lung dysfunction eventually causes all the lung volumes and capacities to become decreased. Because the distensibility of the lung is decreased, the inspiratory reserve volume

Table 5-1 Examples of restrictive and obstructive lung disease with general presentation and symptoms.

Obstructive lung disease		Restrictive lung disease	
Diagnoses	**Cardinal presentation**	**Diagnoses**	**Cardinal presentation**
Chronic bronchitis	Air trapping	IPF	Decreased compliance
Emphysema	Increased RV/TLC	Lung cancer	Decreased lung volume*
Asthma	Decreased FEV_1/FVC	Musculoskeletal causes	Decreased lung capacity*
Cystic fibrosis (mixed)	Decreased FEV_1	Neuromuscular causes	FEV_1/FVC preserved
	CO_2 retention	PE/pulmonary edema	Decreased diffusion capacity*
	DLCO decreased	Sarcoidosis	Tachypnea*
	Cyanotic	Pneumonia	Hypoxemia*
	Wheezing	Connective tissue causes	Decreased breath sounds*
	Dyspnea	Traumatic causes	Dyspnea**
	Cough	Obesity/DM	Cough**
			Cor pulmonale*
			Weight loss**

* Six classic signs of RLD.
** Classic symptoms of RLD.
CO_2, carbon dioxide; DLCO, diffusing capacity of lung for carbon monoxide; FEV_1, forced expiratory volume in 1 second; FVC, total amount of air exhaled during the FEV test; IPF, idiopathic pulmonary fibrosis; RV, residual volume; TLC, Total lung capacity.

Table 5-2 Clinical manifestation of respiratory distress syndrome

		Findings
Signs	Pulmonary function tests	←↑ RR
		↓ Lung compliance
		↓ Lung volumes (FRC, VC)
		←↑ Work of breathing
	Chest radiograph	Diffuse, hazy reticulogranular densities[1]
		In severe RDS, air bronchograms are prominent
		In severe RDS, cardiothymic silhouette indistinct (diffuse microatelectasis)
	Arterial blood gases	Marked ↓ in PaO_2
		←↑ $Paco_2$
		↓ pH (acidosis)
		←↑ Dead space ventilation and ↓ alveolar ventilation, with V/Q mismatch
	Breath sounds	Presence of expiratory grunt
		Fine inspiratory crackles and/or ↓ breath sounds due to atelectasis[1]
	Cardiovascular	Possible bradycardia
		Possible cerebral, pulmonary, or intraventricular hemorrhage
Symptoms	Respiratory pattern	Rapid and labored
		Significant intercostal, sternal, and substernal retractions
	Nasal flaring	
	Grunting	
	Crying: decreased in volume and strength	
	May be cyanotic	

FRC, functional residual capacity; $Paco_2$, arterial partial pressure of CO_2; PaO_2, arterial partial pressure of O_2; RDS, respiratory distress syndrome; RR, respiratory rate; VC, vital capacity; V/Q, ventilation–perfusion.

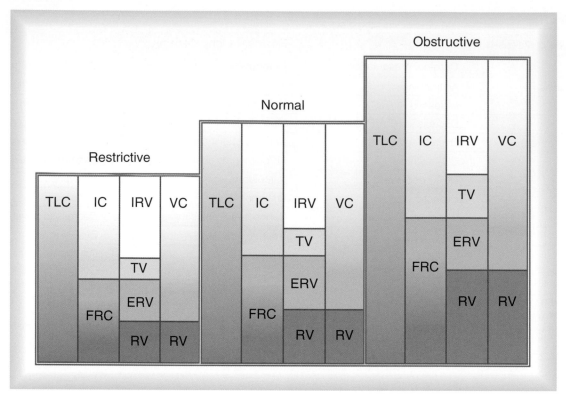

Figure 5-2 Changes in lung volumes and capacities with pulmonary disease. *ERV*, expiratory reserve volume; *FRC*, functional residual capacity; *IC*, inspiratory capacity; *IRV*, inspiratory reserve volume; *RV*, residual volume; *TLC*, total lung capacity; *TV*, tidal volume; *VC*, vital capacity. (From Kacmarek R, Stoller J, Heuer A: *Egan's Fundamentals of Respiratory Care*, ed 10, St. Louis, 2013, Mosby.)

(IRV) is diminished. Although the body tries to preserve the tidal volume (TV) in RLD, the compliance gradually decreases and the work of breathing increases; thus the TV decreases. The expiratory reserve volume (ERV) is the volume of air or gas that can be exhaled following a normal exhalation. No matter the etiology, RLD effects a reduction in the ERV; this reduction is particularly pronounced if a decrease in lung compliance is the principal etiologic factor. The residual volume (RV) is usually decreased, but with some causes of RLD (spinal cord injury, amyotrophic lateral sclerosis [ALS], and other neuromuscular disorders), it may be increased. This results in decreasing the dynamic lung volumes. The most marked decreases in lung volumes are seen in the IRV and ERV.

Because all lung volumes are decreased with RLD, all lung capacities are also decreased. Total lung capacity (TLC) and vital capacity (VC) are the two most common spirometric measurements used in the identification of RLD. Decreases in TLC and functional residual capacity (FRC) are a direct result of a decrease in lung compliance. At TLC, the force of the inspiratory muscles is balanced by the inward elastic recoil of the lung. Because the recoil pressure is increased if lung compliance is decreased, this balance occurs at a lower volume, and thus the TLC is diminished. At FRC, the outward recoil of the chest wall is balanced by the inward elastic recoil of the lung. Because this elastic recoil is increased, the balance is achieved at a lower lung volume and so the FRC is decreased (see Fig. 5-2).[3]

Work of Breathing

With RLD, the work of breathing is increased. The respiratory system normally fine-tunes the respiratory rate and the VT to minimize the mechanical work of breathing. As previously mentioned, a greater transpulmonary pressure is required to achieve a normal VT. The result is that the patient's work of breathing is increased and a new equilibrium, with a decreased VT and an increased respiratory rate, is sought in an effort to reduce energy expenditure. However, if the respiratory rate is too high, energy is wasted in overcoming airway resistance and in ventilating the anatomic dead space. Furthermore, if the TV is larger than required, energy is wasted overcoming the natural recoil of the lung and in expanding the chest wall. Anything that increases airway resistance, increases flow rates, or decreases lung or chest wall compliance increases the work of breathing. In RLD, both lung and chest wall compliance and lung volumes may decrease. These changes can significantly affect the work of breathing.[4] To overcome the decrease in pulmonary compliance, the respiratory rate is usually increased; the normal inspiratory muscles, especially the diaphragm, work harder; and the accessory muscles of respiration, the scaleni and the sternocleidomastoid (see Chapters 1 and 2), are recruited to assist in expanding the thorax.[5] These additional efforts require additional oxygen (O_2) expenditure. In normal persons at rest, the body uses less than 5% of the oxygen consumption per minute (O_2), or 3 to 14 mL O_2/min, to support the work of breathing.[4,6] With RLD, the percentage of O_2 needed to support the work of breathing can reach and exceed 25%.[4,6] This change is usually very insidious as the RLD progresses and is countered by the concurrent decrease in activity seen in these patients. Although the respiratory muscle pump is very resistant to fatigue, these patients can experience respiratory muscle fatigue, overuse, and failure as RLD progresses.

Clinical Manifestation

Signs

Six classic signs often indicate and are always consistent with RLD (see Table 5-1). The first is tachypnea, or an increased respiratory rate. Because the inspiratory muscles have to work so hard to overcome the decreased pulmonary compliance, an involuntary adjustment is made to increase the respiratory rate and decrease the volumes so that the minute ventilation is maintained. Early in the course of RLD, there may be overcompensation, with the respiratory rate increasing to the point that minute ventilation is increased and alveolar hyperventilation occurs, resulting in greater exhalation of carbon dioxide (CO_2).

Ventilation–perfusion mismatching, an invariable finding in RLD, leads to the second classic sign: hypoxemia. This mismatching may be due to changes in the collagenous framework of the lung, scarring of capillary channels, distortion or narrowing of the small airways, compression from tumors within the lung or bony abnormalities of the chest wall, or a variety of other causes. Even if patients are not hypoxemic at rest, they may quickly become hypoxemic with exercise.

The third classic sign of RLD is decreased breath sounds with dry inspiratory crackles, which are thought to be caused by atelectatic alveoli opening at end inspiration, and are most often heard at the bases of the lungs.

The fourth and fifth classic signs are apparent from PFT. The decrease in lung volumes and capacities, determined by spirometry, is the fourth classic sign of RLD. The fifth classic sign is the decreased diffusing capacity of lung for carbon monoxide (DLCO). This arises as a consequence of a widening of the interstitial spaces as a result of scar tissue, fibrosis of the capillaries, and ventilation–perfusion abnormalities. In RLD, the DLCO has been measured at less than 50% of predicted.[7]

The sixth classic sign usually apparent with RLD is cor pulmonale. This right-sided heart failure is due to hypoxemia, fibrosis, and compression of the pulmonary capillaries, which leads to pulmonary hypertension. The rise in pressure in the pulmonary circulation increases the work of the right ventricle. Because the pulmonary capillary bed is fibrotic, it is also less able to distend to handle the ordinary increase in cardiac output expected with exercise. Therefore during exercise, hypoxemia may occur earlier or be more pronounced. Other signs include a decrease in chest wall expansion and possible cyanosis or clubbing (see Table 5-1).

Symptoms

Three hallmark symptoms are usually experienced with RLD (see Table 5-1). The first is dyspnea, or shortness of breath. This symptom typically manifests itself with exercise, but as RLD progresses, dyspnea at rest may also be experienced. The second symptom, and the one that usually brings the patient into the physician's office, is an irritating, dry, and nonproductive cough. The third hallmark symptom of RLD is the wasted, emaciated appearance these patients present as the disease progresses. With the work of breathing increased as much as 12-fold over

normal, these individuals are using caloric requirements similar to those necessary for running a marathon 24 hours a day.[4] Additionally, because breathing is such hard work and eating makes breathing more difficult, these patients usually are not eager to eat and often report a decrease in appetite. Because their energy expenditure is up and their caloric intake is down, they are very often in a continual weight loss cycle, which becomes more severe as the RLD progresses.

Treatment

Treatment interventions for RLD are discussed briefly for each disease. Generally, however, if the etiologic factors that are causing RLD are permanent (spinal cord injury) or progressive (idiopathic pulmonary fibrosis), the treatment consists primarily of supportive measures (Box 5-1). Supportive interventions include supplemental oxygen to support the arterial partial pressure of oxygen (PaO_2), antibiotic therapy to fight secondary pulmonary infection, measures to promote adequate ventilation and prevent the accumulation of pulmonary secretions, and good nutritional support. However, if the changes that are causing the RLD are acute and reversible (pneumothorax) or chronic but reversible (Guillain–Barré syndrome), the treatment consists of specific corrective interventions (e.g., chest tube placement) and supportive measures (e.g., temporary mechanical ventilation) to assist the patient to maintain adequate ventilation until he or she is again able to be independent in this activity. Each section discusses the pathology that would apply to each condition.

Maturational Causes of Restrictive Lung Dysfunction

Abnormalities in Fetal Lung Development

- Agenesis is the total absence of the bronchus and the lung parenchyma. Unilateral agenesis is rare.[8]
- Aplasia is the development of a rudimentary bronchus without the development of the normal lung parenchyma. This condition is also rare.[8]
- Hypoplasia is the development of a functioning although not always normal bronchus with the development of reduced amounts of lung parenchyma. This developmental abnormality is much more common and may affect one lung or one lobe of a lung. It is often present in infants born with a large diaphragmatic hernia and displaced abdominal organs.[8]

Clinical Manifestation

Depending on the amount of lung parenchyma lost, these infants can be asymptomatic or can exhibit severe pulmonary insufficiency. The pulmonary impairment is restrictive, in that the volumes are decreased even though the lung compliance may be normal.

Respiratory Distress Syndrome

Respiratory distress syndrome (RDS), also known as *hyaline membrane disease* (HMD), is a disorder of prematurity or lack of complete lung maturation in the human fetus. It usually takes 36 weeks of normal gestation to achieve lung maturity in the fetus. Infants born with a gestational age less than 36 weeks often exhibit respiratory distress and may develop the full complement of signs and symptoms associated with RDS.[9]

Etiology

Insufficient maturation of the lungs is the cause of RDS, and it is usually linked directly to the gestational age of the fetus at birth. The incidence of RDS in infants with a gestational age of 26 to 28 weeks at birth is approximately 75%.[8] In contrast, the incidence of RDS in infants with a gestational age of 36 weeks at birth is less than 5%.[9] Other factors that seem to contribute to the development of RDS are gender, race, abruptio placentae, and maternal diabetes. Premature male infants are more at risk to develop RDS than are premature female infants. White premature infants have a greater incidence of RDS than black premature infants. Fetal lung maturation is delayed in pregnant women with diabetes, so infants born of diabetic mothers are at increased risk of developing RDS. Worldwide, 1% of infants are affected by RDS.[8] In the United States, 60,000 to 70,000 are affected.[1,10]

Pathophysiology

Respiratory distress syndrome is caused primarily by abnormalities in the surfactant system and inadequate surfactant production. Structural abnormalities within the immature lung, such as alveolar septal thickening, may also contribute to the pathophysiology of this syndrome. The surfactant dysfunction causes the overall retractive forces of the lung to be greater than normal, which decreases lung compliance, increases the work of breathing, and leads to progressive diffuse microatelectasis, alveolar collapse, increased ventilation–perfusion mismatching, and impaired gas exchange (Fig. 5-3). In addition, alveolar epithelial and endothelial permeability are abnormal in the immature lung. Therefore when these premature infants are mechanically ventilated without sufficient normal surfactant, the bronchiolar epithelium is disrupted. This leads to pulmonary edema and the generation of hyaline membranes. Further, because the proximal and distal airways in the infant are very compliant and the alveoli may be less compliant due to atelectasis and the formation of hyaline membrane, the mechanical ventilator pressures used can disrupt, dilate, and deform the airways. Mechanical ventilator pressures can also cause air leaks, tension pneumothorax, and extensive pulmonary interstitial emphysema.

Another cause of decreased gas exchange is the often severe pulmonary hypertension evident in infants with RDS. These

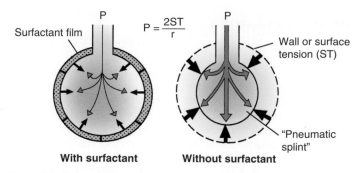

$$P = \frac{2ST}{r}$$

Figure 5-3 Surfactant abnormalities.

infants have hypoxemia and are acidotic, both of which cause vasoconstriction. This response is exaggerated in the infant and causes severe pulmonary hypertension, increased ventilation–perfusion mismatching, and decreased gas exchange. Restrictive lung dysfunction may be complicated further by persistent patency of the ductus arteriosus, resulting in a left-to-right shunt within the infant's heart. The patent ductus arteriosus increases pulmonary pressures and blood flow and could allow plasma proteins to leak into the alveolar space, causing pulmonary edema and further interfering with surfactant function.

Complications common in infants with RDS include intracranial hemorrhage, sepsis, pneumonia, pneumothorax, pulmonary hemorrhage, and pulmonary interstitial emphysema. This syndrome can also result in the development of bronchopulmonary dysplasia. Recovery in RDS is usually preceded by an abrupt unexplained diuresis.[9]

Many infants still die or have chronic effects from RDS. However, over the past three decades the death rate has significantly decreased, and most deaths are limited to infants who are 24 to 26 weeks' gestation weighing 500 to 800 g at birth.[1]

Diagnostic Tests

Definitive diagnosis for RDS usually is made by chest radiograph (Fig. 5-4).

Clinical Manifestation

The clinical manifestation of RDS can be found in Table 5-2.

Treatment

Traditional treatment for RDS entails continuous positive airway pressure (CPAP) and positive end expiratory pressure (PEEP). Surfactant replacement therapy and high-frequency ventilation (HFV) have also been added as traditional treatment approaches. A trial of CPAP using nasal prongs is indicated. If oxygenation does not improve or the infant's clinical condition deteriorates, mechanical ventilation with PEEP should be instioued.[1]

Surfactant replacement is currently the standard of care in treating infants with RDS. The artificial surfactant is given as a liquid suspension in saline and delivered to the infant by aerosol via endotracheal intubation. The results of this therapeutic intervention are immediate reduction in oxygen requirements, a major decrease in pulmonary complications such as pneumothoraces or pulmonary interstitial emphysema, and rapid weaning from mechanical ventilation, often within 12 to 24 hours.[10]

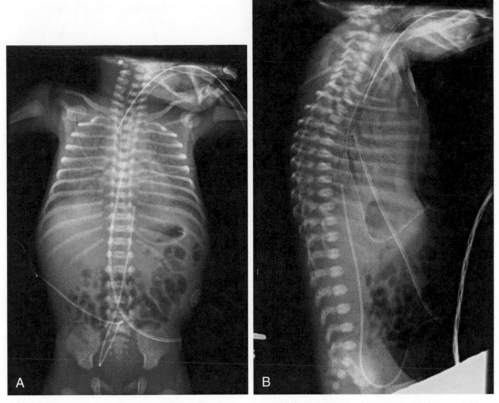

Figure 5-4 Radiopaque appearance of severe respiratory distress syndrome. Anteroposterior **(A)** and lateral **(B)** radiographs show diffuse hazy appearance with low lung volumes and air bronchograms that extend into the periphery. (From Kacmarek R, Stoller J, Heuer A: *Egan's Fundamentals of Respiratory Care*, ed 10, St. Louis, 2013, Mosby.)

If the infant does not adequately respond to surfactant administration, then the infant, if large enough, may be treated with extracorporeal membrane oxygenation (ECMO) or nitric oxide administration delivered in the inspiratory gas to cause pulmonary vasodilation.[10]

An alternative to treatment is prevention of the disease by maternal/fetal treatment with corticosteroids. Administration of corticosteroids to the mother before delivery can accelerate fetal lung maturation by stimulating surfactant synthesis, inducing changes in the elastic properties of the fetal lung, stimulating alveolarization, and decreasing the permeability of the airway and alveoli epithelium.[9,10]

Bronchopulmonary Dysplasia

Bronchopulmonary dysplasia (BPD) is a chronic pulmonary syndrome in neonates that occurs in some survivors of RDS who have been ventilated mechanically and have received high concentrations of oxygen over a prolonged period. Other names used for this syndrome are *pulmonary fibroplasia* and *ventilator lung*.[8,9]

Etiology

The incidence of BPD following RDS varies from 2% to 68% in different studies.[9] The incidence increases in neonates who had low birth weights (< 1000 g); required mechanical ventilation, particularly using continuous positive pressure; received inspired oxygen concentrations (Fio_2) at 60% or higher; or received supplemental oxygen for more than 50 hours.[8,9] In fact, BPD almost invariably develops in neonates

who received oxygen at an Fio_2 of 60% or higher for 123 hours or more.[8] See Chapter 6 for more details on BPD.

Normal Aging

Maturation of the various body systems is a natural process that takes place throughout a lifetime. Normal aging usually refers to physiologic changes that occur with regularity in the majority of the population and can therefore be predicted. Physiologic changes that commonly are considered part of the aging process can begin as early as 20 years of age.[11]

Etiology

The normal aging process in the pulmonary system is very slow and insidious, and because we have great ventilatory reserves, the changes are often not felt functionally until the sixth or seventh decade of life.[12] Universally, the normal aging process in the lungs is complicated by the fact that throughout life the lungs have had to cope with the external environment. This includes general pollution, noxious gases, specific occupational exposures, inhaled drug use, and, of course, cigarette smoking.[11]

Physiology

The compliance of the pulmonary system starts to decrease at about age 20 and decreases approximately 20% over the next 40 years.[11] Maximum voluntary ventilation decreases by 30% between the ages of 30 and 70.[11] Vital capacity also drops by about 25% between 30 and 70 years of age.[12] However, functional status often is not affected until the sixth and seventh decades.

AGING

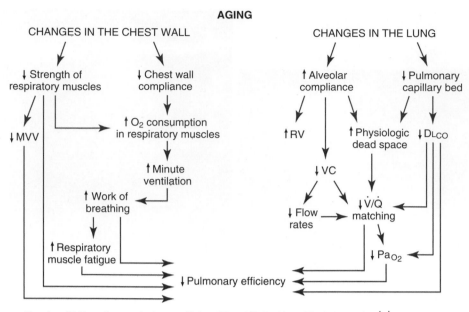

Figure 5-5 Respiratory changes with aging. *MVV*, maximum voluntary ventilation; *RV*, residual volume; *VC*, vital capacity; *V̇/Q̇*, ventilation–perfusion; *PaO₂*, arterial partial pressure of oxygen; *DL_CO*, diffusing capacity of the lungs for carbon monoxide.

The control of ventilation undergoes significant change (Fig. 5-5). The peripheral chemoreceptors are not as responsive to hypoxia, and the central receptors are not as responsive to acute hypercapnia. These changes mean that the ventilatory response mediated by the central nervous system is significantly depressed.[4,9] The normal PaO_2 in a 70-year-old is 75, a measurement that is not interpreted as hypoxia by the central nervous system.[11]

The thorax undergoes a number of changes, including decalcification of the ribs, calcification of the costal cartilages, arthritic changes in the joints of the ribs and vertebrae, dorsal thoracic kyphosis, and increased anteroposterior diameter of the chest (barrel chest). The effects of these changes combine to decrease the compliance of the chest wall and increase the work of breathing. Oxygen consumption in the respiratory muscles is increased, causing an increase in the minute ventilation. The strength and endurance of the inspiratory muscles gradually diminishes, which results in a decreased maximal ventilatory effort.[3] The forced expiratory volume in 1 second (FEV_1) is reduced by about 40 mL per year.[11]

The lung tissue itself shows enlargement of the air spaces due to enlargement of the alveolar ducts and terminal bronchioles. The alveolar surface area and the alveolar parenchymal volume are decreased. The alveolar walls become thinner, and the capillary bed incurs considerable loss, with an increase in ventilation–perfusion mismatching. Distribution of inspired air and pulmonary blood flow becomes less homogeneous with age. Diffusing capacity is therefore reduced, and physiologic dead space is increased.[11]

The static elastic recoil of the alveolar tissue decreases, which means that alveolar compliance is increased and the lungs do not empty well. The lung compliance curve is shifted to the left in the elderly. Thus although TLC may not change with age, RV increases and dynamic volumes therefore decrease.[11,12] Closing volumes are increased, which results in early closure of the small airways, particularly in the dependent lung regions. By approximately age 55, small airways are closed at or above FRC in the supine position. In

the upright position, with the attendant increase in FRC, this change occurs at approximately age 70.[11]

Of course, normal concomitant aging changes take place in the cardiovascular system, including a decrease in maximum heart rate and cardiac output. These changes combine with the decreased oxygen exchange capability of the lungs and result in a decrease in the maximum oxygen uptake with exercise and therefore a decrease in the anaerobic threshold. After 50 years of age, the maximum oxygen uptake usually declines at a rate of 0.45 mL/kg/min for each year.[4,9]

Ventilation during sleep is altered in the elderly. Electroencephalographic (EEG) studies have shown that total nocturnal sleep time is shorter, with more frequent and longer nocturnal awakenings in the elderly. The pattern of ventilation during sleep is irregular more often in the elderly than in young adults. Repetitive periodic apneas occur in 35% to 40% of the elderly, predominantly in males during sleep stages 1 and 2.[9]

Clinical Manifestation

The clinical manifestation of normal aging can be found in Table 5-3.

Treatment

Biological aging is a process of change affecting tissues and organs. However, a healthy lifestyle choice, including avoidance of health-damaging behaviors, may slow functional decline. Existing evidence also supports the need to keep aerobically exercising and possibly adding strength training into one's daily regimen.[13–15]

The elderly should be encouraged to remain active and fit. Although even with regular activity about 0.45 mL/kg/min of oxygen consumption is lost each year, the fit elderly person has a greater maximum oxygen consumption than the sedentary person. In addition, a sedentary elderly person beginning regular exercise can improve maximum oxygen consumption by 5% to 25% and can regain the exercise capability that was present as much as 5 to 10 years earlier.[11]

Table 5-3 Comparison of obstructive and restrictive types of pulmonary diseases

Characteristic	Obstructive disease	Restrictive disease
Anatomy affected	Airways	Lung parenchyma, thoracic pump
Breathing phase difficulty	Expiration	Inspiration
Pathophysiology	Increased airway resistance	Decreased lung or thoracic compliance
Useful measurements	Flow rates	Volumes or capacities

Pulmonary Causes of Restrictive Lung Dysfunction

Interstitial Causes

Idiopathic Pulmonary Fibrosis

Idiopathic pulmonary fibrosis (IPF) is a chronic, progressive, irreversible, and usually lethal lung disease. It occurs mostly in older adults, and the cause is unknown.[16] It is characterized by progressive worsening of dyspnea and lung function.[17] It affects all of the components of the alveolar wall, including epithelial and endothelial cells, the cellular and noncellular components of the interstitium, and the capillary network. These components are supported by the connective tissue framework made up of collagen and elastic fibers and contain a milieu of ground substance. Prevalence estimates have varied from 2 to 29 cases per 100,000 in the general population, and more men have been reported with IPF than women.[17]

Etiology

The cause of IPF is unknown; however, it appears to be a disease that likely arises from the interplay between genetic and environmental factors.[16] Initially, the disease was thought to be a chronic inflammatory process. Research now is revealing that it likely is due to a fibrotic response driven by abnormally activated alveolar epithelial cells.[16] The most important environmental risk factors are cigarette smoking and exposure to metal and wood dust.[16] Other potential risk factors include microbial agents and gastroesophageal reflux.[17] Genetic transmission occurs in about 0.5% to 3.7% of cases.[16]

Pathophysiology

The pathogenesis remains largely unknown. Over the past decade, research has changed the perspective on IPF. Rather than primarily a proinflammatory disorder, IPF now appears to be the result of an atypical reparative process that occurs after an injury to the lung epithelium. The disease is, therefore,

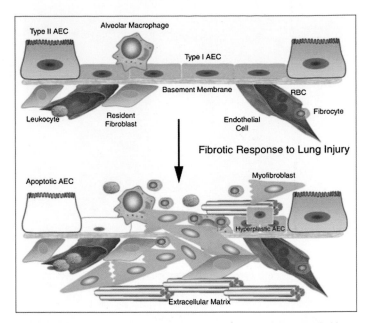

Figure 5-6 Pathogenic alterations in IPF. (From Loomis-King H, Flaherty KR, Moore BB: Pathogenesis, current treatments and future directions for idiopathic pulmonary fibrosis, *Curr Opin Pharmacol* 13(3):377-385, 2013.)

marked by proliferation and accumulation of fibroblasts or myofibroblasts and excessive deposition of extracellular matrix. This results in scarring and destruction of the lung architecture (Fig. 5-6).[16,18,19]

Along with a steady decline in lung function, the course includes acute exacerbations characterized by rapid deterioration in lung function not due to infections or heart failure. The acute exacerbations include low-grade fever, worsening dyspnea and cough, worsening gas exchange, and appearance of new opacities on radiology.[20]

Idiopathic pulmonary fibrosis is associated with a median survival rate of 2 to 3 years after initial diagnosis.[21]

Diagnostic Tests

Diagnosis of IPF requires a detailed review of the patient's clinical history, as well as the exclusion of other known causes of interstitial lung disease (drug toxicity, occupational environmental exposures).[17] Testing by high-resolution computerized tomography (HRCT) of the chest is also indicated, and if this is not definitive, surgical lung biopsy may be needed (Fig. 5-7).[22]

Clinical Manifestation

The clinical manifestation of IPF can be found in Table 5-4.

Treatment

At present, there is no effective standard treatment.[23] However, based on research over the past 10 years and new understanding of the pathogenesis, the pharmacologic approach to the disease has changed. Trials previously were focused on the efficacy of drugs that would suppress the inflammatory or immune response, such as corticosteroids. Currently, treatment approaches and trials are now geared toward agents with antifibrotic properties. At present, pirfenidone is the only antifibrotic drug approved for treatment of IPF.[23]

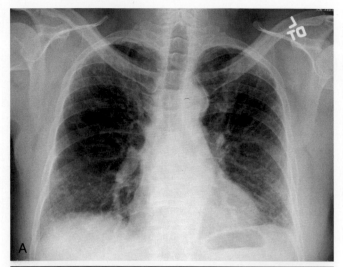

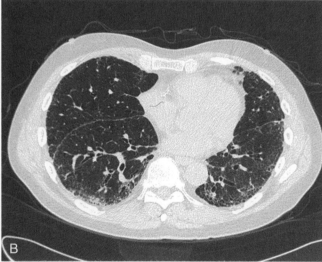

Figure 5-7 A, Posteroanterior chest radiograph showing the characteristic features of idiopathic pulmonary fibrosis, a common interstitial lung disease. Notice the bilateral lower zone reticulonodular infiltrates and the loss of lung volume in the lower lobes. **B,** Chest CT image shows the peripheral nature of the fibrosis. (From Kacmarek R, Stoller J, Heuer A: *Egan's Fundamentals of Respiratory Care,* ed 10, St. Louis, 2013, Mosby.)

Other supportive therapies include provision of supplemental oxygen for hypoxemia, pulmonary rehabilitation, and lung transplantation in appropriate candidates.[22]

The number of lung transplants for IPF is steadily rising, especially in the United States, where IPF now represents the leading indication for lung transplantation. Five-year survival rates after lung transplantation in IPF are estimated at 50% to 56%. Additional evidence suggests that patients with pulmonary fibrosis undergoing lung transplantation have favorable long-term survival compared with other disease indications.[18] However, this surgical therapeutic intervention is not without risks (see Chapter 12), including restrictive lung dysfunction, namely, bronchiolitis obliterans.

Sarcoidosis

Sarcoidosis is an idiopathic granulomatous inflammatory disorder that affects many organ systems, including the lungs, heart, skin, central nervous system, and eyes, among others.[24] Clinically, the lung is the most involved organ (Fig. 5-8).[25–27]

Table 5-4 Clinical manifestation of idiopathic pulmonary fibrosis		
		Findings
Signs	Pulmonary function tests	↓ TLC, ↓ VC, ↓ FRC, ↓ RV
		Normal or ↓ flow rates
		↓ DLCO
		As disease progresses, VT ↓ and RR ↑←
	Chest radiograph	Diffuse reticulonodular patterns throughout both lungs
		Predominance of abnormal markings in lower lung fields
	Computed tomography (HRCT)	Presence of reticular opacities with a subpleural basal predominance, honeycombing with or without traction bronchiectasis[21]
	Arterial blood gases	↓ PaO_2
		$Paco_2$ normal
		Hypoxemic with exercise early in disease, hypoxemic at rest as disease progresses
	Breath sounds	Bibasilar end-inspiratory dry rales
		↓ Breath sounds[22]
	Cardiovascular	One-third of IPF patients develop pulmonary hypertension[22]
		With pulmonary hypertension, right ventricular dysfunction, and cor pulmonale
		Late in course: cyanosis, clubbing of digits[24]
Symptoms		Dyspnea on exertion progresses to dyspnea at rest in late disease
		Repetitive nonproductive cough (some have mucus hypersecretion and expectoration)[28]
		Weight loss, decrease in appetite
		Fatigue
		Sleep disturbances with loss of rapid eye movement sleep[24,29]

DLCO, diffusing capacity of the lungs for carbon monoxide; *FRC,* functional residual capacity; *HR,* heart rate; *HRCT,* high-resolution computed tomography; *IPF,* idiopathic pulmonary fibrosis; *Paco₂,* arterial partial pressure of CO₂; *PaO₂,* arterial partial pressure of O₂; *RR,* respiratory rate; *RV,* residual volume; *TLC,* total lung capacity; *VC,* vital capacity; *VT,* tidal volume.

Etiology

Despite extensive research, the etiology of sarcoidosis is unknown. Infectious agents, chemicals or drugs, allergy, autoimmunity, and genetic factors have all been researched as possible causes.[30] Sarcoidosis most commonly affects young adults, with 70% of the cases diagnosed in persons 20 to 40 years of age. Sarcoidosis is more common in women than in men. The incidence is increased tenfold in black Americans compared with whites. It is rare in Native Americans.[31]

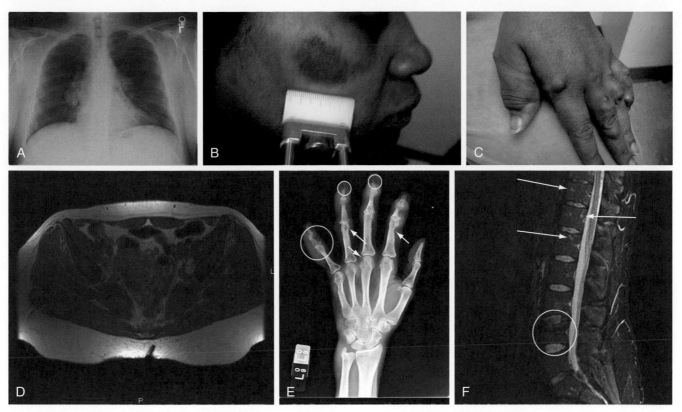

Figure 5-8 Various manifestations of sarcoidosis. **A,** Bilateral hilar adenopathy and right paratracheal lymph node enlargement demonstrated on a posterior anterior chest roentgenogram, Scadding stage 1. **B,** Facial lesion consistent with lupus pernio. **C,** Hand changes consistent with sarcoidosis in the fingers. **D.** Noncontrast magnetic resonance image of the pelvis demonstrating bone marrow replacement by granulomatous tissue. **E,** Cystic changes (*arrows*) within the bones of the fingers of a patient with sarcoidosis. **F,** Gadolinium enhancement of lesions of the spine seen on magnetic resonance image of a sarcoidosis patient. (From Firestein G, Budd R, Gabriel SE, et al: Kelley's Textbook of Rheumatology, ed 9, Saunders, St. Louis, 2013.)

Pathophysiology

This disease presents with three distinctive features within the lung: alveolitis, formation of well-defined round or oval granulomas, and pulmonary fibrosis.[25] The alveolitis usually appears earliest and is an infiltration of the alveolar walls by inflammatory cells, especially macrophages and T lymphocytes. The core of the sarcoid granuloma contains epithelioid cells and multinucleated giant cells; there is rarely any necrosis in the core. The core is surrounded by monocytes, macrophages, lymphocytes, and fibroblasts. These granulomas may resolve without scarring, but many go on to become obliterative fibrosis, which is characterized by the accumulation of fibroblasts and collagen around the granuloma. Diffuse fibrosis of the alveolar walls is not typical in this disease, although it can occur late in the disease progression. Approximately 25% of patients with pulmonary sarcoidosis experience a permanent decrease in lung function, which over time proves fatal in 5% to 10% of patients.[25] This loss of lung function is due to restrictive lung impairment primarily, but this disease also has an obstructive component. Prognosis seems to be better if the onset of pulmonary symptoms is acute. If the onset is insidious, with progressive dyspnea, then the prognosis is worse (patients will have more impairments, less function, and may have higher mortality rates).

Sarcoidosis is a multisystem disease, and although the pulmonary system is the most commonly involved (90%), other systems are affected also. Seventeen percent of patients have ocular involvement, which can lead to blindness.[25] The most common ocular presentation is granulomatous uveitis, which causes redness and watering of the eyes, cloudy vision, and photophobia.[32] Five percent of patients have neurologic involvement, which can include encephalopathy, granulomatous meningitis, or involvement of the cranial nerves.[25] Other organ systems that can be involved are the liver (60% to 80%), the lymphatics (50% to 75%), the heart (30%), the skin (30%), the spleen (15%), the kidney, muscles, joints, and the immune system.[3,8,25,26,31,33]

The progression of this disease is extremely variable. It can be active and resolve spontaneously, or it can be inactive and stable for long periods. About 30% of patients with sarcoidosis develop chronic progressive disease.[2] Mortality in sarcoidosis is less than 5%.[2] Neurologic and cardiac involvement may present acutely and portend a poor prognosis. Progressive pulmonary fibrosis is the most common cause of death.[32]

Clinical Manifestation

The clinical manifestation of sarcoidosis can be found in Table 5-5.

Treatment

Most patients require no treatment. When treatment is necessary, patients usually improve with moderate doses of corticosteroids. Steroid-sparing agents often are administered to minimize the long-term side effects of systemic corticosteroids.[32] In treating the three pulmonary manifestations of this disease, corticosteroids are used early to suppress the alveolitis and granuloma formation, especially if the patient has

Table 5-5 Clinical manifestation of sarcoidosis

		Findings
Signs	Pulmonary function tests	↓ TLC, ↓ all lung volumes, ↓ RV, ↓ lung compliance
		↓ DLCO due to ←↑ ventilation/perfusion mismatching
		Late in disease may find obstructive deficits with ↓ flow rates and/or 20% to 30% ↓ in PFT values[28]
	Chest radiograph	Bilateral hilar lymphadenopathy
		Lung parenchyma show diffuse infiltrates with interstitial reticulo-nodular pattern
	Arterial blood gases	Remain in normal limits until late in disease when ↓ PaO₂
	Breath sounds	Chest expansion ↓, ←↑ RR
		Auscultation: bibasilar rales and ↓ sounds in apices as a result of bullae with occasional wheezing
	Cardiovascular	15% develop pulmonary hypertension[24]
		Dysrhythmias, CHF, and papillary muscle dysfunction
Symptoms		One-third develop dyspnea during course of disease[33]
		Cough (±sputum)
		Complaint of vague retrosternal discomfort
		Fever, fatigue, weight loss, erythema nodosum

CHF, congestive heart failure; *DLCO*, diffusing capacity of the lungs for carbon monoxide; *PaO₂*, arterial partial pressure of O2; *PFT*, pulmonary function testing; *RR*, respiratory rate; *RV*, residual volume; *TLC*, total lung capacity.

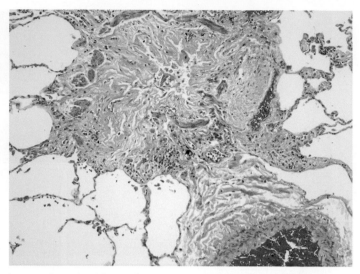

Figure 5-9 Bronchiolitis obliterans. The lumen is obliterated by the fibrosis. The bronchiole is identifiable only by the presence of smooth muscle bundles or discontinuous elastic tissue around a central scar. (From Husain A: *Thoracic Pathology*, St. Louis, 2013, Saunders.)

respiratory symptoms and/or a 20% to 30% reduction in PFT values.[10,28] Established granulomas with pulmonary fibrosis are relatively fixed lesions and do not respond to therapy.

Bronchiolitis Obliterans

Bronchiolitis obliterans is a fibrotic lung disease that affects the smaller airways. It can produce restrictive and obstructive lung dysfunction. This syndrome has been known and discussed under a variety of names, including bronchiolitis, bronchiolitis obliterans with organizing pneumonia (BOOP), bronchiolitis fibrosa obliterans, follicular bronchiolitis, and bronchiolitis obliterans with diffuse interstitial pneumonia.[25]

Etiology

Bronchiolitis obliterans was first recognized in children, usually those under the age of 2 years. Pediatric bronchiolitis obliterans is often caused by a viral infection, most commonly by the respiratory syncytial virus (RSV), parainfluenza virus, influenza virus, or adenovirus.[32] An adult form of the disease has now been recognized that can occur in persons from 20 to 80 years of age and has a wider variety of causes. In the adult, bronchiolitis obliterans may be caused by toxic fume inhalation (nitrogen dioxide) or by viral, bacterial, or mycobacterial infectious agents, particularly *Mycoplasma pneumoniae*. It may be associated with connective tissue diseases, such as rheumatoid arthritis (RA); related to organ transplantation and graft versus host reactions; or allied with other diseases, such as IPF. It also may be idiopathic, with no known cause.[25]

Pathophysiology

Bronchiolitis obliterans is characterized by necrosis of the respiratory epithelium in the affected bronchioles. This necrosis allows fluid and debris to enter the bronchioles and alveoli, causing alveolar pulmonary edema and partial or complete obstruction of these small airways. With complete obstruction, the trapped air is absorbed gradually and the alveoli then collapse, causing areas of atelectasis. When the destruction of the respiratory epithelium is severe or widespread, it may be followed by a significant inflammatory response. This causes fibrotic changes in the adjacent peribronchial space, the alveolar walls, and the air spaces. The fibrotic changes are patchy and usually occur primarily within the bronchial tree and alveoli rather than in the interstitial lung tissue, as happens in IPF. All these changes combine to increase ventilation–perfusion mismatching; decrease lung compliance; impair gas transport; and, in some patients, cause demonstrable airway obstruction (Fig. 5-9).[25]

Clinical Manifestation

The clinical manifestation of bronchiolitis obliterans can be found in Table 5-6.

Treatment

In children, treatment is supportive, usually consisting of hydration and supplemental oxygen. If the child is unable to clear secretions, postural drainage and suctioning are employed. Mechanical ventilation is rarely needed. If RSV is the causative pathogen, then the antiviral agent ribavirin may be administered via aerosol.[32] Corticosteroids, antibiotics, and bronchodilators are not recommended in the

Table 5-6 Clinical manifestation of bronchiolitis obliterans		
		Findings
Signs	Pulmonary function tests	Lung volumes normal or ↓, flow rates normal or ↓
		↓ DLCO, ←↑ RR
	Chest radiograph	Variable depending on cause and extent of BO
		Pediatric BO:
		Hyperinflation and ←↑ bronchial markings
		With subsegmental consolidation and collapse
		Some have patchy alveolar infiltrates, some with diffuse nodular or reticulonodular pattern and interstitial inflammation and scarring
		Adults:
		Pulmonary edema and bilateral patchy alveolar infiltrates.
		Late in course
		Nodular pattern with fibrotic changes in bronchi and alveoli
	Arterial blood gases	Hypoxemia (↓ PaO$_2$)
		Paco$_2$ normal or ←↑
	Breath sounds	Rales and expiratory wheezing. Some areas of ↓ sounds
	Cardiovascular	Tachycardia
Symptoms		Dyspnea, ←↑ RR and hacking, nonproductive cough
		Infants: chest wall retractions
		Cyanosis in some patients, chronic infections in others

BO, bronchiolitis obliterans; *DLCO*, diffusing capacity of the lungs for carbon monoxide; *RR*, respiratory rate.

treatment of pediatric bronchiolitis obliterans. In adults, supplemental oxygen and proper fluid balance are also very important. Corticosteroids have proved very effective in treating adult bronchiolitis obliterans that is idiopathic, caused by toxic fume inhalation, or associated with connective tissue disease.

Environmental/Occupational Causes

Coal Workers' Pneumoconiosis

Coal workers' pneumoconiosis (CWP), an interstitial lung disease, is defined as the accumulation of coal dust in the lungs and the subsequent reaction by the surrounding tissue. Coal workers' pneumoconiosis is classified into two categories based on radiographic findings: simple CWP with small opacities (<1 cm in size) and complicated CWP, or pulmonary massive fibrosis (PMF), with one or more large opacities (>1 cm).[34]

Etiology

Coal workers' pneumoconiosis is caused by repeated inhalation of coal dust over a long period; usually, 10 to 12 years of underground work exposure is necessary for the development of simple CWP.[35] Complicated CWP usually occurs only after even longer exposure to coal dust. Anthracite coal is more hazardous than bituminous in the development of this disease.[32]

Pathophysiology

The pathologic hallmark of CWP is the coal macule, which is a focal collection of coal dust with little tissue reaction either in terms of cellular infiltration or fibrosis. These coal macules are often located at the division of respiratory bronchioles and are often associated with focal emphysema.[35] Lymph nodes are enlarged and homogeneously pigmented and are firm but not fibrotic. The pleural surface appears black due to the deposits of coal dust. Simple CWP is a benign disease if complications do not develop. Less than 5% of cases progress to complicated CWP.[31]

Complicated CWP results in large confluent zones of dense fibrosis that are usually present in apical segments in one or both lungs. These zones are made up of dense, acellular, collagenous, black-pigmented tissue. The normal lung parenchyma can be completely replaced, and the blood vessels in the area then show an obliterative arteritis. These fibrous zones can completely replace the entire upper lobe.[35]

Other conditions that may result from complicated CWP include emphysema, chronic bronchitis, tuberculosis, cor pulmonale, and pulmonary thromboembolism.

Although CWP is preventable, it continues to occur at a disturbing rate, which leads to significant morbidity and mortality in coal miners.[34] The main cause of death is progression of lung disease and then development of respiratory failure.[34]

Diagnostic Tests

The diagnosis of CWP can be made by an adequate history of exposure to coal mine dust and characteristic chest radiograph.[34]

Clinical Manifestation

The clinical manifestation of CWP can be found in Table 5-7.

Treatment

Complicated CWP with pulmonary fibrosis is nonreversible; there is no cure for it. Supportive treatment includes cessation of exposure to coal dust, good nutrition, interventions to ensure adequate oxygenation and ventilation, and progressive exercise training to maximize the remaining lung function and tolerance to activity. Lung transplantation may be an option for those with advanced disease (Fig. 5-10).[36]

Silicosis

Silicosis, one of the occupational pneumoconioses, is a fibrotic lung disease caused by the inhalation of free crystalline silicon dioxide or silica.[37]

Table 5-7 Clinical manifestation of coal workers' pneumoconiosis (CWP)

		Findings
Signs	Pulmonary function tests	Spirometric tests often normal or slight ↓ VC and ↓ RV with ↓ DLCO
		Complicated
		↓ TLC, ↓ VC, ↓ FRC, ↓ lung compliance, ↓ DLCO, ←↑ RR
	Chest radiograph	Simple
		Small discrete densities more nodular than linear
		Predominantly in upper regions
		Complicated
		Coalescent opacities of black fibrous tissue
		Usually in posterior segments of upper lobes or superior segments of lower lobes. Cavities may be present as a result of superimposed TB or secondary to ischemic necrosis
	Arterial blood gases	↓ PaO₂
	Breath sounds	Simple
		Slightly diminished breath sounds, rhonchi due to concomitant bronchitis
		Complicated
		Abnormal bronchial breath sounds above compressed atelectatic areas and rhonchi or rales with bronchitis
	Cardiovascular	Complicated
		Fibrotic pulmonary hypertension
		Cor pulmonale
Symptoms		Severe dyspnea and cough
		Copious amounts of black sputum
		Barrel chest
		Progressive weight loss

DLCO, diffusing capacity of the lungs for carbon monoxide; *FRC,* functional residual capacity; *PaO₂,* arterial partial pressure of O₂; *RR,* respiratory rate; *RV,* residual volume; *TB,* tuberculosis; *TLC,* total lung capacity; *VC,* vital capacity.

Etiology

Free crystalline silicon dioxide is very common and widely distributed in the earth's crust in a variety of forms, including quartz, flint, cristobalite, and tridymite.[35] Industries in which silicon dioxide exposure can occur include mining, tunneling through rock, quarrying, grinding and polishing rock, sandblasting, ship building, and foundry work.[29] More recent exposure hazards now include hydraulic fracturing (fracking) of oil and gas wells.[38] The most

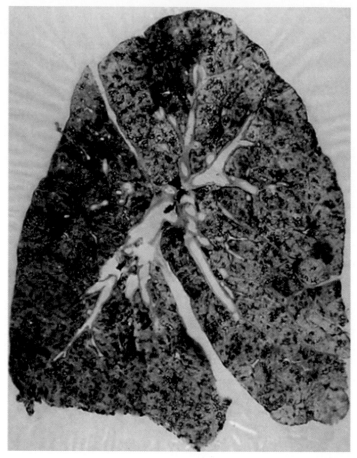

Figure 5-10 Coal workers' pneumoconiosis. The lungs show increased black pigmentation. (From Danjanov I: *Pathology: a color atlas,* St. Louis, 2000, Mosby.)

important factor in developing silicosis is the cumulative dose of silica inhaled.[38] Even after the patient is no longer exposed, lung function impairment worsens as the disease progresses.[37]

Currently, about 2 million U.S. workers are exposed to silica. According to the National Institute for Occupational Safety and Health, there has been a decrease in U.S. death rates due to silicosis, from about 1200 in 1968 to fewer than 100 per year in the early 2000s. Aside from a few states having their own, there is no national surveillance system.[38]

Pathophysiology

Inhaled silica causes macrophages to enter the area to ingest these particles. But the macrophages are destroyed by the cytotoxic effects of the silica. This process releases lysosomal enzymes that then induce progressive formation of collagen, which eventually becomes fibrotic. Another characteristic of silicosis is the formation of acellular nodules composed of connective tissue called *silicotic nodules.* Initially, these nodules are small and discrete, but as the disease progresses, they become larger and coalesce. Silicosis normally affects the upper lobes of the lung more than the lower lobes. Silicosis also seems to predispose the patient to secondary infections by mycobacteria, including *Mycobacterium tuberculosis.*

Complicated silicosis follows a steadily deteriorating course that leads to respiratory failure.[3,33]

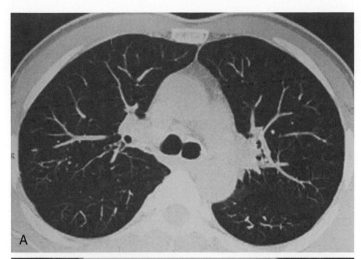

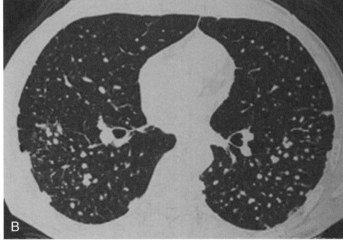

Figure 5-11 Axial high-resolution computed tomography sections of two patients with silicosis. Early silicosis with sparse and small silicotic nodules **(A)** and silicosis with many nodules of varying sizes **(B)**. (From Leung CC, Tak Sun Yu I, Chen W: Silicosis, *Lancet* 379(9830):2008 - 2018, 2012.)

Diagnostic Tests

Diagnosis is made based on a history of substantial exposure to silica, exclusion of other competing diagnoses, and chest radiography (Fig. 5-11).[37]

Clinical Manifestation

The clinical manifestation of silicosis can be found in Table 5-8.

Treatment

No curative treatment exists, but comprehensive management strategies help to improve quality of life and slow deterioration. Supportive therapy includes avoidance of further exposure, provision of adequate oxygenation, ventilation, and nutrition. It has been shown that physical training can improve functional exercise capacity, shortness of breath, and quality of life in patients with interstitial lung disease. Another therapeutic option for those with advanced lung disease is lung transplantation, especially for young patients with acute silicosis.[37]

Table 5-8 Clinical manifestation of silicosis

		Findings
Signs	Pulmonary function tests	↓ TLC, ↓ VC, ↓ pulmonary compliance, ↓ FEV$_1$
	Chest radiograph	Small rounded opacities or nodules that enlarge over time (more in upper lung fields)
		Some may have diffuse interstitial pattern of fibrosis without the typical nodular opacities.[37]
		Hilar lymph nodes enlarged and calcified
	Arterial blood gases	↓ PaO$_2$ with exercise
	Breath sounds	Decreased breath sounds in upper lobes
		Rhonchi may be present
	Cardiovascular	No specific changes
Symptoms		Shortness of breath and cough (may be productive)

FEV$_1$, forced expiratory volume in 1 second; *PaO$_2$*, arterial partial pressure of O$_2$; *TLC*, total lung capacity; *VC*, vital capacity.

Asbestosis

Asbestosis is a pneumoconiosis caused by the inhalation of asbestos.[32,39] Occupational asbestos exposure is also associated with an increased incidence of primary cancer of the larynx, oropharynx, esophagus, stomach, and colon.[35]

Etiology

There are six naturally occurring fibrous silicate minerals that are referred to as *asbestos fibers*.[39] They include chrysotile, which accounts for more than 70% of the asbestos used in the United States; crocidolite; amosite; tremolite; anthophyllite; and actinolite (amphiboles). There is another naturally occurring silicate called *vermiculite*, which may be contaminated with asbestos fibers, therefore also posing a health risk.[39]

Asbestos was initially used due to its exceptional fireproof and insulation properties. The most common trades known for asbestos exposure include aircraft mechanics and manufacturers, aerospace/missile production, electrical workers, power plant employees, telephone linemen, shipyard workers (e.g., insulators, laggers, painters, pipefitters), building supply manufacturers, railroad and sheet metal workers, operational navy and coast guard personnel, and asbestos mining and transport.[39]

Pathophysiology

How asbestos causes a fibrotic reaction is not understood. It is hypothesized that the asbestos fiber causes an alveolitis in the area of the respiratory bronchioles, which then progresses to peribronchiolar fibrosis due to the release of chemical mediators. Plaques, which are localized fibrous thickenings of the parietal pleura, are common and are usually seen posteriorly, laterally, or on the pleural surface of the diaphragm. Pleural effusions may also occur with asbestosis. Also, "asbestos bodies," or ferruginous bodies, appear in the lungs and sputum of these patients. These rod-shaped bodies with clubbed ends seem to be an asbestos fiber coated by macrophages with an iron–protein complex.[3,8,32,35]

There is often a dormancy period of 20 to 30 years for asbestos-related lung disease to reveal itself. Prevalence in the United States is unknown.[39]

Studies have shown conclusively that cigarette smoking has a multiplicative effect in the development of primary lung cancer in persons who have been exposed to asbestos.[35] Complications of asbestosis include bronchiectasis, pleural mesothelioma, and bronchogenic carcinoma.[8]

Diagnostic Tests

Diagnosis can be made based on a history of respiratory symptoms and occupational exposure, including type of work and duration of exposure. A complete history on smoking is also important. The posteroanterior chest radiograph remains the standard for evaluation and classification of asbestosis.[39]

Clinical Manifestation

The clinical manifestation of asbestosis can be found in Table 5-9.

Treatment

There is no curative treatment for asbestosis and the disease progresses even though exposure to asbestos has ceased. Symptomatic support includes cessation of smoking, good nutrition, exercise conditioning to maximize lung function, and prompt treatment of recurrent pulmonary infections. For those with advanced diseases, lung transplant may be an option.[36]

Infectious Causes

Pneumonia

Pneumonia is an inflammatory process of the lung parenchyma that usually begins with an infection in the lower respiratory tract. Causative agents include bacteria, viruses, fungi, or mycoplasmas.

There are four categories of pneumonias: community-acquired pneumonias, hospital-acquired pneumonias (HAPs), health care–associated pneumonia (HCAP), and ventilator-associated pneumonia (VAP). The latter three were known as nosocomial.[1]

The World Health Organization estimates that lower respiratory tract infection is the most common infectious cause of death in the world (the third most common cause overall), with almost 3.5 million deaths yearly.[2] Together, pneumonia and influenza constitute the ninth leading cause of death in the United States, resulting in 50,000 estimated deaths in 2010.[40]

Etiology

Community-acquired pneumonias can be divided into two types: acute and chronic. The group depends on the clinical presentation. Acute pneumonia generally appears with sudden onset over a few hours to several days.[1] Chronic is more insidious, often with gradually worsening of symptoms over days, weeks, or even months.[1] *Streptococcus pneumonia*, also called *pneumococcus*, has been found to be the most common cause of community-acquired pneumonia, accounting for 20%

Table 5-9 Clinical manifestation of asbestosis

		Findings
Signs	Pulmonary function tests	↓ lung compliance, ↓ lung volumes: ↓ TLC, ↓ VC, ↓ RV
		↓ FEV_1 and ↓ DLCO
	Chest radiograph	Irregularities or linear opacities are distributed throughout lung fields in lower zones. Advanced asbestosis often reveals upper lobe involvement and honeycombing.[39]
		Loss of distinct heart and diaphragm borders (shaggy appearance)
		Diaphragmatic and pericardial calcification
		Late in disease: cyst formation, honeycomb appearance
	Arterial blood gases	↓ PaO_2 with exercise; late in disease ↓ PaO_2 at rest
		$Paco_2$ within normal limits
	Breath sounds	Fine end-inspiratory crackles at the bases and ↓ breath sounds[39]
		Percussion dull at bases
	Cardiovascular	Pulmonary hypertension develops as pulmonary capillary bed destroyed: ←↑ work on RV Right-sided heart failure[39]
		Clubbing present; may develop cyanosis and cor pulmonale
Symptoms		Dyspnea on exertion: progresses to dyspnea at rest
		Recurrent infections, chronic cough with or without sputum
		Weight loss, ↓ appetite, and ↓ exercise tolerance

DLCO, diffusing capacity of the lungs for carbon monoxide; *FEV_1*, forced expiratory volume in 1 second; *RV*, residual volume; *TLC*, total lung capacity; *VC*, vital capacity.

to 70% of cases. Other causative organisms include *Haemophilus influenzae, Staphylococcus aureus*, and gram-negative bacilli, each accounting for 3% to 10% of cases. *Legionella* spp., *Chlamydophila pneumonia*, and *M. pneumonia* together account for 10% to 20% of cases and are considered atypical.[1] Although there are many infectious agents in the environment, few pneumonias develop because of the efficient defense mechanisms in the lung. Those who develop community-acquired pneumonias usually have been infected with an exceedingly virulent organism or a particularly large inoculum or have impaired or damaged lung defense mechanisms.[32]

Health care–associated pneumonia, HAP, and VAP are often caused by different microorganisms than community-acquired pneumonia (Table 5-10). Hospital-acquired pneumonia is a common clinical problem and represents the second most common nosocomial infection in the United States and accounts

Table 5-10 Pneumonia transmission and treatment

Pneumonia type	Transmission route	Susceptible populations	Preferred drug
Bacterial			
Streptococcus pneumonia	Droplet inhalation Direct contact with infected respiratory secretions Indirect contact with articles soiled by infected respiratory secretions	Infants, elderly Patients having congestive heart failure, COPD, splenectomy, alcoholism, multiple myeloma, or a predisposing viral infection	Penicillin G Tetracyclines Ampicillin
Legionella pneumophila	Inhalation of an aerosolized infected water source (drinking water, air conditioning, shower heads, lakes)	Elderly Patients having diabetes, COPD, AIDS, renal ransplantation, malignancy, and alcoholism Smokers	Erythromycin
Haemophilus influenzae	Droplet inhalation Direct contact with infected respiratory secretions Indirect contact with articles soiled by infected respiratory secretions	Elderly Patients having chronic bronchitis, AIDS, alcoholism, splenectomy, chronic debilitation, or a predisposing viral infection	Ampicillin Cephalosporins
Klebsiella pneumoniae	Droplet inhalation Direct contact with infected respiratory secretions Indirect contact with articles soiled by infected respiratory secretions	Elderly in nursing homes Patients having COPD, alcoholism, diabetes, malignancy, chronic renal failure, and chronic debilitation	Aminoglycosides Cephalosporins
Pseudomonas aeruginosa	Droplet inhalation Direct contact with infected respiratory secretions Indirect contact with articles soiled by infected respiratory secretions Hematogenously Wound infection	Patients having cystic fibrosis, ARDS, or neutropenia Patients on mechanical ventilation	Carbenicillin Aztreonam Aminoglycosides
Staphylococcus aureus	Droplet inhalation Direct contact with infected respiratory secretions Indirect contact with articles soiled by infected respiratory secretions Hematogenously Aspiration	Patients having cystic fibrosis, drug addictions, splenectomy, or a predisposing viral infection	Antistaphylococcal penicillin Cephalosporins Vancomycin Clindamycin Gentamicin
Mycoplasmal			
Mycoplasma pneumoniae	Droplet inhalation Direct contact with infected respiratory secretions Indirect contact with articles soiled by infected respiratory secretions	School children College students Patients with AIDS	Erythromycin Tetracycline Streptomycin
Viral			
Respiratory syncytial virus	Droplet inhalation Direct contact with infected respiratory secretions Indirect contact with articles soiled by infected respiratory secretions	Infants 2-5 months of age and school-aged children	Ribavirin
Adenovirus	Droplet inhalation Direct contact with infected respiratory secretions or infected feces Indirect contact with articles soiled by infected respiratory secretions or feces	Children 6 months to 5 years and military recruits	None
Cytomegalovirus	Contact with infected body fluids, including tears, saliva, blood, breast milk, urine, semen Can be infected in utero and by infected transplanted organs	Fetuses Patients having malignancy, AIDS, major organ transplantation, or chronic debilitation	Acyclovir analogue

Continued

Table 5-10 Pneumonia transmission and treatment—cont'd

Pneumonia type	Transmission route	Susceptible populations	Preferred drug
Influenza virus	Droplet inhalation Direct contact with infected respiratory secretions Indirect contact with articles soiled by infected respiratory secretions	Women in the third trimester of pregnancy Elderly Patients having malignancy, heart disease, COPD, diabetes, chronic renal failure, neuro-muscular disorders, or chronic debilitation	Amantadine
Fungal			
Pneumocystis carinii	Unknown, probably droplet inhalation	Premature infants Patients with AIDS, or chronic debilitation	Trimethoprimsulfa-methoxazole Pentamidine
Chlamydial			
Chlamydia psittaci	Inhalation of infected droplets, droplet nuclei, or dust from the desiccated dropping of infected birds (parrots, parakeets, turkeys, pigeons, chickens)	Persons with pet birds and workers on poultry farms and in poultry processing plants	Tetracycline Chloramphenicol

AIDS, acquired immunodeficiency syndrome; *ARDS*, adult respiratory distress syndrome; *COPD*, chronic obstructive pulmonary disease.
From Cottrell GP, Surkin HB: *Pharmacology for Respiratory Care Practitioners.* Philadelphia, 1995, FA Davis.

for 15% to 18% of all such infections.[9] The patients most likely to develop a nosocomial pneumonia have one or more of the following risk factors: nasogastric tube placement; intubation; dysphagia; tracheostomy; mechanical ventilation; thoracoabdominal surgery; lung injury; diabetes; chronic cardiopulmonary disease; intraabdominal infection; uremia; shock; history of smoking; advanced age; poor nutritional status; or certain therapeutic interventions, such as the administration of broad-spectrum antibiotics, corticosteroids, antacids, or high oxygen concentrations.

Pathophysiology

Bacteria and other microbes commonly enter the lower respiratory tract. It has been estimated that during sleep, 45% of healthy people aspirate oropharyngeal secretions into the lower respiratory tract.[9] However, because of the elaborate defense mechanisms within the pulmonary system, pneumonia usually does not develop. The mechanical defenses include cough, bronchoconstriction, angulation of the airways favoring impaction and subsequent transport upward, and action of the mucociliary escalator. The immune defenses include bronchus-associated lymphoid tissue; phagocytosis by polymorphonuclear cells and macrophages; immunoglobulins A and G; and complement, surfactant, and cell-mediated immunity by T lymphocytes.[32]

The most common routes for infection leading to pneumonia are inhalation and aspiration (see Table 5-10). When the causative agent is bacterial, the first response to infection is an outpouring of edema fluid. This is followed rapidly by the appearance of polymorphonuclear leukocytes that are involved in active phagocytosis of the bacteria, and then fibrin is deposited in the inflamed area. Usually by day 5, specific antibodies are in the area fighting the bacterial infection. Clinically, bacterial pneumonia usually has an abrupt onset and is characterized by lobar consolidation, high fever, chills, dyspnea, tachypnea, productive cough, pleuritic pain, and leukocytosis.[2,35,41] When the causative agent is viral, the virus first localizes in respiratory epithelial cells and causes destruction of the cilia and mucosal surface, leading to the loss of mucociliary function. This impairment may then predispose the patient to bacterial pneumonia. If viral infection reaches the level of the alveoli, there may be edema, hemorrhage, hyaline membrane formation, and possibly the development of adult RDS. Primary viral pneumonia is a serious disease with diffuse infiltrates, extensive parenchymal injury, and severe hypoxemia. Clinically, viral pneumonia usually has an insidious onset and is characterized by patchy diffuse bronchopulmonary infiltrates, moderate fever, dyspnea, tachypnea, nonproductive cough, myalgia, and a normal white blood cell count.[32]

Diagnostic Tests

Radiographic appearances of new or progressive pulmonary infiltrates, as well as clinical symptoms, are seen in Table 5-9.

Clinical Manifestation

The clinical manifestation of pneumonia can be found in Table 5-11.

Treatment

Drug therapy is the primary focus in the treatment of pneumonia, particularly antibiotics for treating bacterial pneumonia. Antibiotic therapy should be pathogen specific if the pathogen can be determined; if not, an empiric regimen of multiple antibiotics may be needed. Oxygen and temporary mechanical ventilation or noninvasive ventilation may be necessary in patients with refractory hypoxemia (PaO_2 < 60 mm Hg). Other supportive therapy includes postural drainage, percussion, vibration, and assisted coughing techniques for patients who are producing more than 30 mL per day of mucus or have an impaired cough mechanism.[32] Adequate hydration and nutrition are also important. These infections can also be prevented by rigorous environmental controls in hospitals, such as strict guideline adherence for the prevention of contamination of ventilators and other

Table 5-11	Clinical manifestation of pneumonia	
		Findings
Signs	Pulmonary function tests	↓ lung volumes, ↓ lung compliance, ↓ gas exchange ←↑ RR, ←↑ inspiratory pressure, ↑ work of breathing
		←↑ ventilation–perfusion mismatching, ↓ oxygen uptake
		Pulmonary capillary leakage
		Resolution of pneumonia may result in fibrosis and scarring
	Chest radiograph	Bacterial:
		Lobar consolidation in one or more lobes
		Viral:
		Bilateral bronchopneumonia: diffuse scattered fluffy shadows indicating patchy alveolar infiltrates
		Necrotizing pneumonia: when cavities present
	Arterial blood gases	↓ PaO$_2$, may have ↓ Paco$_2$ as a result of breathing pattern blowing off CO$_2$
	Breath sounds	May have bronchial sounds above lobar pneumonia, absent breath sounds over pneumonia and dull to mediate percussion
		May also have bubbling rales, rhonchi, decreased or absent sounds, egophony, and whispering pectoriloquy
	Cardiovascular	Usually have ←↑HR, especially in presence of fever
Symptoms		Bacterial: high fever, chills, dyspnea, tachypnea, productive cough, pleuritic pain
		Viral: moderate fever, dyspnea, tachypnea, nonproductive cough, myalgias

HR, heart rate; *Paco$_2$*, arterial partial pressure of CO$_2$; *PaO$_2$*, arterial partial pressure of O$_2$; *RR*, respiratory rate.

respiratory equipment, careful aseptic patient care practices, and surveillance of infections and antibiotic susceptibility patterns in high-risk areas.

Pneumonia is simply an inflammatory process of some part of the lung where gas exchange occurs that progresses beyond inflammation and develops into infection. The key to treatment of pneumonia is to first identify the microbe (virus vs. gram-positive or gram-negative bacteria). Specific medical treatment (specific antibiotic) is based on identification of the microbe, although broad-spectrum medications may be initiated before identification has been made.

Specific Pneumonias

Bacterial Pneumonias

Streptococcus pneumoniae.

S. pneumoniae is more common in the elderly; in alcoholics; and in those with asplenia, multiple myeloma, congestive heart failure (CHF), or chronic obstructive lung disease. Seventy percent of patients report a preceding viral illness.[32] This type of pneumonia occurs more frequently during the winter and early spring. Specific signs and symptoms include rusty-colored sputum, hemoptysis, bronchial breath sounds, egophony, increased tactile fremitus, pleural friction rub, severe pleuritic chest pain, pleural effusion in 25% of patients, and slight liver dysfunction.[30,32] Complications can include lung abscess, atelectasis, delayed resolution in the elderly, pericarditis, endocarditis, meningitis, jaundice, and arthritis.[35] Streptococcal pneumonia is treated with penicillin G, ampicillin, or tetracyclines.[42] There is also a pneumococcal vaccine; this injection provides lifetime protection against serotypes of the pneumococcus that account for 85% of all cases of pneumococcal pneumonia.[32,42]

Legionella pneumophila.

Legionella pneumophila can occur in epidemic proportions because the organism is water borne and can emanate from air-conditioning equipment, drinking water, lakes, river banks, water faucets, and shower heads. *L. pneumophila* accounts for 7% to 15% of all community-acquired pneumonias.[32] It is found commonly in patients who are on dialysis; in persons who have a malignancy, a chronic obstructive pulmonary disease (COPD), a smoking history, or are older than 50 years; and in persons who are alcoholics or diabetics. Transplant recipients of any organ are at the highest risk.[30] Signs and symptoms in addition to those characteristic of bacterial pneumonias include headache, myalgias, preceding diarrhea, mental confusion, hyponatremia, bradycardia, and liver function abnormalities. Productive coughs with purulent sputum and hemoptysis can develop in 50% to 75% of patients.[30] However, most patients (90%) begin with a nonproductive cough.[30] The chest radiograph may show lobar consolidation or unilateral or bilateral bronchopneumonia; rounded densities with cavitation may also be seen. Fifteen percent of these patients have pleural effusions. The antibiotic of choice is erythromycin. Rifampin may also be used in addition to erythromycin.[32]

Haemophilus influenzae.

H. influenzae causes pneumonia, particularly in children who have had their spleen removed, in patients with COPD, in alcoholics, in AIDS patients, in those with lung cancer, in patients with hypogammaglobulinemia, and in the elderly.[10] In addition to the expected signs and symptoms of bacterial pneumonia, *H. influenzae* often causes a sore throat. The chest radiograph may show focal lobar, lobular, multilobar, or patchy bronchopneumonia or segmental pneumonia that usually involves the lower lobes. Complications can include empyema, lung abscess, epiglottitis, otitis media, pericarditis, meningitis, and arthritis. The preferred antibiotic is ampicillin; however, 20% of patients have been shown to be resistant to ampicillin. In these cases, cephalosporins, trimethoprim–sulfamethoxazole, and chloramphenicol are used.[32,35]

Klebsiella pneumoniae.

Klebsiella pneumoniae may cause either a community-acquired pneumonia or nosocomial pneumonia. The community-acquired *Klebsiella* pneumonia is seen most commonly in men over the age of 40 who are alcoholic or diabetic or who have underlying pulmonary disease. These patients may show purulent blood-streaked sputum, hemoptysis, cyanosis, and hypotension. Chest radiographic findings most frequently show right-sided involvement of the posterior segment of the upper lobe or the lower lobe segments. There may be outward bulging of a lobar fissure as a result of edema, and 25% to 50% of these patients have lung abscesses.[35] Complications include empyema, lung abscess, pneumothorax, chronic pneumonia, pericarditis, meningitis, and anemia. Treatment includes a two-drug therapy: an aminoglycoside and a cephalosporin. Oxygen is also used to maintain an oxygen saturation level of 80% to 85%. The mortality rate for this gram-negative pneumonia is 20%.[35]

Nosocomial *Klebsiella* pneumonia is a fulminant infection that causes severe lung damage and has a 50% mortality rate.[32] It affects debilitated patients in hospitals and nursing homes, middle-aged or older, who suffer from concomitant alcoholism, diabetes, malignancy, or chronic renal or cardiopulmonary disease. Their sputum is thick, purulent, and bloody or is thin and has a "currant jelly" texture. Tachycardia is common. The chest radiograph can show lobar consolidation, usually in the upper lobes, with lung abscesses, cavities, scarring, and fibrosis. A bronchopneumonia appearance may also occur. Complications are the same as those in community-acquired *Klebsiella* pneumonia. Drug therapy includes the use of aminoglycosides, cephalosporin, and antipseudomonal penicillin.[32,35]

Pseudomonas aeruginosa.

Pseudomonas aeruginosa is a gram-negative bacillus and is the most common cause of nosocomial pneumonias. It causes 15% of all HAPs and affects 40% of all mechanically ventilated patients.[32] Those at most risk for this infection are patients with cystic fibrosis, bronchiectasis, tracheostomy, or neutropenia or those who are on mechanical ventilation or corticosteroid therapy. This necrotizing pneumonia causes alveolar septal necrosis, microabscesses, and vascular thrombosis and has a mortality rate of 70% in postoperative patients.[32] Signs and symptoms include confusion, bradycardia, and hemorrhagic pleural effusion. The chest radiograph shows bilateral patchy alveolar infiltrates, usually in the lower lobes, with nodular infiltrates and cavitation.[32] Treatment always involves two drugs. Aminoglycosides, carbenicillin, and aztreonam are used to overcome this bacterium.[42]

Staphylococcus aureus.

S. aureus causes approximately 5% of community-acquired pneumonias.[32] This type of pneumonia is usually seen in infants and children under the age of 2 years, in patients with cystic fibrosis or COPD, or in patients who are recovering from influenza. The hallmark lesion seen in this pneumonia is ulcerative bronchiolitis with necrosis of the bronchiolar wall.[42] Signs and symptoms include cough with dirty salmon-pink purulent sputum, high fever, dyspnea, and pleuritic chest pain.[42] Other manifestations commonly seen in children are cyanosis, labored breathing, grunting, flaring of the nostrils, and chest wall retractions. The chest radiograph shows a diffuse bronchopneumonia, with bilateral infiltrates, cavitary lung abscesses, pneumatoceles, and pleural effusions. Complications include pneumothorax, lung abscess, endocarditis, and meningitis. Treatment is with antistaphylococcal penicillin, cephalosporin, vancomycin, clindamycin, and gentamicin.[32,35,42]

Mycoplasma pneumonias.

Mycoplasmas are the smallest free-living organisms that have yet been identified. This class of organisms is intermediate between bacteria and viruses. Unlike bacteria, they have no rigid cell wall, and unlike viruses, they do not require the intracellular machinery of a host cell to replicate.

Mycoplasma pneumoniae.

M. pneumoniae is seen in all age groups but is more common in persons less than 20 years old. Mycoplasma pneumonias account for 20% of all community-acquired pneumonias.[32] This infection is common year round, but usually the incidence increases in the fall and winter. Mycoplasma pneumonia has also been termed *walking pneumonia* because the respiratory symptoms are often not severe enough for people to seek medical attention. The course of the disease is approximately 4 weeks, and it is very infectious; whole families may become ill once a child brings it into the home. The signs and symptoms often include many extrapulmonary manifestations that are not common in bacterial or viral pneumonias. Patients may have fever, shaking chills, dry cough, headache, malaise, sore throat, earache, arthralgias, arthritis, immune dysfunction with an autoantibody response, meningoencephalitis, meningitis, transverse myelitis, cranial nerve palsies, Guillain–Barré syndrome, myocarditis, pericarditis, gastroenteritis, pancreatitis, glomerulonephritis, hepatitis, generalized lymphadenopathy, and erythema multiforme, including Stevens–Johnson syndrome.[30] The chest radiograph shows interstitial infiltrates, usually unilateral in the lower lobe; 20% of patients have a pleural effusion. Treatment is with erythromycin, tetracycline, or streptomycin.[32,42]

Viral Pneumonias

Cytomegalovirus, varicella zoster, and herpes simplex cause viral pneumonias most commonly in immunocompromised hosts, such as patients who have had major organ transplants or who have AIDS or malignancy. The respiratory syncytial virus and the parainfluenza virus cause viral pneumonias in children. The adenovirus is a source of viral pneumonias in children and in military recruits. Viral pneumonias in the debilitated elderly are most commonly caused by the influenza virus. Persons most at risk for a viral pneumonia are those who have an underlying cardiopulmonary disease or who are immunosuppressed or pregnant. Complications of viral pneumonias include secondary bacterial infections, bronchial hyperreactivity and possibly asthma, chronic air flow obstruction, tracheitis, bronchitis, bronchiolitis, and acellular hyaline membrane formation.

Some antiviral agents are now available. Acyclovir is used against herpes simplex and varicella-zoster. Amantadine is the drug of choice for influenza A. Ribavirin is used in children to treat the respiratory syncytial virus. Cytomegalovirus is treated with the acyclovir analog dihydroxyphenylglycol (DHPG). No drug therapy is available for all the varieties of viral agents, so treatment is often limited to supportive measures.[32,35]

Fungal Pneumonias

Pneumocystis jiroveci.

Previously called *Pneumocystis carinii* and originally described as a protozoan, this is now thought to be a fungal organism.[30] *Pneumocystis carinii* pneumonia (PCP) is closely associated with AIDS because nearly 75% of AIDS patients have at least one episode of PCP during their lifetime.[30] Patients with AIDS have impairment of T-cell function, as well as humoral immune dysfunction, and thus are susceptible to infection from bacteria, viruses, fungi, and parasites. *Pneumocystis carinii* pneumonia is also seen in transplant patients, especially those on cyclosporine, and in patients with lymphoreticular hematologic malignancies.[10] The chest radiograph most commonly shows bilateral diffuse interstitial or alveolar infiltrates, more prominent in the perihilar regions, and a solitary pulmonary nodule.[10] *Pneumocystis carinii* pneumonia damages the parenchymal cells within the lung and alters the alveolar–capillary permeability. This type of pneumonia usually has a subacute course of fever, dyspnea, cough, chest pain, malaise, fatigue, weight loss, and night sweats, but the symptoms can progress to include tachypnea, reduced PaO_2, and cyanosis.[10] Treatment is with trimethoprim-sulfamethoxazole. If this drug is not tolerated, then pentamidine is prescribed.[10,12,32]

Chlamydial Pneumonias

Chlamydia psittaci.

C. psittaci causes approximately 12% of the community-acquired pneumonias in the student population and about 6% of the community-acquired pneumonias in the elderly.[32] The onset is usually insidious, with cough, sputum, hemoptysis, dyspnea, headache, myalgia, and hepatosplenomegaly.[10,30] Complications include laryngitis, pharyngitis, encephalitis, hemolytic anemia, bradycardia, hepatitis, renal failure, and macular rash. Treatment is with tetracycline or chloramphenicol.[10,30]

Neoplastic Causes

Bronchogenic Carcinoma

Lung cancer, collectively called *bronchogenic carcinoma*, is a growth of abnormal epithelial cells in the tracheobronchial tree.[32,43] As the tumor enlarges, irritation occurs in the airways and alveoli, causing swelling, fluid buildup in adjacent alveoli, mucus production, and eventual obstruction.[43] This growth or tumor may spread by infiltrating surrounding tissues, such as the mediastinum, chest wall, ribs, or diaphragm, or by metastasizing to other body organs, or both (Fig. 5-12).[7] Currently, the International Association for the Study of Lung Cancer (IASLC) has defined two main types of lung cancer: small cell cancer and non–small cell lung cancer, which includes squamous cell, adenocarcinoma, and large cell, undifferentiated.[44] With more than 221,000 new

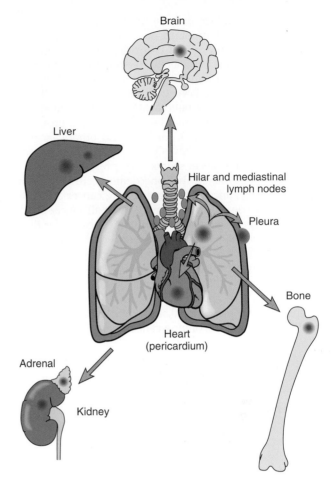

Figure 5-12 Primary lung cancer metastasizes to pleura, lymph, bone, brain, kidney, and liver. (From Damjanov I: *Pathology for the Health Professions*, ed 3, St. Louis, 2006, Saunders.)

cases annually (as estimated for 2015), lung cancer is the leading cause of cancer deaths, accounting for 27% (Fig. 5-13).[43-45]

Etiology

The causes of lung cancer are numerous. It has now been well established through numerous studies that the primary causative factor is tobacco use. Approximately 80% to 90% of lung cancers are caused by tobacco, and heavy smokers are 25% more likely to develop a neoplasm compared with nonsmokers.[30,43,44] The average cigarette smoker has ten times the risk of developing lung cancer as the nonsmoker, as there are 4000 different carcinogenic chemicals in tobacco smoke. Most disturbing is the finding that lung cancer risk is closely related to initiating smoking at an early age. When children start smoking at 15 years of age or younger and continue smoking, after 50 years, they have a 100-fold increased risk of lung cancer over that of a nonsmoker.[30] Passive smoking, or secondhand smoking—exposure to cigarette smoke exhaled by a smoker—as well as side-stream smoke have also been shown to increase the incidence of lung cancer by approximately 30%. Like active smoking at an early age, passive smoking during childhood and adolescence may pose a significantly increased risk.[30,43]

Occupational agents have also been implicated in the development of bronchogenic carcinoma. The known carcinogens present in the workplace include radioactive material, asbestos, chromates, nickel, mustard gas, isopropyl oil, hydrocarbons, arsenic, hematite, vinyl chloride, diesel exhaust, and bis(chloromethyl) ether.[32,43] Increased exposure to radon or significant air pollution also increases the incidence of lung cancer, although the relationship is very difficult to quantify. It is interesting that diets containing beta carotene (found in many green, yellow, and orange fruits and vegetables) have been shown to modestly decrease the risk for lung and other cancers.[28] In some individuals and families, a genetic predisposition for the development of lung cancer seems to be present.

Globally, it is estimated that one death occurs each minute as a result of lung cancer.[30] Currently, lung cancer accounts for 33% of all cancer deaths in men and 23% of all cancer deaths in women and is the second most common cancer. Over the past 20 years, the male–female ratio of lung cancer deaths has dropped from 5.7:1 to 1.4:1 as a result of the striking increase in lung cancer among women, which began about 1965.[10] It is now the leading cause of death from cancer in both men and women, surpassing breast cancer. In 2008 approximately 159,400 Americans died of lung cancer: 88,900 men and 70,500 women.[29] In the same year, almost 219,000 new cases of lung cancer were diagnosed.[32]

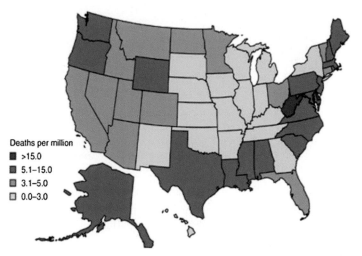

Deaths per million
- ■ >15.0
- ■ 5.1–15.0
- ■ 3.1–5.0
- □ 0.0–3.0

Figure 5-13 Age-adjusted mortality rates for asbestosis in US residents aged 15 or older by state (1990-1999). Delaware and West Virginia had the highest asbestosis mortality rates during 1990-1999. States in the second highest mortality rate category were predominantly coastal states. All states in these 2 groups had asbestosis mortality rates above the US average rate of 5.4 per million. (From NIOSH 2002 IN Lazarus AA, Philip A: Asbestosis. *Disease-a-Month.* 2011; 57(1):14-26.)

Pathophysiology

Each of the four major types of bronchogenic carcinoma is discussed separately (Table 5-12).[43,45]

Small cell carcinoma, also called *oat cell carcinoma*, accounts for 10% to 15% of all lung cancer.[3,45] It may arise in any part of the bronchial tree; however, 75% of the time it presents as a centrally located proximal lesion.[32] It often has hilar or mediastinal lymph node involvement. This tumor usually does not extend into the bronchial lumen, but spreads through the submucosa and can cause obstructive and restrictive dysfunction through compression of the surrounding lung tissue. This type of lung cancer rapidly involves the vascular channels, lymph nodes, and soft tissue. It is known to metastasize widely and early, and in most patients has metastasized by the time the diagnosis is made. This tumor rarely cavitates, but commonly produces hormones that can lead to a wide variety of symptoms in many different body systems not involved in direct metastasis.

A number of body organs, however, are involved in direct metastasis. Seventy-five percent of small cell carcinoma metastasizes to the central nervous system, 65% to the liver, 58% to the adrenal gland, 30% to the pancreas, 28% to bone, 20% to the genitourinary system, 10% to the thyroid, and 10% to the spleen.[32] The metastases to the central nervous system and the bone often produce clinical symptoms such as hemiplegia, epilepsy, personality changes, confusion, speech deficits, headache, bone pain, and pathologic fractures. Metastases to the liver and the adrenal glands are often clinically silent.[9] Other clinical symptoms caused by tumor hormone production that are of particular interest to the physical therapist include abnormalities in the neurologic or musculoskeletal systems. These complications of small cell carcinoma can include progressive dementia, ataxia, vertigo, sensory neuropathy with numbness and loss of reflexes, motor neuropathy with progressive muscle weakness and wasting, atrophic paresis of the proximal limb-girdle musculature, marked fatigability, osteoarthropathy, arthralgia, and peripheral edema.[32]

Squamous cell carcinoma accounts for 25% to 30% of all lung cancer.[45] It arises from the bronchial mucosa after repeated inflammation or irritation caused by cancer stimuli. Squamous cell carcinoma often arises in the segmental or subsegmental bronchi, but can also cause a hilar tumor. It is considered a centrally located tumor and occurs in the peripheral lung only about 30% of the time. Squamous cell tumors are bulky. They cause obstructive dysfunction because they extend into the bronchial

Table 5-12 Descriptions of types of Bronchogenic Carcinoma					
	Cell type/location	**Prevalence**	**Growth rate**	**Metastasis**	**Unique feature**
Small Cell/Oat Cell	Bronchial epithelium, near hilar region	10% to 15% of all lung cancers	Very rapid (doubles in 30 days)	Early, to mediastinum or distal lung	Oval shape, strongest correlation with smoking
Squamous Cell	Bronchial epithelium Near hilar and project into bronchi	25 to 30% More common in men	Slow (doubles in 100 days)	Late, to hilar lymph nodes	Presents with obstructive pattern due to location
Adenocarcinoma	Mucous glands Tracheobronchial tree	40% Most common More common in women	Moderate	Early	Glandular configuration, mucus production
Large Cell (undifferentiated)	Central or peripheral but often in trachea/large airways	10% to 15%	Rapid	Early and widespread	No evidence of differentiation

populations.[52] Also recently updated was the term *ALI*. Previously, the term was used to describe the milder end of the spectrum; however, now the term used is *mild ARDS*.[51]

Etiology

Approximately 150,000 cases of ARDS are diagnosed annually in the United States.[32] Table 5-15 presents the most common pulmonary and extrapulmonary triggers of ARDS.

Table 5-15 Triggers of ARDS	
Pulmonary	**Extra pulmonary**
• Pneumonia	• Sepsis
• Inhalation injury	• Major trauma
• Aspiration of gastric contents	• Burns
•	• Pancreatitis
• Chest trauma/pulmonary contusion	• Fat embolism
•	• Hypovolaemia
• Near drowning	• Transfusion-related acute lung injury (TRALI)
	• Cardiopulmonary bypass

Pathophysiology

Acute respiratory distress syndrome is a widespread inflammatory condition affecting the pulmonary tissue. It includes a three-stage process: exudative, proliferative, and fibrotic. In the exudative phase, a capillary leak causes the alveoli to fill with a neutrophilic infiltrate and protein-rich edema. This cycle of leakage and inflammation is worsened by the release of inflammatory mediators from the activated neutrophils. If the syndrome develops into the proliferative and fibrotic phases, chronic inflammation will subsequently lead to scar formation. Inflammatory debris in the early phase will cause diffusion abnormalities, ventilation–perfusion mismatch, and reduced compliance. Thrombus formation within the pulmonary capillaries increases dead space ventilation, and hypoxic pulmonary vasoconstriction may contribute to right-sided heart failure. This will ultimately lead to respiratory failure (Fig. 5-19).[51]

Diagnostic Tests

Arterial blood gas analysis, as well as chest radiograph and/or CT scan, are required. Bilateral opacities consistent with pulmonary edema are the defining criteria (Fig. 5-20).[51]

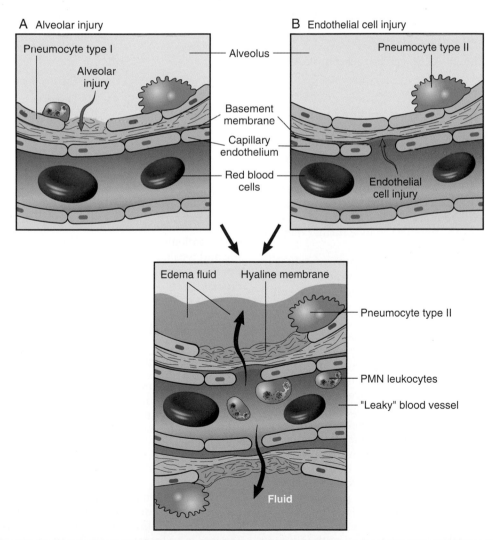

Figure 5-19 Pathogenesis of adult respiratory distress syndrome. **A,** Alveolar cell injury. **B,** Endothelial cell injury. Regardless of the initial injury, the established lesions appear identical and comprise hyaline membranes, ruptured alveolar walls, and intraalveolar edema fluid. *PMN,* polymorphonuclear neutrophil. (From Damjanov I: *Pathology for the Health Professions,* ed 3, St. Louis, 2006, Saunders.)

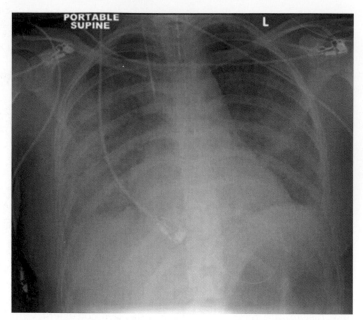

Figure 5-20 Pulmonary edema (From Mettler F: Essentials of radiology, ed 2, St. Louis, 2014, Saunders.)

Clinical Manifestation

The clinical manifestation of ARDS can be found in Table 5-16.

Treatment

The first area is treatment of the precipitating cause of the ARDS. A wide range of treatment protocols are used to address the many underlying causes. The second area of treatment is mechanical ventilation. A treatment strategy called *lung protective ventilation* is utilized where the goal is to achieve adequate gas exchange with the lowest possible TVs (4 to 8 mL/kg of ideal body weight), airway pressures (goal plateau pressures 30 cm H_2O or less), and oxygen concentrations.[52] This has been shown to reduce further damage due to mechanical ventilation.[52]

Positive end expiratory pressure of approximately 5 to 15 cm H_2O is often utilized. Positive end expiratory pressure will increase oxygenation by inflating collapsed alveoli.[51] Also, because the dependent areas of the lung are often more severely affected, positioning the patient in a prone position is recommended. This will improve oxygenation by altering the dependent area of lung to areas less severely affected.[51] Thus oxygenation will improve. The next area of treatment is supportive: managing the patient's nutritional status and fluid balance. Fluid and electrolyte balance is very important in these patients. Management may mean monitoring input and output and using diuretics. Or, because ARDS can be associated with multiorgan failure, it may mean the use of highly technical interventions such as continuous arteriovenous hemofiltration (CAVH) or dialysis in patients with chronic renal insufficiency.[9] The final focus of treatment is to prevent and treat complications of the patient's condition, along with intensive care measures. The prognosis in ARDS is always guarded; mortality can be as high as 50% to 70%, especially if this syndrome is associated with failure in other organ systems or is complicated by serious or repeated infections.[9,32]

Table 5-16 Clinical manifestation of adult respiratory distress syndrome

		Findings
Signs	Pulmonary function tests	↓ FRC, ↓ VC, ↓ VT and ↓ lung compliance with ←↑ work of breathing and ←↑ RR
		Flow rates normal or ↓ slightly, ↓ DLCO
	Chest radiograph	Symmetric bilateral diffuse fluffy infiltrates
		May coalesce into diffuse haze or lung white out
		May also have findings of COPD, atelectasis, or pneumonia
	Arterial blood gases	↓ PaO_2 (<60 mm Hg),[9] ↓ $Paco_2$ unless patient had previous CO_2 retention issues; then $Paco_2$ is ←↑
	Breath sounds	↓ breath sounds over fluid-filled areas of lungs, wet rales, wheezing and rhonchi may also be heard
	Cardiovascular	Tachycardia, may have arrhythmias due to hypoxemia
Symptoms		Appear acutely ill; dyspneic at rest and with any activity
		Breathing pattern fast and labored
		Cyanotic
		May have impaired mental status, restlessness, headache, and ←↑ anxiety

COPD, chronic obstructive pulmonary disease; *DLCO*, diffusing capacity of the lungs for carbon monoxide; *FRC*, functional residual capacity; *Paco₂*, arterial partial pressure of CO_2; *PaO₂*, arterial partial pressure of O_2; *RR*, respiratory rate; *VC*, vital capacity; *VT*, tidal volume.

All patients with ARDS suffer some degree of muscle wasting and weakness, which continues past 1-year postdischarge. For this reason, when appropriate to initiate, early mobility is crucial.

Cardiovascular Causes

Pulmonary Edema

Pulmonary edema is an increase in the amount of fluid within the lung resulting from excessive fluid movement from the pulmonary vascular system to the extravascular system. Usually, the pulmonary interstitium is affected first and then the alveolar spaces.[32,43,53]

Etiology

Pulmonary edema has two main categories: cardiogenic pulmonary edema and noncardiogenic pulmonary edema. Cardiogenic pulmonary edema, which is discussed in this section, is an increase in the pulmonary capillary hydrostatic pressure, often secondary to left ventricular failure (see Fig. 4-8). Cardiogenic pulmonary edema is also known as *high-pressure pulmonary edema, hydrostatic pulmonary edema,* or *hemodynamic pulmonary edema.* Common causes of cardiogenic pulmonary edema include arrhythmias producing low cardiac output, congenital heart defects, excessive fluid administration, left ventricular failure, mitral or aortic disease, myocardial infarction, pulmonary embolus, renal failure, rheumatic heart disease or myocarditis, and systemic hypertension.

Noncardiogenic pulmonary edema has a multitude of causes, including increased capillary permeability, lymphatic insufficiency, decreased intrapleural pressure, or decreased oncotic pressure. Pulmonary edema can also be caused by increased alveolar capillary membrane permeability secondary to various causes. This type of pulmonary edema is also named *ARDS* and was discussed under the section "Pulmonary Causes of Restrictive Lung Dysfunction."[9,32,43]

Pathophysiology

As the left ventricle fails, its ability to contract and pump blood into the systemic circulation efficiently is diminished. This results in an increase in left atrial pressure, which is transmitted back to the pulmonary circulation. Because of this impedance to blood flow, the pressure in the microcirculation of the lung is increased, which increases the transvascular flow of fluid into the interstitium of the lung. When the pulmonary vascular hydrostatic pressure rises above 25 to 30 mm Hg, the oncotic pressure loses its holding force and fluid is allowed to spill into the interstitial space. The interstitial space can accommodate a small amount of excess fluid, approximately 500 mL.[32] The lymphatic drainage can be enhanced to move some excess fluid out of the thorax. However, when the left atrial pressure rises above 30 mm Hg, these protective mechanisms are overcome.[32] The interstitial edema fluid disrupts the tight alveolar epithelium, floods the alveolar spaces, and moves through the visceral pleura, causing pleural effusions. The pulmonary edema fluid in cardiogenic pulmonary edema is characterized by low protein concentrations. This finding is in contrast to that in ARDS in which the pulmonary edema fluid has elevated protein concentrations. With fluid in the alveoli and the interstitium, lung compliance is decreased, ventilation–perfusion mismatching is increased, gas exchange is disrupted, the work of breathing is increased, and there is restrictive lung dysfunction.[9,32,53] As a result of gravity, as well as the pulmonary perfusion pressure and pulmonary venous pressure from the apex to the base, excess fluid gathers in the dependent areas of the lung.[54]

Prognosis for patients with pulmonary edema does not directly correlate with the edema itself, but rather the impact of the edema. Adequate treatment of the fluid buildup is critical for treatment. Correct diagnosis of cardiogenic pulmonary edema and therefore adequate treatment can aid in improving prognosis.[53,54]

Diagnostic Tests

Pulmonary edema is usually seen as basilar infiltrates with pulmonary vascular redistribution and with increased upper lobe appearance. In the context of patients with CHF, the cardiac silhouette is often visualized as large. Brain natriuretic peptide (BNP) levels can increase in relation to factors beyond pressure, and volume overload may be elevated.[54]

Table 5-17	Clinical manifestation of pulmonary edema	
		Findings
	Laboratory values	BNP > 1200 pg/mL (likely to be cardiogenic pulmonary edema vs. ARDS)
Signs	Pulmonary function tests	↓ Lung volumes, ←FEV1 normal or ↑ but FVC ↓,↑ RR ↑, Flow rates normal, DLCO normal or ↓
	Chest radiograph	←↑ Vascular markings in hilar region to peripheral borders, may see cardiomegaly
		Kerley B lines present (short, thin, horizontal lines extending inward from pleural space)
		Interstitial and alveolar infiltrates are diffuse and pleural effusions common, fluffy opacities
	Arterial blood gases	↓ PaO$_2$, ↓ Paco$_2$, ↑ pH Respiratory alkalosis
		Possible ← Paco$_2$ ↑ late in clinical course
	Breath sounds	Wet rales with ↓ breath sounds
		Some patients present with bronchospasm and wheezing
	Cardiovascular	Most have significant cardiac dysfunction[28]
		Arrhythmias common in this population
Symptoms		Appear in respiratory distress, report sense of suffocation
		Short of breath, cyanotic, ←↑ RR, labored breathing, pallor, diaphoresis
		Cough: pink frothy sputum

DLCO, diffusing capacity of the lungs for carbon monoxide; *PaO$_2$,* arterial partial pressure of O$_2$; *PFT,* pulmonary function test; *RR,* respiratory rate.

Clinical Manifestation

The clinical manifestation of pulmonary edema can be found in Table 5-17 and Fig. 5-21.

Treatment

Treatment is aimed at decreasing the cardiac preload and maintaining oxygenation of the tissues. To decrease cardiac preload, venous return to the heart is decreased, which decreases the left ventricular filling pressure. Venodilators, such as morphine sulfate or sodium nitroprusside, and diuretics, such as furosemide, are used to decrease the venous return and decreased afterload. Angiotensin-converting enzyme (ACE) inhibitors may also be used to decrease afterload in more chronic cases. Positive inotropes,

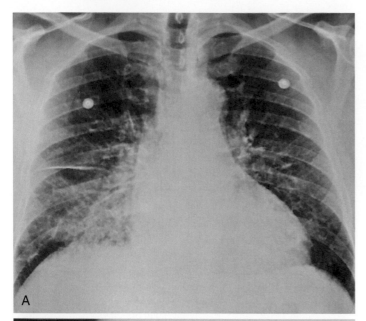

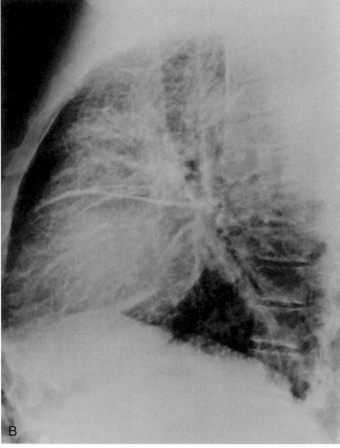

Figure 5-21 Cardiogenic pulmonary edema following myocardial infarction in a 52-year-old man, illustrating widespread fissural thickening and lack of clarity of the intrapulmonary vessels. There is frank alveolar edema in the right lower zone. The fissural thickening caused by subpleural edema is particularly striking. **A,** Frontal view. **B,** Lateral view. (From Armstrong P, Wilson AG, Dee P, et al: *Imaging of diseases of the chest,* ed 3, St. Louis, 2000, Mosby.)

such as dopamine, dobutamine, amiodarone, and digitalis, may be given to improve cardiac contractility and increase cardiac output. To maintain oxygenation, supplemental oxygen is provided. Intubation with mechanical ventilation may also be necessary.[28] Bronchial hygiene treatments may be used to assist with clearance of secretions. Furthermore, albumin or mannitol may be used to increase osmotic pressure to combat the increased hydrostatic forces.

Pulmonary Emboli

Pulmonary emboli are a complication of venous thrombosis in which blood clots or thrombi travel from a systemic vein through the right side of the heart and into the pulmonary circulation, where they lodge in branches of the pulmonary artery (Fig. 5-22).[3,26,43]

Etiology

Pulmonary embolism is the most common acute pulmonary problem among hospitalized patients in the United States. Each year it is estimated that 300,000 to 600,000 Americans have a pulmonary embolic event.[32,43,55] Many of these events may go unnoticed because they are clinically silent, with only 20% presenting with the classic triad of symptoms: dyspnea, hemoptysis, and pleuritic chest pain. However, approximately 10% to 30% of pulmonary embolisms result in the patient's death within 1 month of diagnosis.[32] About one-third of the deaths occur within 1 hour of the acute event, and more than half of these fatalities occur in patients in whom the diagnosis was not clinically suspect.[32,43]

In more than 95% of the cases, the thrombi that caused the pulmonary emboli were formed in the lower extremities.[3,43] In the remaining 5% of the cases, the thrombi may be formed in the pelvis, the arms, or the right side of the heart. Numerous risk factors increase the likelihood of thrombus formation in the lower extremities (Box 5-2). The highest risk group for thrombophlebitis is orthopedic patients. Studies have shown that the frequency of deep vein thrombosis (DVT) perioperative is 80% in patients after hip or knee surgery.[28,43]

Pathophysiology

The pathophysiologic changes that occur following pulmonary embolism affect the pulmonary system and the cardiovascular system. First, the occlusion of one or more pulmonary arterial branches causes edema and hemorrhage into the surrounding lung parenchyma. This is known as *congestive atelectasis.* Second, the lack of blood flow causes coagulative necrosis of the alveolar walls; the alveoli fill with erythrocytes, and there is an inflammatory response. Third, there is an increase in the alveolar dead space because a portion of the lung is being ventilated but no longer perfused. Pneumoconstriction of the affected area occurs, with a marked decrease in alveolar carbon dioxide due to the lack of gas exchange and the patient's respiratory pattern of hyperventilation. In addition, the alveolar surfactant decreases over a period of approximately 24 hours, which results in alveolar collapse and regional atelectasis. These changes combine to cause an acute increase in ventilation–perfusion mismatching, a decrease in lung compliance, and impaired gas exchange. If the oxygen supply is completely cut off to a portion of the lung, then frank necrosis and infarction of